Structural Interfaces and Attachments in Biology

Stavros Thomopoulos • Victor Birman
Guy M. Genin
Editors

Structural Interfaces and Attachments in Biology

Springer

Editors
Stavros Thomopoulos
Department of Orthopedic Surgery
Washington University
St. Louis, MO, USA

Victor Birman
Engineering Education Center
Missouri University of Science and Technology
St. Louis, MO, USA

Guy M. Genin
Mechanical Engineering
and Materials Science
Washington University
St. Louis, MO, USA

ISBN 978-1-4614-3316-3 ISBN 978-1-4614-3317-0 (eBook)
DOI 10.1007/978-1-4614-3317-0
Springer New York Heidelberg Dordrecht London

Library of Congress Control Number: 2012946721

Printed on acid-free paper

Springer is part of Springer Science+Business Media (www.springer.com)

Preface

Attachment of dissimilar materials in engineering and surgical practice is a perennial challenge. Bimaterial attachment sites are common locations for initial and repeated injury and mechanical failure. Nature presents several highly effective solutions to the challenge of bimaterial attachment that differ from those currently adopted in engineering practice. The goal of this text is to simultaneously elucidate natural bimaterial attachments and outline engineering principles underlying successful attachments as a guide to the communities of tissue engineers, structural engineers, and surgeons.

We assembled this book with the hope of generating a cross-disciplinary dialogue among our biomedical and engineering communities. The intended readership includes orthopaedic surgeons, researchers in the areas of orthopaedic biomechanics and tissue engineering, senior undergraduate and beginning graduate students in mechanical and biomedical engineering, and structural engineers. We expect that the book will be of value to orthopaedic surgeons, who are regularly presented with the challenge of attaching dissimilar materials (e.g., tendon-to-bone repair for rotator cuff tears or anterior cruciate ligament reconstruction). The lessons learned from the study of biological attachments may be useful for developing new surgical strategies for improved patient outcomes. We also anticipate that this book will be of interest to structural engineers. Understanding the mechanisms by which the body solves the problem of attaching dissimilar materials may enable engineers to design better structural attachments (e.g., for connecting an airplane wing to the fuselage). Attachment schemes in nature provide established and time-proven strategies for bimaterial attachment, and our goal is for this text to provide engineers with an entry point into the study of these.

A key objective of the text is to make the current body of work on attachments accessible in a concise format and across disciplines. The book can be used as a textbook for a graduate level course cross-listed among orthopaedics, mechanical engineering, biomedical engineering, and materials programs. The background readings for such a course have not yet been assembled elsewhere. A comprehensive treatment is presented of physiologic attachments from the engineering perspective and engineering attachments in the context of schemes observed in nature. In such a course, we expect that students of different educational backgrounds will emerge with both a broad comprehensive picture and in-depth knowledge of topics that build upon their individual foundations.

The editors thank their families for their support during the preparation of the book. The editors also acknowledge Washington University in St. Louis, Missouri University of Science and Technology, and the National Science Foundation (CAREER 844607) for their support of this effort.

St. Louis, MO, USA

Stavros Thomopoulos
Victor Birman
Guy M. Genin

Contents

Contributors

Victor Birman Engineering Education Center, Missouri University of Science and Technology, St. Louis, MO, USA

Brenda S. Bohaty Department of Pediatric Dentistry, University of Missouri-Kansas City, Kansas City, MO, USA

Steven R. Caliari Department of Chemical and Biomolecular Engineering, University of Illinois at Urbana-Champaign, Urbana, IL, USA

Michael Detamore Department of Chemical and Petroleum Engineering, University of Kansas, Lawrence, KS, USA

Kathryn F. Farraro Department of Bioengineering, University of Pittsburgh, Pittsburgh, PA, USA

Virginia L. Ferguson Department of Mechanical Engineering, University of Colorado, Boulder, CO, USA

Leesa M. Galatz Department of Orthopaedic Surgery, Washington University in St. Louis, St. Louis, MO, USA

Huajian Gao School of Engineering, Brown University, Providence, RI, USA

Guy M. Genin Department of Mechanical Engineering and Materials Science, Washington University in St. Louis, St. Louis, MO, USA

Haimin Yao School of Engineering, Sun Yat-sen University, Guangzhou, China

Brendan A.C. Harley Department of Chemical and Biomolecular Engineering, University of Illinois-Urbana Champagne, Urbana, IL, USA

Serhat Hosder Department of Mechanical and Aerospace Engineering, Missouri University of Science and Technology, Rolla, MO, USA

Kei Kamino Biotechnology Center, National Institute of Technology and Evaluation, Kisarazu, Chiba, Japan

Tyler Keil Sandia National Laboratories, Albuquerque, NM, USA

Jennifer S. Laurence Department of Pharmaceutical Chemistry, University of Kansas, Lawrence, KS, USA

Jennifer Lei George W. Woodruff School of Mechanical Engineering, Georgia Institute of Technology, Atlanta, GA, USA

Yanxin Liu Department of Mechanical Engineering and Materials Science, Washington University in St. Louis, St. Louis, MO, USA

Orestes Marangos Bioengineering Research Center, University of Kansas, Lawrence, KS, USA

Anil Misra Department of Civil, Environmental, and Architectural Engineering, Bioengineering Research Center, University of Kansas, Lawrence, KS, USA

Neethu Mohan Department of Chemical and Petroleum Engineering, University of Kansas, Lawrence, KS, USA

Rachel C. Paietta Department of Mechanical Engineering, University of Colorado, Boulder, CO, USA

Jonggu Park Bioengineering Research Center, University of Kansas, Lawrence, KS, USA

Ranganathan Parthasarathy Bioengineering Research Center, University of Kansas, Lawrence, KS, USA

Scott A. Rodeo Department of Orthopaedic Surgery, Sports Medicine and Shoulder Service, Hospital for Special Surgery/Weill Cornell Medical College, New York, NY, USA

Andrea Schwartz Department of Orthopaedic Surgery, Washington University, St. Louis, MO, USA

Viraj Singh Department of Mechanical Engineering, University of Kansas, Lawrence, KS, USA

John M. Solic Sports Medicine and Shoulder Center, Triangle Orthopaedic Associates, Durham, NC, USA

Paulette Spencer Department of Mechanical Engineering, Bioengineering Research Center, University of Kansas, Lawrence, KS, USA

Matteo M. Tei Department of Bioengineering, University of Pittsburgh, Pittsburgh, PA, USA

Johnna S. Temenoff Department of Biomedical Engineering, Georgia Institute of Technology, Atlanta, GA, USA

Stavros Thomopoulos Department of Orthopaedic Surgery, Washington University in St. Louis, St. Louis, MO, USA

Talila Volk Department of Molecular Genetics, Weizmann Institute, Rehovot, Israel

Jizeng Wang Key Laboratory of Mechanics on Disaster and Environment in Western China, Lanzhou University, Lanzhou, Gansu, China

Daniel W. Weisgerber Department of Materials Science and Engineering, University of Illinois at Urbana-Champaign, Urbana, IL, USA

Savio L.-Y. Woo Department of Bioengineering, University of Pittsburgh, Pittsburgh, PA, USA

Haimin Yao Department of Mechanical Engineering, The Hong Kong Polytechnic University, Hung Hom, Kowloon, Hong Kong

Qiang Ye Bioengineering Research Center, University of Kansas, Lawrence, KS, USA

Part I
Attachment of Dissimilar Materials: Challenges and Solutions

Chapter 1
The Challenge of Attaching Dissimilar Materials

Stavros Thomopoulos, Victor Birman, and Guy M. Genin

1.1 Introduction

Interfaces between dissimilar structural materials have existed since our first multicellular ancestors evolved. Attachments and joints between dissimilar materials are commonly found throughout nature, physiology, and engineering. A difference in material properties may be realized as either a step-wise change from one material to the other or as a gradual variation across a short distance, as is the case with functionally graded interfaces. A mismatch between material properties at the interface raises unique problems related to strength, stiffness, and fracture behavior of the attachment. For example, the difference in stiffness between bone and tendon, where the modulus of elasticity varies by almost two orders of magnitude over a short distance, could cause severe problems at the tendon-to-bone attachment; the potential stress concentrations are alleviated in part through gradation of properties at the interface. Fracture along the bondline between a metal hip replacement and bone is driven by a mismatch in the properties of these materials. Issues related to interfaces between dissimilar materials arise in many engineering applications as well. For example, high thermal stresses are problematic in electronic packaging along the junction between the chip and the substrate due to the different thermal expansion coefficients of the two materials.

S. Thomopoulos (✉)
Department of Orthopaedic Surgery, Washington University in St. Louis, St. Louis, MO, USA
e-mail: thomopouloss@wudosis.wustl.edu

V. Birman
Engineering Education Center, Missouri University of Science and Technology, Rolla, MO, USA
e-mail: vbirman@mst.edu

G.M. Genin
Department of Mechanical Engineering and Materials Science, Washington University in St. Louis, St. Louis, MO, USA
e-mail: gening@seas.wustl.edu

S. Thomopoulos et al. (eds.), *Structural Interfaces and Attachments in Biology*,
DOI 10.1007/978-1-4614-3317-0_1,

Although the mechanics of attachment for dissimilar materials can be studied using many standard engineering methodologies, biological systems present additional challenges (e.g., biocompatibility requirements for total joint replacements). On the other hand, in contrast to numerous engineering applications, biological systems typically operate in a well-defined environment where the range of temperature, hydration, and pH is tightly regulated. The effects of these variations can therefore be neglected in most analyses of biologic attachments.

The goal of this introductory chapter is to illustrate examples of representative attachments of dissimilar materials in engineering and biology, and to place into context the deeper treatments of the mechanics and physiology of material attachments studied throughout the rest of the book. While we do not attempt to present a comprehensive list of such attachments, the chosen examples demonstrate typical cases and problems associated with such joints. We include as well a brief discussion of the relevant fracture problem that should be addressed when designing or analyzing attachments of dissimilar materials.

1.2 Examples of Attachments of Dissimilar Materials

1.2.1 Engineering

Attachments of dissimilar materials in engineering are usually adhesively bonded or bolted, and have presented challenges to generations of engineers. Beginning in the 1950s, a series of rigorous treatments of the mechanical responses of such attachments have been developed. These have increased in sophistication in recent years, so that estimating the toughness of simple engineering materials is now possible. This is in stark contrast to frameworks for understanding biological attachment. Chap. 3 presents an overview of some of the established models for understanding the bonded attachment of engineering materials, and places the attachment of tendon to bone into the context of these models.

Adhesively bonded attachments possess a number of advantages, such as sealing against corrosion, damage tolerance, and reasonably good fatigue behavior. On the other hand, these attachments are characterized by high residual stresses, they cannot be disassembled or easily inspected, and they are sensitive to peeling and transverse shear stresses that lead to debonding. Bolted connections are less sensitive to peeling and transverse shear stresses and they can easily be inspected or disassembled. However, bolted assemblies also introduce stress concentrations and a degree of compliance, and their fatigue behavior is generally inferior to adhesively bonded attachments. We concentrate here on several examples of bonded attachments.

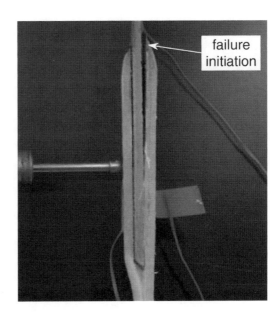

Fig. 1.1 Failure of a metal-composite joint. The cracks are clearly visible. The onset of failure at the edge of the joint is identified by a white arrow (adapted, with permission, from [3])

1.2.1.1 Metal-to-Composite Components

A classical problem in mechanics involves the strength of adhesively bonded joints. In particular, this problem is relevant to numerous applications found in hybrid metal-composite structures in aerospace engineering, naval architecture, and other fields. The properties of metal and composite adherends are typically different, magnifying the complexity of the analysis, as the joints involve three vastly different materials (i.e., metal, composite, and adhesive). The extensive literature on adhesive joints and methods of their analysis is summarized in several reviews, such as [1] and [2]. Failure is usually initiated by a crack in the adhesive layer between the metal and the composite, originating from the edge of the joint as a result of a local concentration of peeling and transverse shear stresses (Fig. 1.1). These high local stresses result in the onset of a Mode I fracture, which subsequently propagates along the interface and unzips the joint.

1.2.1.2 Electronic Packaging Problems

A typical interface between dissimilar materials in electronics is the die (chip)-substrate assembly. Failure often occurs due to an elevated temperature, in which case a mismatch between the coefficients of thermal expansion leads to delamination cracking along the interface between the heat sink (substrate) and the chip. An example of such crack between a copper heat sink and a laser diode is shown in Fig. 1.2. One of the materials in such bimaterial assemblies exhibits low thermal expansion and is brittle, increasing the vulnerability of the joint [4]. The underfill

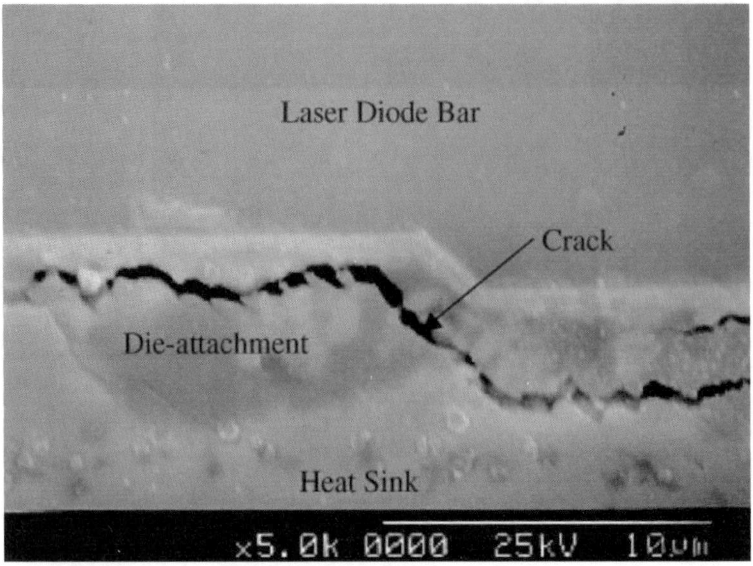

Fig. 1.2 Crack propagating along the diode-to-heat sink attachment (adapted, with permission, from [5])

(i.e., epoxy adhesive between the chip and substrate) may somewhat relieve the effect of thermal loading, but the problem of fracture along the interface of dissimilar materials remains a critical issue in electronic packaging. The highest stress singularity occurs at the corner of electronic packages, as is evidenced by experimental results (Fig. 1.3).

1.2.1.3 Sandwich Structures: Facing-to-Core Bond

Sandwich structures represent an extrapolation of the concept of an I-beam or a truss, combining two predominantly load-carrying flanges with one relatively underloaded web to maximize the bending strength and stiffness. In a sandwich panel, the flanges are replaced with facings that are typically fiber-reinforced composites or metallic, while the core is solid polymeric, foam, or honeycomb. In the latter case, the honeycomb core is either composite or metallic. The vast majority of sandwich structures utilize heavier and stiffer materials in the facings and lighter materials with a lower strength and stiffness in the core (in case of honeycomb cores, "lighter" typically refers to the weight density, rather than the weight of a bulk core material). In these cases, debonding of facings from the core represents a major failure mode that is also difficult to detect by inspection.

An example, of a sandwich panel with facings and a solid polymeric core experiencing interfacial debonding as a result of a low-velocity (5 m/s) impact with a 25 mm hemispherical indenter is shown in Fig. 1.4. The facings

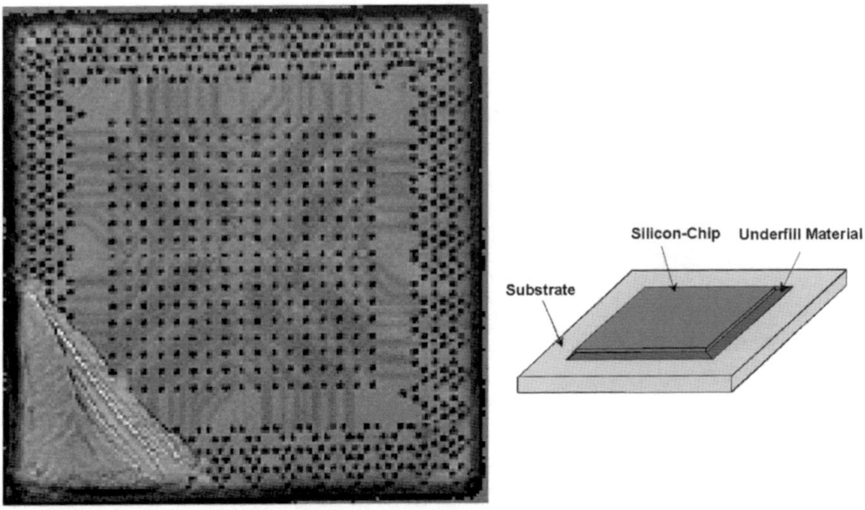

Fig. 1.3 Acoustic microscopy image of a crack initiating from a corner at the interface between a silicon die and the epoxy underfill in a flip chip package (adapted, with permission, from [6])

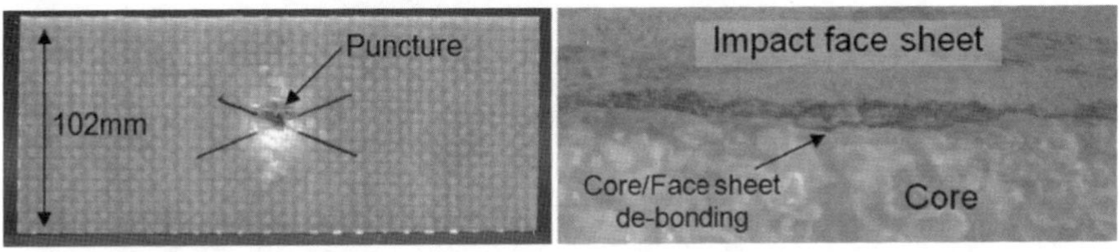

Fig. 1.4 Low-velocity impact damage in a sandwich panel. *Left*: Facing subject to impact. *Right*: facing-core debonding (adapted, with permission, from [7])

were manufactured from E-glass/vinylester, while the solid polymeric core was manufactured from Corecell A800. The central region of punctured material is surrounded by a lighter colored region with an area nearly three times that of the puncture. This corresponds to a region of debonding between the face sheet and the core material. As will be discussed in Chap. 3, the opening of a free edge between the face sheet and the core can introduce stresses sufficiently large to drive a crack between face sheet and core.

A possible approach to alleviate facing-core debonding in sandwich structures utilizes graded interfaces, where the volume fractions of facing and core materials vary over a short distance from pure facing to pure core material. A modification of this concept is based on using a graded core, where the properties vary throughout its entire depth to achieve a desired response, while eliminating a sharp property mismatch along the interface (Fig. 1.5). It has been experimentally shown that, while damage in conventional sandwich structures involves a facing-core debonding, such a mode can be eliminated through the use of a graded core. For

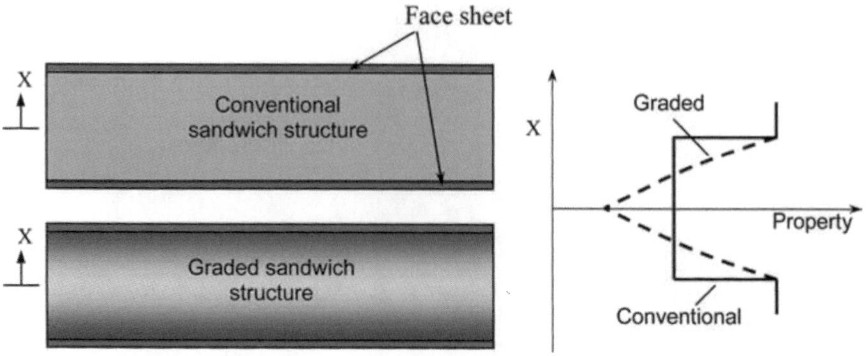

Fig. 1.5 Schematic illustration of the concept of a functionally graded core or graded facing-core interface (adapted, with permission, from [8])

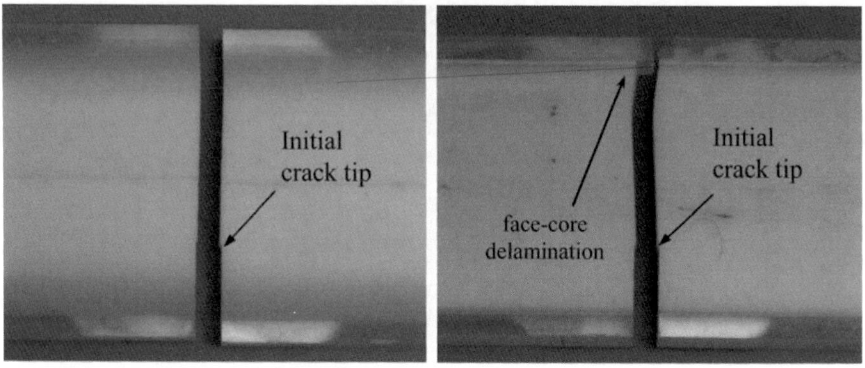

Fig. 1.6 Photograph of graded (*left*) and conventional (*right*) sandwich specimens from optical tests (adapted, with permission, from [8])

example, the crack growth in the pre-cracked core of sandwich structures with and without a graded core was monitored in one study (Fig. 1.6). In the conventional design, the crack generated interfacial debonding upon reaching the facing-to-core interface. Such damage was absent in the counterparts with a graded core.

In conclusion of this section, it is noted that grading is often adopted in engineering applications at the interface between dissimilar materials for an enhanced macromechanical response of the structure. A review of functional grading in engineering applications can be found in Chap. 2.

1.2.2 Biology and Medicine

A wide variety of attachment systems can be found in nature. These systems may be instructive for engineering and medical practice. In the human musculoskeletal system, these include the attachment of tendon/ligament to bone (Chap. 4) and the attachment of cartilage to bone (Chap. 5). These junctions effectively transfer load between two dissimilar materials through complex transitions in composition, architecture, and mechanical properties. They develop through a well-orchestrated developmental process via gradients of biologic factors to produce efficient natural attachments (Chaps. 6 and 11). Similar mechanisms of attachment have been described at interfaces found in teeth (Chap. 7).

Numerous organisms have evolved novel attachment systems to interact with their environments and to enhance their physiologic function. The attachment between muscle and tendon in fruit flies is discussed in Chap. 6, with a discussion of the origin and development of tendon in the embryo of the fly. Furthermore, the myotendinous junction and the molecular pathways driving embryonic development are considered.

A diverse set of material designs is described in Chap. 9 for organisms that need to attach to surfaces in aqueous environments. By studying the attachment systems of mussels, barnacles, and tubeworms, the mechanisms of underwater adhesion are elucidated. A fascinating attachment system is exhibited by geckos, enabling them to easily form and release attachments to surfaces (Chap. 10). Both attachment and detachment are achieved by changing the pulling angles at an interface and manipulating an anisotropic adhesion mechanism. In addition, it is shown that the fractal gecko hair system is highly damage-tolerant, being able to withstand extensive cracking.

Chapter 8 reviews the mechanics of cellular attachment to surfaces. As cell adhesion is critical for many biological functions, including cell migration, proliferation, differentiation, and growth, a better understanding of cell adhesion mechanisms has broad implications in biology and biophysics.

In the current chapter, we present an introductory overview of several biologic examples where dissimilar materials with a large mismatch in mechanical properties attach over a relatively short distance. The cases considered include dental tissues, metal-to-bone orthopedic interfaces, and tendon-to-bone attachments.

1.2.2.1 Dental Attachments

An archetypal example of the attachment of dissimilar materials is found at the interface between the tooth and alveolar bone. As described in [9], this attachment involves two distinct interfaces: one between the alveolar bone and the cementum (through periodontal ligament (PDL) collagen fibers) and one between the cementum and the root dentin (through the cementum-dentin junction (CDJ)). The attachment structure and the variation in modulus throughout the attachment are shown in Fig. 1.7. It is interesting to observe that both interfaces possess lower stiffnesses than those of adjacent materials. A similar observation was made in the course of research at the tendon-to-bone insertion site; this is discussed below, where it is hypothesized that such a dip in the stiffness is beneficial for reducing stress concentrations. Chap. 7 further explores the adhesive mechanisms in teeth and Chap. 3 explores the mechanics of attaching tendon to bone.

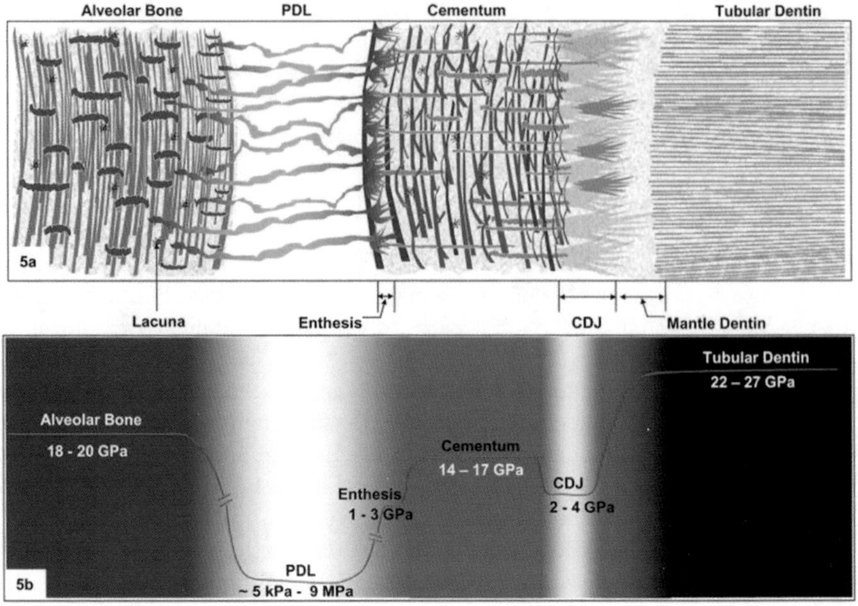

Fig. 1.7 Schematics of the tissues and interfaces responsible for tooth attachment. (**a**) Structure and (**b**) variation of the modulus of elasticity, reflecting the presence of graded regions between bone, PDL, cementum, and root dentin (adapted, with permission, from [9])

Notably, the surface structure, in particular the surface roughness, and the surface chemistry of oral implants influence their anchoring in jaw bones. In one study, the metal-to-bone interface between an implant surface and a jaw was modified by sandblasting the metal component with different particles [10]. The surface modification of the titanium implant was produced by blasting it with particles of Al_2O_3 or of bioceramics; these treatments resulted in improvements in attachment. This illustrates that an artificially developed roughness on the implant surface may benefit attachments for tooth implants. Nevertheless, caution should be exercised using this approach, since local damage may be introduced in the material during the blasting process. Additionally, the mechanisms by which this improvement is attained are not understood. The presence of local roughness may serve as a source of microscopic stress concentrations; a macroscopic crack may originate from one of these local areas. Alternatively, the roughness might serve as a cue for living cells within the jaw to produce material more conducive to an effective metal-to-bone interface.

1.2.2.2 Metal-to-Bone Orthopedic Interfaces

Metal-to-bone interfaces in orthopedic total joint implants have been extensively investigated. A mismatch in the stiffness along the interface can cause both pain and eventual loosening or failure, requiring replacement of the artificial joint. A second issue that can lead to negative outcomes is the biocompatibility of the metal.

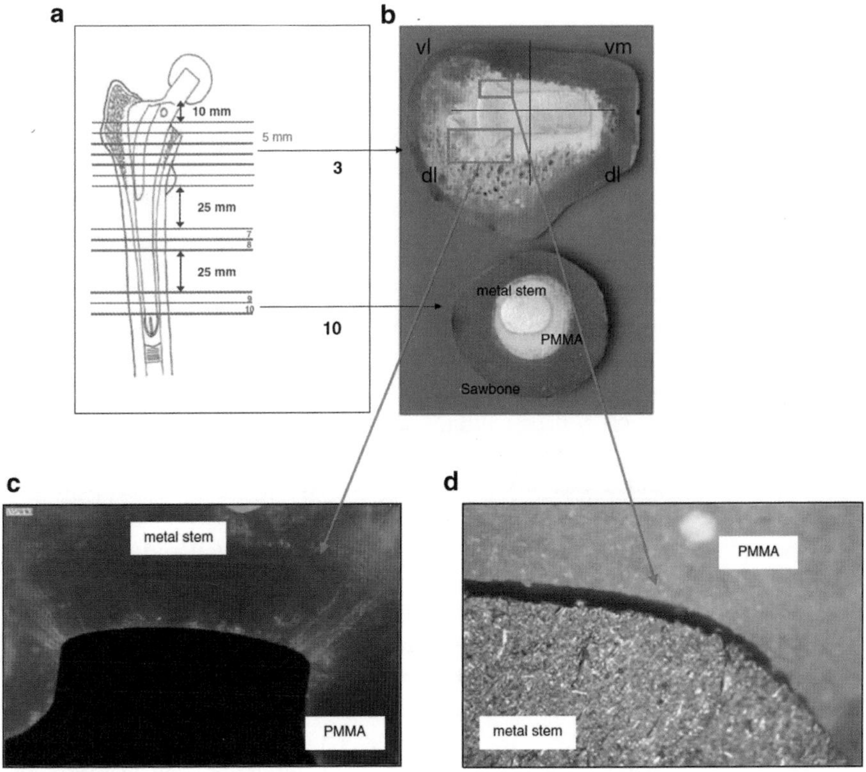

Fig. 1.8 (**a**) Schematic of implant in a femur. (**b**) Representative slices of the implanted stem surrounded by bone cement. (**c**) Cement mantle cracks generated from "sharp-edge" corners. (**d**) Debonding along the metal-bone cement interface (adapted, with permission, from [13])

Consider, for example, the attachment of stems to the femur for total hip arthroplasty. Stress shielding can result in bone loss if stresses are poorly distributed along the bone–metal interface. In the case of a noncemented stem, this problem can be alleviated if the fixation is implemented along the entire length of the stem surface [11]. The use of hydroxyapatite coatings may enhance bone ingrowth and reduce bone resorption, without a detrimental effect on the stress distribution. One of the solutions proposed to alleviate the problem of attaching metal to bone employed a graded interface between the metal and bone materials as is exemplified by cemented hips (Fig. 1.8). The cement (polymethylmethacrylate) is first applied to the hip to avoid a direct linking between the bone cement and metal of the artificial hip. The tendency of the metal–cement interface to debond is alleviated through the use of a silane-coupling coating of metal that enhances the hydrolytic stability [12]. The metal-to-cement bond can further be improved using an additional silica oxide interlayer that adheres to the oxide on the surface of metal [13]. In the experiments reported in this study, femur stems covered with a silica/silane interlayer coating were cemented into artificial femur bones and subject to standard torsional fatigue loading. A comparison between coated and uncoated (control) specimens demonstrated a significant improvement of the bond strength available using a silica/silane coating. Thus, introduction of a coating between metal and bone may improve contact and reduce loosening in hip arthroplasty. Notably, while the dental interface discussed in Sect. 2.1 was graded, satisfactory results in the present case were achieved by merely introducing an interface, without a direct intentional grading. Ways that an interlayer might be beneficial in the context of alleviating stress singularities are discussed in Chap. 3.

1.2.2.3 Tendon-to-Bone Attachment

As an example case of a clinically relevant attachment, the mechanics of the tendon-to-bone insertion will be explored in the remainder of this chapter. Later chapters will review the current surgical approaches for repairing tendon to bone, and the lackluster clinical outcomes that have been achieved to date (Chap. 12 will review the repair of the rotator cuff to the humeral head and Chap. 13 will review anterior cruciate ligament reconstruction, which requires tendon graft healing in a bone tunnel). Chapter 3 will discuss the mechanics of this attachment in greater detail. The mechanical properties of tendon and bone are vastly different; bone has a modulus on the order of 20 GPa and tendon has an axial modulus on the order of 450 MPa and a transverse modulus on the order of 45 MPa. This material mismatch presents significant challenges for stress transfer between the two tissues. These issues are directly relevant to surgical considerations as well as for potential engineering biomimetic designs. Surgical and rehabilitation considerations as well as future biologic approaches are discussed in Chaps. 11, 12, and 13. Several subsequent chapters then address the potential for biomimetic designs for enhanced tendon-to-bone repair. Chapter 14 reviews functionally graded approaches for interface tissue engineering. Chapter 15 presents approaches for synthesizing fibrous tissues for attachment of tendons and ligaments to bone. Finally, Chap. 16 discusses fabrication of layered scaffolds for the formation of tendon/ligament- and cartilage-to-bone insertions. The methods discussed in these chapters include designs based on the optimization of cell types, development of scaffolds, and the use of exogenous factors (including soluble growth factors and bioreactors) to successfully regenerate both tendons/ligaments and their interfaces with bone.

The transfer of the load between tendon and bone has been considered in a number of studies (e.g., [14–16]). The studies were motivated by the observation that once damaged, a resilient tendon-to-bone insertion is not regenerated after healing. This is reflected in the extraordinary high re-tear rate after surgical repair of rotator cuffs, ranging from 20% to 94% (with the range dependent on the extent of the initial injury and the age of the patient) [17]. While the uninjured tendon-to-bone insertion site is characterized by variations in properties from tendon to bone that are highly anisotropic, the scar tissue forming at healed attachments is isotropic. Furthermore, the compliant region that is present at the uninjured attachment site, as discussed below, is not regenerated during healing. These differences between the natural and postsurgical attachments likely explain the mechanical inferiority of the latter tissue. These differences also motivate further study of the mechanisms of load transfer between the natural tendon-to-bone insertion site.

Four strategies have been identified as contributing to the effectiveness of the natural tendon-to-bone insertion site [18]. They include: (1) a shallow attachment angle at the insertion of transitional tissue and bone, (2) shaping of gross tissue morphology of the transitional tissue, (3) interdigitation of bone with the transitional tissue, and (4) functional grading of transitional tissue between tendon and bone. These mechanisms are further discussed in the next section of this chapter and in Chaps. 3 and 11.

In one study, experimentally measured collagen fiber orientations and mineral concentration data were used in micromechanically based models to monitor the stiffness distribution along the insertion site. This distribution complied with the above-mentioned drop in the stiffness, the lower stiffness region being closest to the tendon [15]. The same model predicted an abrupt increase in the stiffness of the insertion between the mineral percolation threshold and the bone. The rationale for a decrease in the stiffness remained unclear, however. Subsequent studies were necessary to demonstrate that the compliant region optimizes distribution of stresses to reduce stress concentrations [19]. Using an example of an idealized rotator cuff insertion site, it was demonstrated that a biomimetically inspired compliant and functionally graded interface between tendon and bone can lead to a drastic reduction and even elimination of stress concentrations [19].

1.3 Prevention of Fracture at the Interface of Dissimilar Materials: Engineering and Biological Solutions

The interface between dissimilar materials presents a number of challenging problems to medical doctors, researchers, and engineers alike. In theory, a stress singularity at the corner of such an interface (Fig. 1.9) could cause the onset of cracking at a stress level that would be benign to each material considered individually [20]. The effect of material property mismatches was demonstrated for the interface between bone-like isotropic and tendon-like orthotropic materials [18]. The contributions of functional grading, local and gross morphology, and interdigitation were studied and discussed in detail in [18]. The order of the singularity was shown to be a function of the property mismatch, and to approach a constant order in the case of a relatively stiff isotropic material attaching to an orthotropic material. The singularity could be avoided only in the case of a relatively compliant isotropic material, the observation being interesting for potential applications, but irrelevant for the tendon-to-bone attachment.

While the previous results refer to fracture along the interface between dissimilar materials, an improvement in the stress distribution and fracture characteristics of the attachment may be possible using an interfacial layer. The beneficial

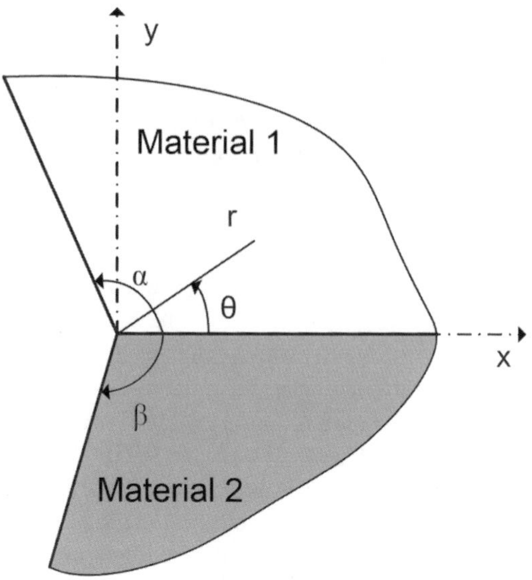

Fig. 1.9 Geometry in the vicinity of the free edge at the attachment between two dissimilar materials (the z-axis is perpendicular to the plane)

effect of such a layer in dental and metal-to-bone interfaces and at the tendon-to-bone insertion site has already been discussed. While the stiffness and stress analyses could be conducted along the lines of previously cited studies, the fracture problem is more challenging. One complication is related to several possible scenarios of the crack propagation. For example, cracking can occur along the bondline between the interfacial layer and one of the dissimilar materials or alternatively, cracking can occur within the interfacial layer itself. Finally, it is also possible for the crack to "depart" from the interfacial region and propagate into one of the joined materials.

The orientation of the crack may be predicted adopting one of several available criteria applicable to fracture in a functionally graded material. For example, such criteria can include [21]:

- The maximum hoop stress criterion, i.e., the crack propagates along the axis of the maximum hoop stress.
- The maximum strain energy release rate criterion, i.e., the crack propagates along the axis corresponding to the maximum strain energy release rate.
- The maximum strain energy density criterion, i.e., crack propagation occurs with the direction corresponding to the smallest strain energy density.

The previous discussion implies that an optimum interface is likely to be graded in the direction perpendicular to the surfaces of joined dissimilar materials. The case of a uniform interface can be treated as a particular case of the more general graded counterpart. Numerous relevant problems have been considered in engineering science (e.g., [22–24]), although the optimization of the interface arresting the crack propagation has not been attempted.

A possible enhancement of the concept of functionally graded interfaces between dissimilar materials suggested here is an in-plane graded interface or an interface graded in two or three dimensions. In-plane grading in such interfaces may be designed to deflect or arrest a crack.

It is noted that fracture referred to in the above-referenced studies is concerned with cracks propagating in continuous materials and interfaces. The problem is different if the material is discontinuous, e.g., it consists of a family of fibers interconnected by discontinuous "bridges." For example, evidence exists that collagen fibers in tendons are discontinuous, requiring connections between fibers for load transfer [25]. These connections may involve chemical cross-links between molecules, bridging proteins between fibers (e.g., decorin proteoglycans), or mineral platelets large enough to cross from one fiber to another. Such a model complicates the analysis of failure; classical fracture analysis approaches in this case should be replaced with a nano- or micro-mechanical stress analyses that trace the degradation of connections between adjacent fibrils.

1.4 Conclusions

An outline of typical attachments of dissimilar materials in engineering and biology was presented, demonstrating a remarkable diversity of attachment mechanisms. One general conclusion that can be made from the studies discussed above relates to the advantages of graded interfaces between dissimilar materials. Interfacial gradings in engineering and biology reduce local stress concentrations, enhance the toughness of the attachment, and reduce fracture trends. When designing an optimum interface between two materials, one should be aware of material limitations. Mechanical properties should be derived from mechanical analyses based on the distribution and geometry of constituent materials forming the interface. This understanding is necessary in order to translate theoretical attachment designs to practical use. These analyses must also consider multiscale modeling approaches, as many of the attachment systems are hierarchical in nature, from the nano- to the millimeter scales. A second observation related to functional grading at the interface between dissimilar materials is that the design criteria should satisfy several requirements, including strength, fracture, toughness, and stiffness. This may require prioritization of mechanical property behavior (e.g., sacrificing strength for improved toughness). Further study of biological attachments may provide biomimetic lessons for medical and engineering applications. For example, the advantages of a compliant zone between the attachment of a compliant orthotropic material with a stiff isotropic material would not have been realized without careful experimental and modeling studies of tendon, ligament, and meniscal attachments to bone.

References

1. Tong L, Steven GP (1999) Analysis and design of structural bonded joints. Kluwer, Hingham, MA
2. Palazotto AN, Birman V (1995) Environmental and viscoelastic effects on stresses in adhesive joints. J Aerosp Eng 8:107–118
3. Tsouvalis NG (2011) An investigation of the tensile strength of a composite-to-metal adhesive joint. Appl Compos Mater 18:149–163
4. Suhir E (2009) Predictive analytical thermal stress modeling in electronics and photonics. Appl Mech Rev 62(4):040801–040820
5. Dhamdhere AR, Malshe AP, Schmidt WF, Brown WD (2003) Investigation of reliability issues in high power laser diode bar packages. Microelectron Reliab 43(2):287–295
6. Nied HF (2003) Mechanics of interface fracture with applications in electronic packaging. IEEE T Dev Maters Reliab 3(4):129–143
7. Jackson M, Shukla A (2011) Performance of sandwich composites subjected to sequential impact and air blast loading. Compos Part B 42(2):155–166
8. Kirugulige MS, Kitey R, Tipput HV (2005) Dynamic fracture behavior of model sandwich structures with functionally graded core: a feasibility study. Compos Sci Technol 65:1052–1068
9. Ho SP, Marshall SJ, Ryder MI, Marshall GW (2007) The tooth attachment mechanism defined by structure, chemical composition and mechanical properties of collagen fibers in the periodontium. Biomaterials 28(35):5238–5245
10. Müeller W-D, Gross U, Fritz T, Voigt C, Fischer P, Berger G, Rogaschewski S, Lange K-P (2003) Evaluation of the interface between bone and titanium surfaces being blasted by aluminium oxide or bioceramic particles. Clin Oral Implants Res 14(3):349–356
11. Huiskes R, van Rietbergen B (1995) Preclinical testing of total hip stems. The effects of coating placement. Clin Orthop Relat Res 319:64–76
12. Yerby SA, Paal AF, Young PM, Beaupre GS, Ohashi KL, Goodman SB (2000) The effect of a silane coupling agent on the bond strength of bone cement and cobalt-chrome alloy. J Biomed Mater Res 49:127–133
13. Mumme T, Marx R, Mueller-Rath R, Siebert C, Wirtz D (2008) Surface coating to improve the metal-cement bonding in cemented femur stems. Arch Orthop Trauma Surg 128(8):773–781
14. Thomopoulos S, Marquez JP, Weinberger B, Birman V, Genin GM (2006) Collagen fiber orientation at the tendon to bone insertion and its influence on stress concentrations. J Biomech 39(10):1842–1851
15. Genin GM, Kent A, Birman V, Wopenka B, Pasteris JD, Marquez PJ, Thomopoulos S (2009) Functional grading of mineral and collagen in the attachment of tendon to bone. Biophys J 97 (4):976–985
16. Thomopoulos S, Das R, Birman V, Smith L, Ku K, Elson E, Pryse KM, Marquez P, Genin GM (2011) Fibrocartilage tissue engineering: the role of the stress environment on cell morphology and matrix expression. Tissue Eng Part A 17(7–8):1039–1053
17. Galatz LM, Ball CM, Teefey SA, Middleton WD, Yamaguchi K (2004) The outcome and repair integrity of completely arthroscopically repaired large and massive rotator cuff tears. J Bone Joint Surg Am 86-A(2):219–224
18. Liu Y, Birman V, Chen C, Thomopoulos S, Genin GM (2011) Mechanisms of bimaterial attachment at the interface of tendon to bone. J Eng Mater Technol 133(1):art no. 011006
19. Liu YX, Thomopoulos S, Birman V, Li J-S, Genin GM (2012) Bi-material attachment through a compliant interfacial system at the tendon-to-bone insertion site. Mech Mater 44:83–92
20. Delale F (1984) Stress singularities in bonded anisotropic materials. Int J Solids Struct 20:31–40
21. Kim J-H, Paulino GH (2007) On fracture criteria for mixed-mode crack propagation in functionally graded materials. Adv Mech Maters 14:227–244

22. Paulino GH, Jin ZH (2001) A crack in a viscoelastic functionally graded material layer embedded between two dissimilar homogeneous viscoelastic layers—antiplane shear analysis. Int J Fract 111(3):283–303
23. Wang Y-S, Huang G-Y, Gross D (2004) On the mechanical modeling of functionally graded interfacial zone with a Griffith crack: plane deformation. Int J Fract 125(1):189–205
24. Tvergaard V (2002) Theoretical investigation of the effect of plasticity on crack growth along a functionally graded region between dissimilar elastic–plastic solids. Eng Fract Mech 69:1635–1645
25. Redaelli A, Vesentini S, Soncini M, Vena P, Mantero S, Montevecchi FM (2003) Possible role of decorin glycosaminoglycans in fibril to fibril force transfer in relative mature tendons—a computational study from molecular to microstructural level. J Biomech 36(10):1555–1569

Chapter 2
Functionally Graded Materials in Engineering

Victor Birman, Tyler Keil, and Serhat Hosder

2.1 Introduction

Functionally graded materials (FGM) are composite materials formed of two or more constituent phases with a continuously variable distribution. The variations in the phase distribution may be reflected in their volume or weight fraction, orientation, and shape. In the majority of studies of FGM in engineering, the authors aim to achieve their goals with only one of these factors, the volume fraction being a typical variable. The variation of the phase volume fractions may be exclusively through the thickness of the structure and/or in any other direction, such as in-surface coordinates of a plate or shell.

The present chapter approaches the issue of FGM in engineering from the point of view of the classification and mathematical formulation for typical FGM, identification of characteristic problems addressed using these materials, methodology of the analysis, obstacles to the application of FGM, and the potential for these material systems in biomedical applications. The chapter does not attempt to present a comprehensive review of the subject, as the number of references addressing miscellaneous aspects of mechanics, manufacturing, and applications of FGM amount to hundreds per year, but rather concentrates on the most recent and typical problems and studies.

V. Birman (✉)
Engineering Education Center, Missouri University of Science and Technology, St. Louis, MO, USA
e-mail: vbirman@mst.edu

T. Keil
Sandia National Laboratories, Albuquerque, NM, USA
e-mail: tjkq35@mail.mst.edu

S. Hosder
Department of Mechanical and Aerospace Engineering, Missouri University of Science and Technology, Rolla, MO, USA
e-mail: hosders@mst.edu

S. Thomopoulos et al. (eds.), *Structural Interfaces and Attachments in Biology*,
DOI 10.1007/978-1-4614-3317-0_2,

FGM are often considered in thermomechanical applications, such as ceramic-metal composite structures where a higher ceramic concentration at the surface exposed to an elevated temperature or heat flux may be beneficial. As most biological applications serve in a narrow temperature range, we intentionally exclude thermal FGM problems from this chapter. The chapter introduces the concept of FGM, demonstrates a mathematical approach to their analysis, and presents a review of representative modern studies. Finally, we illustrate an example where grading the facings of a sandwich panel results in an impressive improvement in its stability and vibration characteristics.

2.2 Introduction to FGM

FGM were first suggested in Japan in the mid-1980s for thermal barrier coatings in aerospace applications. Since their inception, these materials have experienced a rapid development and found many applications in various fields of engineering. There are a number of reviews outlining the development of FGM, including books [1, 2], review articles [3], and proceedings of conferences dedicated to the field of FGM [4, 5]. The areas where FGM offer potential improvements and advantages in engineering applications include a reduction of in-plane and transverse through-the-thickness stresses, prevention or reduction of delamination tendencies in laminated or sandwich structures, improved residual stress distribution, enhanced thermal properties, higher fracture toughness, and reduced stress intensity factors.

Typical FGM architectures employ a variation of volume fractions of constituent materials in one or several directions. For example, a one-dimensional variation of mineral and metal phases can be employed to improve fracture toughness of prosthesis joints [6] and improve their mechanical strength, while retaining necessary biocompatibility as schematically shown in Fig. 2.1 [7]. Another example of a one-dimensional functional grading is found in sandwich panels where a functionally graded core (e.g., [8]) or a graded facing-core interface can improve fracture characteristics, and in particular, prevent debonding between the facings and core.

Besides a through-the-thickness variation of material volume fractions, the grading and corresponding property tailoring can be achieved through an in-surface variable volume fraction and through a coordinate-dependent orientation and sizing of fibers in a composite material. This type of grading is essentially biomimetic; for example, collagen fibers vary their orientation across the tendon-to-bone insertion site as is discussed below. Bamboo is an interesting example of a natural FGM where both the number and shape of fibers vary from the inner to outer periphery, i.e., the fibers at the outer periphery have a nearly circular cross section and a higher density, while their counterparts in the inner section have an ellipsoidal cross section and a lower volume fraction [9]. Besides grading the volume fraction and/or shape of constituent materials, FGM include materials with graded porosity that can be applied in such dissimilar components as hard tissue implants and diesel engine filters [10].

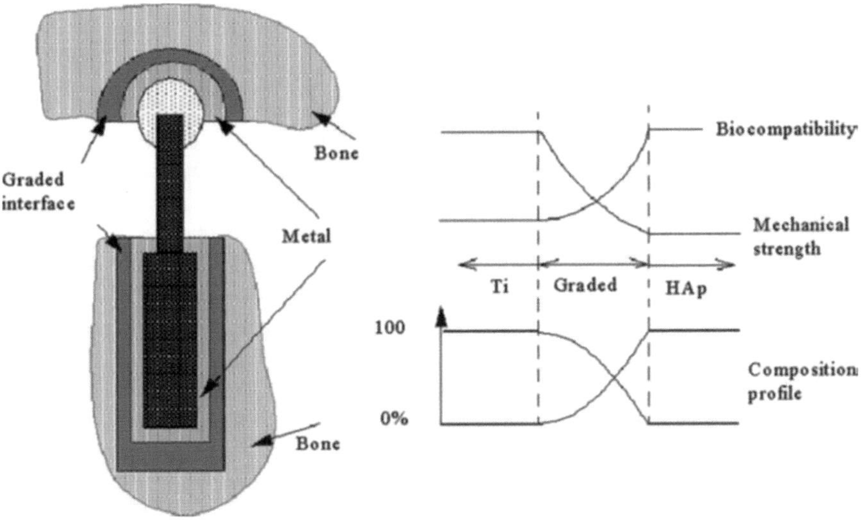

Fig. 2.1 Schematic of a functionally graded materials (FGM) interface within a prosthesis (reproduced, with permission, from [7])

2.3 Mathematical Backgrounds of Micromechanical and Macromechancial Analyses

The analysis of FGM in engineering is often concerned with relatively thin structures where the content of the constituent phases and the properties vary in the thickness direction. This is not always the case in biological applications as is evidenced by a gradual gradation of both the collagen fibers orientation and the mineral content along the tendon-to-bone insertion site (e.g., [11]).

Accordingly, we present here a relevant mathematical formulation that enables the stress analysis for the general case of three-dimensional variations of the volume fractions of the constituent materials. Temperature fluctuations in a human body and other biological systems usually remain within a narrow range, i.e., its explicit effect on the stresses as well as the implicit effect through the influence on the material properties can be disregarded. A possible exception could be cited in the case where an FGM employed in biological or medical applications is manufactured at an elevated temperature, raising a concern for residual stresses. This case, which can be analyzed with a relative ease due to a presumed uniform temperature distribution during the manufacturing process, is omitted from the following mathematical formulation.

Homogenization techniques predict material properties, such as the tensor of stiffness and the strength, in terms of the properties of the constituent phases, their shape and orientation, and their local volume fraction. Such analysis can be conducted using standard homogenization methods that should be modified to account for a gradient in the volume fraction distribution, in case it is sufficiently large to affect the local micromechanical problem (e.g., [12]). In a rather typical situation where the gradient of the volume fraction is sufficiently small to be neglected at the unit cell level, a variety of homogenization techniques that are well researched in mechanics of composites are available [13–15]. Random aspects of micromechanics of FGM can be treated using the corresponding methods developed for heterogeneous media [16].

While a detailed discussion of homogenization techniques is outside the scope of this chapter, the comprehension of the general approach is available based on the principles established by Hill [17]. Consider an FGM where the properties do not noticeably vary at the scale of a representative volume element (RVE). All constituent materials are assumed to remain in the elastic range. Then the average stress and strain vectors of this composite are related by

$$\boldsymbol{\sigma} = \mathbf{L}(\bar{x})\boldsymbol{\varepsilon}, \quad \boldsymbol{\varepsilon} = \mathbf{M}(\bar{x})\boldsymbol{\sigma} \tag{2.1}$$

where $\mathbf{L}$ and $\mathbf{M} = \mathbf{L}^{-1}$ are the overall tensors of stiffness and compliance, respectively, that should be specified according to a homogenization theory. Note that in FGM the stiffness and compliance vary with the coordinates of the RVE, i.e., $\bar{x}$.

Both stresses and strains in each constituent phase can be expressed in terms of the local average stress and strain:

$$\boldsymbol{\sigma}_n = \mathbf{A}_n(\bar{x})\boldsymbol{\sigma}, \quad \boldsymbol{\varepsilon}_n = \mathbf{B}_n(\bar{x})\boldsymbol{\varepsilon} \tag{2.2}$$

where n is the phase identifier number, while $\mathbf{A}_n$ and $\mathbf{B}_n$ are the stress and strain concentration tensors, respectively.

By the definition of the average stress and strain,

$$\sum_n c_n(\bar{x})\mathbf{A}_n(\bar{x}) = \mathbf{I}, \quad \sum_n c_n(\bar{x})\mathbf{B}_n(\bar{x}) = \mathbf{I} \tag{2.3}$$

where $c_n(\bar{x})$ is the volume fraction of the corresponding phase and $\mathbf{I}$ is a 6×6 identity matrix.

If the ith constituent phase is locally dominant, the tensors of stiffness and compliance can be determined by

$$\begin{aligned} \mathbf{L}(\bar{x}) &= \mathbf{L}_i(\bar{x}) + \sum_j c_j(\bar{x})[\mathbf{L}_j(\bar{x}) - \mathbf{L}_i(\bar{x})]\mathbf{A}_j(\bar{x}) \\ \mathbf{M}(\bar{x}) &= \mathbf{M}_i(\bar{x}) + \sum_j c_j(\bar{x})[\mathbf{M}_j(\bar{x}) - \mathbf{M}_i(\bar{x})]\mathbf{B}_j(\bar{x}) \end{aligned} \tag{2.4}$$

where index j covers the same range as n, except for $n = i$.

According to the approach illustrated above, given the stress and strain concentration tensors, one can determine the average local tensors of stiffness and compliance. The concentration tensors depend on such objective factors as the shape, volume fraction, and orientation of the inclusions as well as on the subjective aspect of the analysis, i.e., the choice of the micromechanical theory. In particular, if the volume fractions of all constitutive materials, except for the locally dominant material, are small enough to neglect their interaction, the tensor of stiffness obtained by the effective field method is [18]

$$\mathbf{L}(\bar{x}) = \mathbf{L}_i(\bar{x}) + \sum_j c_j(\bar{x})[\mathbf{L}_j(\bar{x}) - \mathbf{L}_i(\bar{x})]\mathbf{T}_j(\bar{x})[c_i(\bar{x})\mathbf{I} + c_j(\bar{x})\mathbf{T}_j(\bar{x})] \tag{2.5}$$

where tensors $\mathbf{T}_j(\bar{x})$ relate the average strain in the i-phase to the average strain to the j-phase inclusions. While the previous micromechanical formulation is three-dimensional, not being constrained by geometry of the structure or solid, the following discussion concentrates on relatively thin-walled structures that are typical in engineering applications.

The stiffness tensor is the outcome of the homogenization procedure. This tensor can be employed to determine the extensional, coupling, and bending stiffness matrices that are necessary for the macromechancial analysis of FGM structures. This procedure requires us to transform a local stiffness tensor to the global coordinate system employed in the analysis. If a relatively thin structure consists of a number of layers, each of them with its unique material grading, the transformation equation for the local stiffness tensor $\mathbf{L}_k$ that governs the response of the kth layer located at $z_k < z < z_{k+1}$ where z is the coordinate counted from the middle surface of the structure is

$$\mathbf{Q}_k(x_1, x_2, z) = \mathbf{P}(\theta_k)\mathbf{L}_k(x_{1k}, x_{2k}, z) \tag{2.6}$$

In (2.6), x_1 and x_2 are in-surface coordinates and $\mathbf{P}(\theta_k)$ is the transformation tensor that depends on the angle θ_k between the global (x_1, x_2, z) and local (x_{1k}, x_{2k}, z) coordinate systems. Examples of in-surface global coordinates are the length and width coordinates in the Cartesian system or the axial and circumferential coordinates in the cylindrical coordinate system.

The matrices of extensional, coupling, and bending stiffness are now evaluated following the standard mechanics of composite materials approach:

$$\{\mathbf{A}(x_1,x_2) \quad \mathbf{B}(x_1,x_2) \quad \mathbf{D}(x_1,x_2)\} = \int_z \mathbf{Q}_k(x_1, x_2, z)\{1 \quad z \quad z^2\}\,\mathrm{d}z \tag{2.7}$$

where the integration is conducted over the entire thickness of the structure. Note that the stiffness matrices in the left side of (2.7) are dependent on in-surface coordinates. In "conventional" composite materials such dependence is absent, but if the volume fraction, shape, or orientation of constituent phases of an FGM structure vary with the x_1 and x_2 coordinates, the stiffness of the structure is variable over the surface.

The constitutive relations for thin-walled structures are reduced from three-dimensional to two-dimensional formulation by integrating the stresses given by (2.1) over the thickness. This integration eliminates the dependence on the z-coordinate and replaces the stresses with a system of equivalent stress resultants, i.e., forces per unit width of the cross section, and stress couples, i.e., moments per unit width of the cross section. Thus the stress resultant and stress couple vectors are defined by

$$\{\mathbf{N} \quad \mathbf{M}\} = \int_z \boldsymbol{\sigma}\{1 \quad z\}\,\mathrm{d}z \tag{2.8}$$

The mathematical formulation should employ assumptions related to the deformed shape of an infinitesimal element detached from the structure. These assumptions reflect kinematics of the structure, i.e., the transformation of the displacement tensor $\mathbf{u}(x)$ in the course of deformation and strain–displacement relationships that can reflect geometrically linear or nonlinear formulations. In particular, in a thin structure characterized by the so-called classical or technical theory, we rely on the Kirchhoff-Love assumptions, i.e., the transverse shear strains as well as the axial strain in the thickness direction are assumed equal to zero. These assumptions imply that the thickness of the structure remains constant, while normal lines to the undeformed middle surface remain straight and perpendicular to this surface upon deformation. The validity of these assumptions becomes questionable for very thick structures or in the vicinity to such discontinuities as cut-outs, rivet holes, etc. In composite materials, the effect of transverse shear strains has to be sometimes accounted for due to low shear stiffness. However, the Kirchhoff-Love assumptions are usually applicable for relatively thin composite plates and shells manufactured from conventional composites, if their in-plane size to thickness ratio is larger than a factor in the range from 30 or 40.

In case of a thin-walled structure characterized by the classical theory, the vector of strain in (2.1) is represented by a sum of two components, i.e., the strains in the middle surface ($\boldsymbol{\varepsilon}_0$) and the changes of curvature and twist $\boldsymbol{\kappa}$:

$$\boldsymbol{\varepsilon} = \boldsymbol{\varepsilon}_0 + z\boldsymbol{\kappa} \tag{2.9}$$

where $\boldsymbol{\varepsilon}_0 = \boldsymbol{\varepsilon}(z = 0)$. The so-called first-order and higher-order theories accounting for the rotation and warping of cross sections perpendicular to the middle surface during deformation include additional terms proportional to integer powers of the z-coordinate.

The substitution of (2.1), (2.7), and (2.9) into (2.8) results in the constitutive relations relating the vectors of stress resultants and stress couples to the vectors of middle surface strains and the changes of curvature and twist:

$$\begin{Bmatrix} \mathbf{N} \\ \mathbf{M} \end{Bmatrix} = \begin{bmatrix} \mathbf{A} & \mathbf{B} \\ \mathbf{B} & \mathbf{D} \end{bmatrix} \begin{Bmatrix} \boldsymbol{\varepsilon}_0 \\ \boldsymbol{\kappa} \end{Bmatrix} \tag{2.10}$$

Equation (2.10) can often be simplified, since the matrices of extensional, coupling, and bending stiffnesses are not fully populated (in other words, some of the elements of these matrices are equal to zero). The matrices are presented for isotropic, specialty orthotropic and generally orthotropic composite laminates in every textbook on composite materials (e.g., [19]). In the case of FGM the properties can vary in three mutually perpendicular directions oriented along the coordinate axes. If the variations of properties within each RVE are negligible, i.e., we account for such variations on the macroscale, rather than on the microscale, the FGM material has three planes of elastic symmetry, each of them perpendicular to the corresponding coordinate axis.

Several possible grading schemes listed below correspond to differently populated matrices of stiffnesses. While the mathematical details are omitted for brevity, we can classify the following cases:

1. Properties vary in three coordinate directions. At the RVE level, the material is generally orthotropic.
2. Properties vary in three coordinate directions. At the RVE level, the material is specially orthotropic.
3. Properties vary in three coordinate directions. At the RVE level, material is isotropic.
4. Properties vary in the thickness direction only. At the RVE level, material is generally orthotropic.
5. Properties vary in the thickness direction only. At the RVE level, the material is specially orthotropic.
6. Properties vary in the thickness direction. At the RVE level, the material is isotropic.

While the first three cases correspond to in-surface variable stiffness, i.e., $\mathbf{A}(\bar{x})$, $\mathbf{B}(\bar{x})$, $\mathbf{D}(\bar{x})$, in the latter three cases the corresponding matrices are constant resulting in a simpler analysis.

Equations of equilibrium and boundary conditions can be derived from the energy principles (e.g., Hamilton's principle) or from the analysis of equilibrium of an infinitesimal element of the thin-walled structure. In both cases, the thickness z-coordinate is eliminated from the analysis, i.e., the equilibrium of an element of the structure is analyzed using a two-dimensional formulation where the stresses that may vary with all three coordinates are replaced with the equivalent system of stress resultants and stress couples via (2.8). The form of equations of equilibrium depends on geometry of the structure, i.e., a doubly curved shell has different equations than a flat plate, etc. For simplicity, we show here static equations for a flat plate utilizing the Cartesian coordinate system, x and y being in-surface coordinates:

$$\begin{aligned} & N_{x,x} + N_{xy,y} = 0 \\ & N_{xy,x} + N_{y,y} = 0 \\ & M_{x,xx} + 2M_{xy,xy} + M_{y,yy} + N_x w_{,xx} + 2N_{xy} w_{,xy} + N_y w_{,yy} = p(x,y) \end{aligned} \tag{2.11}$$

where $w = w(x,y)$ is a deflection and $p(x,y)$ is a pressure applied to the plate.

As is easily observed, the problem formulated in (2.11) is statically indeterminate since there are six unknown stress resultants and stress couples in three equilibrium equations. This is a common feature of mechanics of solids, fluids, and gases. Nevertheless, the problem can be resolved by expressing six stress resultants and couples in (2.11) in terms of three unknown displacements via (2.9), (2.10) and the strain–displacement relations omitted here for brevity. The latter relations can be either linear or nonlinear leading to geometrically linear or nonlinear problems, respectively. The boundary conditions are formulated in terms of displacements and rotations (kinematic conditions) and stress resultants and couples (static conditions).

The major difference between two types of FGM becomes apparent upon the analysis of (2.11). In the case of grading confined to variations of the volume fraction (and/or shapes and orientations of constituent phases) exclusively through the thickness of the structure, the tensor of stiffness is independent of the in-surface coordinates x and y. Accordingly, equations of equilibrium in terms of displacements contain only derivatives of displacements, while the elements of matrices **A**, **B** and **D** are constant. However, if the volume fractions (and/or other grading variables) of constituent phases vary with the in-surface coordinates, i.e., $\mathbf{A}(x, y)$, $\mathbf{B}(x, y)$, $\mathbf{D}(x, y)$, derivatives of stress resultants and stress couples in (2.11) contain derivatives of the corresponding stiffness coefficients. The analytical solution of the corresponding equations of equilibrium becomes impossible, except for simple superficial cases. However, a numerical solution utilizing finite element or finite difference methods is feasible even in this case since in-surface gradients of the properties are relatively small and it is possible to size a mesh where each element can be assigned constant in-surface properties.

An alternative method that is used in the theory of plates and shells, including those from FGM, is based on the introduction of the stress function. In the case of a flat FGM plate, this function (φ) is introduced through the following relations:

$$N_x = \varphi_{,yy}, \quad N_y = \varphi_{,xx}, \quad N_{xy} = -\varphi_{,xy} \tag{2.12}$$

The substitution of the stress function defined by (2.12) into equations of equilibrium (2.11) results in identities for the first two equations. The third equation can be formulated in terms of the stress function and unknown deflection. This equation has to be complemented with the equation expressing compatibility conditions. These conditions guarantee single-valued displacements in case the problem is solved in terms of stresses or stress functions. They do not have to be considered if the problem is solved in terms of displacements since such solution yields unique values of displacements throughout the domain occupied by the structure. In the problem of plane stress the compatibility conditions are reduced to one equation [20]:

$$\varepsilon^0_{x,yy} + \varepsilon^0_{y,xx} - \gamma^0_{xy,xy} = w_{,xy}{}^2 - w_{,xx}\, w_{,yy} \tag{2.13}$$

where ε_x^0 and ε_y^0 are middle surface axial strains and γ_{xy}^0 is the middle surface shear strain.

The considerations discussed with regard to (2.11) remain valid if the problem is solved utilizing the stress function. In the case of in-surface grading the substitution of the stress resultants and stress couples expressed in terms of the stress function and deflection in the third equation (2.11) and in (2.13) results in exceedingly complicated equations. If grading is limited to the through-the-thickness z-coordinate, the corresponding procedure is simplified, essentially coinciding with such procedures for typical laminated composite structures. For example, if an FGM panel is symmetric about the middle surface and the principal axes of the material coincide with the coordinate system (specially orthotropic RVE), the equation of equilibrium and the compatibility condition become:

$$
\begin{aligned}
a_{22}\varphi_{,xxxx} + (2a_{12} + a_{66})\varphi_{,xxyy} + a_{11}\varphi_{,yyyy} &= (w_{,xy})^2 - w_{,xx}\, w_{,yy} \\
D_{11}w_{,xxxx} + 2(D_{12} + 2D_{66})w_{,xxyy} + D_{22}w_{,yyyy} &= p(x,y) + h(\varphi_{,yy}\, w_{,xx} - 2\varphi_{,xy}\, w_{,xy} \\
&\quad + \varphi_{,xx}\, w_{,yy})
\end{aligned}
\tag{2.14}
$$

where the elements of the extensional compliance matrix $[a_{ij}] = [A_{ij}]^{-1}$ and the subscripts comply with standard notation in mechanics of composites.

As is evident from the present discussion, analytical solutions for FGM structures may be possible if grading is limited to the thickness direction. In the general case, the solution has to be numerical. The strain energy of an FGM structure is introduced in the same manner as for any other material, i.e.,

$$
U = \frac{1}{2}\iiint_{\Omega} (\sigma_x\varepsilon_x + \sigma_y\varepsilon_y + \sigma_z\varepsilon_z + \tau_{yz}\gamma_{yz} + \tau_{xz}\gamma_{xz} + \tau_{xy}\gamma_{xy})\, d\Omega \tag{2.15}
$$

where Ω is the volume occupied by the structure. The difference between a conventional composite material and a heterogeneous FGM where grading can vary with in-surface coordinates becomes apparent if we substitute the stress–strain relations (2.1) into (2.15).

It is necessary to emphasize here that assumptions regarding analytical expressions for the tensor of stiffness of FGM should be treated with caution. This is because in realistic situations we can prescribe variations of the volume fraction of constituent materials, i.e., analytical functions $c_n(\bar{x})$. However, analytical expressions for the stiffness, i.e., $\mathbf{A}(x)$, $\mathbf{B}(x)$, $\mathbf{D}(x)$, should be derived based on the adopted micromechanics, reflecting the local volume fraction, shape, and orientation of the inclusions (constituent phases), rather than being assumed arbitrarily. On the other hand, it is possible to develop a reverse scheme starting with the tensor of stiffness of FGM and using micromechanics to specify the corresponding volume fraction and geometry of inclusions.

In conclusion, we outlined fundamental relations involved in the analysis of FGM structures and illustrated the major difference between cases of in-surface and through-the-thickness grading. Two approaches to the micromechanical problem have been identified: a direct approach where the properties, such as the tensor of stiffness, are determined based on the prescribed volume fraction, orientation, and shape of the constituent phases and the reverse approach where the latter volume fractions and geometry are specified based on the prescribed tensor of stiffness.

2.4 Representative Recent Studies of FGM in Engineering

In this section we refer to recent studies in various areas of FGM oriented toward engineering applications. While several comprehensive reviews are cited above, we concentrate here on relatively recent representative additions to the field. The problems anticipated in biomedical and biological applications being mostly limited to a narrow range of temperatures, we eliminate the reference to heat transfer problems and to the effects of temperature on stresses and properties of FGM.

2.4.1 Homogenization of FGM

The homogenization bamboo, a natural FGM, was undertaken using graded finite elements and accounting for a continuous variation of properties through the bamboo wall [21]. A stochastic micromechanical solution utilizing a Mori-Tanaka approach to the evaluation of probabilistic properties of an isotropic FGM was considered in [22] accounting for uncertainties in constituent material properties and their volume fraction. The outcome included the mean and standard deviation of the elastic modulus and Poisson ratio as well as their probability density functions.

The finite-volume theory was developed for modeling of a graded material microstructure with arbitrary shaped cross sections and subsequently applied to the analysis of the conductivity and stiffness matrices [23, 24]. It was found that the proposed approach was competitive with a finite element method.

An additional consideration that may become essential in the micromechanics of FGM with small size RVE or with steep gradients is nonlocal elasticity. Such issues are important if a classical continuum model is not well suited to modeling of the material because of small-scale effects [25]. The concept of nonlocal elasticity is based on the presumption that the stress at a point depends both on the strain at the same point as well as on the strains at other points within the body. As a result, the internal characteristic length, such as the lattice parameter, can be incorporated into constitutive equations. Nonlocal elastic models have been proposed and applied to modeling composite structures incorporating nanotubes, but they may also be useful for the characterization of FGM. These models incorporate the features of both the classical continuum model as well as the internal small-scale length effects.

In general, the main areas where research on the micromechanics and homogenization of FGM is needed include:

1. Accounting for local RVE-scale variations in the properties associated with rapidly varying volume fractions, shapes, and orientation of constituent materials.
2. Multiscale aspects involving an interaction between local and global scales.
3. Random micromechanical formulations reflecting uncertainties of the distribution of constituent phases that may be particularly significant at the microscale as well as uncertainties of constituent material properties.

2.4.2 FGM in Beams, Plates, and Shell Structures

Some of the recent studies of FGM plate structures include analyses of the effect of grading on the nonlinear forced and free response of thin circular plates [26, 27]. Axisymmetric static bending of annular transversely isotropic FGM plates undergoing uniform pressure was considered in [28]. Experimental, numerical, and analytical models of FGM plates subjected to low-velocity impact loading were reflected in optimization formulation yielding material properties of individual layers [29]. A higher-order layer-wise shear-deformation theory for FGM plates was developed and validated for static and dynamic representative cases [30]. A geometrically nonlinear elastic formulation for FGM plates was developed in [31]. While the majority of studies referenced above were confined to grading through the thickness of the structure, elasticity solutions were also developed for FGM beams with the elastic modulus varying both in the thickness and in the axial directions [32].

The bending response of sandwich beams with viscoeleastic FGM facings resting on an elastic foundation was considered in [33]. Various aspects of the response of functionally graded sandwich panels were also considered in recent studies [34, 35].

Dynamic stability of shear-deformable FGM beams, where the length scales of the deformation field and the material microstructure are comparable, was investigated using the couple stress theory [36]. The problem of dynamic stability of FGM shear-deformable shells was considered in [37]. The impact problem of a thick two-dimensionally graded hollow cylinder subject to an internal pressure was investigated in [38] where, predictably, shells with a two-dimensional grading were found superior to one-dimensional counterparts. Buckling of FGM cylindrical shells under axial compression was analyzed, accounting for geometric nonlinearity and initial imperfections [39]. The effect of through-the-thickness grading on the stress distribution in hollow spherical shells was shown to be confined mostly to tangential stresses, while radial stresses remained little affected [40]. A linear through-the-thickness distribution of the shear modulus was found to produce a constant hoop or circumferential stress in elastic FGM hollow cylinders and spheres, respectively [41].

The through-the-thickness grading has a significant effect on buckling of truncated conical FGM shells undergoing hydrostatic pressure [42]. An example of a finite element free vibration analysis of doubly curved shear-deformable shells with through-the-thickness grading is found in [43]. A graded finite element was developed for FGM geometrically nonlinear shells accounting for shear deformability through the first-order theory in [44]. Although thermal problems are avoided in our chapter, it is worth mentioning here the work analyzing thermomechanical behavior of FGM cylindrical shells with flowing fluid; this analysis may relate to problems of blood vessels that are also graded through their thickness [45].

The response of FGM structures with damage has received relatively little attention. Vibrations of FGM beams with cracks of various orientation were analyzed in [46].

Among potential applications of FGM structures wings and thin-walled blades were considered in [47, 48]. In particular the torsional stability of the wing was enhanced using spanwise grading of material properties, rather than through-the-thickness grading. Nonlinear supersonic flutter of FGM plates graded in the thickness direction was considered in [49]. Temperature is often present in aerospace structures; accordingly, we cite here papers accounting for thermal effects that are avoided in the rest of this survey. Among other applications, numerous studies have been conducted on functionally graded coatings; referenced here is paper [50]. A comprehensive review of earlier applications of FGM can be found in [3].

It is emphasized that the study of static and dynamic response of FGM structures should be comprehensive, including a local strength analysis. The latter is particularly important in FGM since their strength is a function of location, varying with the volume fraction, orientation, and shape of inclusions. In addition, fracture toughness of FGM is a function of coordinates and material architecture. These observations further emphasize the necessity of the analysis and design addressing all aspects of the problem, i.e., micromechanics, stiffness, strength, and macromechancial response.

2.4.3 FGM in Smart Structures

Research of smart FGM has mostly been confined to piezoelectrics. Panda and Ray analyzed the effectiveness of a 1–3 piezoelectric composite employed as a constraining layer to control nonlinear vibrations of a functionally graded plate, including an optimum location of a damping patch [51]. The sliding frictional contact problem of a graded piezoelectric half-plane in the state of plane strain was considered by Ke et al. [52]. The displacements and electric potential in a radially graded piezoelectric hollow shaft were found in [53]. Transient dynamic problems in inhomogeneous piezoelectric solids were analyzed by a meshless Petrov-Galerkin method concentrating on the unit step function loading [54]. Free vibrations and static response of doubly curved magneto-electro-elastic FGM shells with grading in the thickness direction were investigated in [55, 56], respectively.

A potentially interesting concept suggested in the present chapter would use superelastic shape memory alloy inclusions for optimum energy dissipation in an FGM composite structure. Superelastic shape memory alloys have an exceptionally high damping potential due to their large hysteresis loop area that can be employed to enhance dynamic response of composites (e.g., [57]).

2.4.4 Waves in FGM

Studies on waves in FGM and on the scattering of waves in FGM structures have gained noticeable popularity in recent years. For example, the effect of grading on the stress and displacement fields generated by Love waves in an FGM layered structure has been recently investigated [58]. The scattering of waves by hollow FGM ZrO_2-Al cylinders submerged in and filled with a nonviscous fluid was analyzed by acoustic resonance scattering theory [59]. A study concerned with the propagation of guided acoustic waves in FGM plates was undertaken in [60].

Propagation of waves in piezoelectric media represents a fascinating theoretical and engineering problem. For example, the problem of wave propagation in piezoelectric FGM structures in contact with viscous fluid was analyzed in [61]. A three-dimensional piezoelastic formulation was employed to study wave propagation in hollow cylinders in [62]. Wave propagation was also considered for transversely isotropic elastic piezoelectric half-sphere with grading in the depth direction [63]. The propagation of antiplane and shear-horizontal planes along the interface between two half-space piezoelectric FGM with properties varying in the direction perpendicular to the interface was analyzed in [64].

Shear wave scattering from a crack in a piezoelectric layer bonded to an FGM half-space was studied yielding normalized dynamic stress intensity factors as well as normalized electric displacement intensity factors [65]. The scattering of electro-elastic waves and the dynamic stress problem in the vicinity of a cavity in an FGM layer bonded to a homogeneous piezoelectric material was considered by Fang [66].

A further degree of complexity is encountered in the problems involving structures composed of piezoelectric and magnetostrictive materials (e.g., such structures are being considered in energy harvesting applications). For example, the propagation of waves in plates composed of graded piezoelectric ($BaTiO_3$) and magnetostrictive ($CoFe_2O_4$) layers was investigated in [67].

2.4.5 Optimization of FGM

An optimization problem in FGM hollow cylinders and spheres with a radial volume fraction variation was considered in [68] aiming either at a constant hoop or circumferential stress or a constant in-plane shear stress (in particular, constant hoop stresses imply an elimination of stress concentration). In the same paper, the radial distribution of constituent volume fractions necessary for a constant through-the-thickness linear combination of the radial and hoop stresses was specified. Although FGM subject to thermal loading are excluded from this review, mentioned here is the work of Bobaru [69], which illustrates that the outcome of the optimization procedure in FGM depends on the micromechanical model employed in the analysis.

It is noted that optimization of FGM may rely on numerous flexible tools, including variations of volume fractions, shapes, and orientations of constituent phases. However, a designer should be aware of limitations superimposed by manufacturability of such materials, including cost considerations.

2.4.6 Fracture, Stress Concentration, and Contact Problems in FGM

Among the many studies on fracture in FGM, fracture in an FGM strip with an arbitrary property variation was considered in [70]. The problem of a crack in an FGM coating inclined relative to a discontinuous interface was analyzed by Li and Lee [71]. An experimental investigation of fracture toughness in FGM consisting of partially stabilized zirconia and austenitic stainless steel was conducted [72], illustrating the benefits of a fine microstructure in FGM. Besides attempts to reduce the fracture tendencies along the interface, nanostructural coatings were shown to significantly increase the hardness of the surface [73].

Numerous studies of fracture in piezoelectric FGM have been published in recent years. The problems of an interfacial crack between an FGM layer and a dielectric substrate was analyzed for three cases, including a crack located near the edge of the interface and cracks far from the interface of a thin or thick piezoelectric layer with the substrate [74]. The interaction between parallel cracks in graded piezoelectric materials was considered in [75]. The mode III fracture of an FGM piezoelectric surface layer bonded to a piezoelectric substrate was studied in the case where cracks were normal to the interface [76]. The mixed-mode fracture in orthotropic FGM loaded by normal and shear tractions applied at the crack surface was also analyzed by Dag et al. using both analytical and finite element methods [77].

Mixed-mode fracture problems for penny-shaped and annular cracks in FGM strips were investigated in [78]. Periodic arrays of cracks in an FGM strip bonded to a homogeneous piezoelectric half-space were considered in [79].

Dynamic fracture problems in FGM are represented by several recent studies. A magnetoelectroelastic half-space with an FGM coating experiencing dynamic interfacial cracking as a result of impact loading was analyzed and a preferable coating grading arrangement was demonstrated [80]. Transient crack propagation along the shear modulus grading direction in an FGM was considered for Modes I and II fracture [81]. A dynamic antiplane fracture problem in magnetoelectroelastic plates with internal or edge cracks oriented in the gradation direction was considered in [82] where it was indicated that the crack propagation can be retarded by an appropriate grading of the material.

A stochastic multiscale approach to the fracture problem in FGM was considered in [83]. The probabilistic crack-driving forces and reliability were assessed employing two stochastic methods, i.e., the dimensional decomposition method and the Monte-Carlo simulation.

The effect of in-plane material grading on the stress concentration factor in an FGM plate with a circular hole was numerically investigated in [84]. It was demonstrated that the stress concentration can be reduced by varying the modulus, gradually increasing it with the distance from the hole.

Contact problems of FGM have also received the close attention of researchers. For example, Lee et al. investigated the effect of modulus of elasticity grading on the indentation produced in an elastic half-space by a rigid indenter [85]. The contact problem for an FGM layer subject to frictional sliding load applied by a flat punch was investigated in [86].

2.4.7 *Manufacturability*

One of the most challenging aspects of engineering FGM is related to the difficulty of manufacturing components with prescribed grading. These complications arise from a very small dimensional scale of property variations. This problem, discussed in a previous review [3] and other references, is particularly severe in case of grading in the thickness direction. If grading occurs with respect to in-surface coordinates, a larger scale usually permits a much easier reproduction of prescribed gradients. Some of the recent studies relevant to the manufacture of FGM components have been discussed in [10, 87, 88].

2.4.8 *Biomedical Applications of FGM*

Biomedical applications of FGM have not been extensively reviewed in the literature (e.g., [3]). Accordingly, we concentrate here on biomedical problems where these materials either may be applied or have been considered.

Erisken et al. investigated viscoelastic and compressive properties of a bovine osteochondral tissue and engineered constructs aiming at a better understanding of grading in properties along the thickness enabling a smooth transition of loads [89]. A bi-phasic model of functionally graded soft tissues was analyzed to describe a response to mechanical loading, accounting for geometric nonlinearities, rate-dependence, and anisotropy in [90]. Willert-Porada reviewed possible applications of biomimetic methods in design and fabrication of both a functionally graded hard tissue implant and, surprisingly, applications such as diesel engine filters [10].

Functional grading at the tendon-to-bone insertion site involves several mechanisms, including variations of the collagen fiber orientation from tendon to bone and a gradual variation of the mineral content. While the fibers that are uniaxially oriented in the tendon exhibit angular variations as they approach the bone, the mineral content varies from high volume fraction at the bone surface to zero at the tendon-insertion boundary. This phenomenon and its implications on the stiffness of the insertion site and the local stress concentration have recently been investigated [11, 91, 92].

Studies of a potential for FGM in hip replacement stems have also been conducted. For example, potential advantages of a 2-D functionally graded stem with variable content of hydroxyapatite, bioglass, and collagen were considered [93]. As was illustrated in this study, stress shielding and interfacial shear stress at the stem-femur interface were dramatically reduced compared to a standard titanium stem.

Dental applications of FGM have also received close attention. In particular, Hedia [94] conducted design of a dental implant coating and illustrated that if it is graded from titanium at the apex to collagen at the root, the von Mises stress in the bone can be reduced by 17% compared to the stress with hydroxyapatite coating. Further studies of the effect of graded implants on the bone can be found in [95].

2.5 Example Problem: Optimization of an FGM Sandwich Panel for Maximum Buckling Load and Fundamental Frequency

Contrary to numerous FGM studies where grading was limited to the thickness direction, it is interesting to quantify potential advantages of in-surface grading in engineering and biomimetic structures. Such analysis is of particular interest since in-surface grading is found in numerous biological systems, such as the previously discussed tendon-to-bone insertion site.

In the present section, we consider the effect of optimized grading of the in-plane stiffness in sandwich plates aiming at an increase in the eigenvalues (buckling load and fundamental frequency), without a penalty in the plate weight. The size of the sandwich plate considered in the study was $1.0 \times 1.0 \times 0.01$ m. Each facing was constructed of 11 cross-ply 0.125 mm thick IM7/977-2 carbon/epoxy layers with the lamination scheme $[0_3/90/0_3/90/0_3]$. The fiber volume fraction in all layers of the original plate (prior to the introduction of grading) was 50%. The 7.25 mm thick foam core was manufactured from Divinycell HT 65.

The boundaries of the plate were simply supported. In the buckling problem, in-plane displacements of the edges loaded by compressive stress resultants were unconstrained in the load direction, while their tangential in-plane displacements (displacements along the edge) were prevented. Such boundary conditions

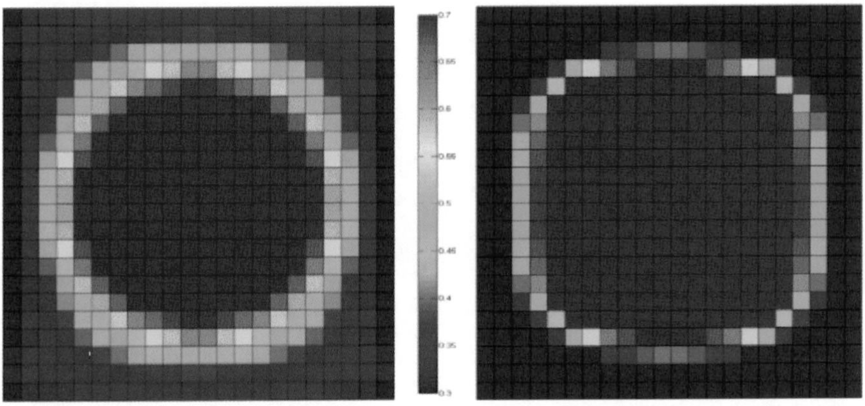

Fig. 2.2 Optimum fiber distribution in the facings of a square sandwich plate resulting in an 18.3% increase of the buckling load (*left*) and in an 8.7% increase of the fundamental frequency (*right*). Different colors correspond to different fiber volume fractions varying from 30 to 70%

resemble the case where the edges are supported by stringers of negligible out-of-plane stiffness and high axial stiffness. The same in-plane boundary conditions were adopted for the couple of unloaded edges. In the vibration problem, all edges were prevented from both tangential and normal in-plane displacements. Such a situation is encountered if the plate is supported by stringers and frames, while being constrained by adjacent structures from expansion or contraction.

The plate was modeled with 1,089 four-node, reduced integration shell elements using the ABAQUS commercial finite element code. Local volume fraction of fibers in the facing layers of the modified FGM plate was varied using the "material properties" module of ABAQUS [96]. A Constrained Minimization (CONMIN) was performed to optimize the plate using the Method of Feasible Directions that is built in the DAKOTA code [97]. The optimization conducted in this study was limited, i.e., while the volume fractions of fibers varied over the surface of the facings, all layers remained identical. Furthermore, the orientation of the layers was not altered. Thus, it may be possible to further improve the outcome of the procedure outlined below.

The optimum distribution of fibers in the layers of the facings is shown in Fig. 2.2 for the buckling problem where the panel is subject to uniaxial compression and for the free vibration problem where we maximize the fundamental frequency. The fiber distribution was changed piecewise in all layers, i.e., further improvements could be possible using different fiber content in different layers, varying the fiber content as a monotonous function of coordinate, or using ellipsoidal boundaries of the regions with different fiber fractions. Nevertheless, even with the present optimization approach, the buckling load was increased by 18.3% and the frequency by 8.7%, without any weight penalty. Furthermore, while the optimization could be refined, the present piecewise optimization complies with technological requirements to

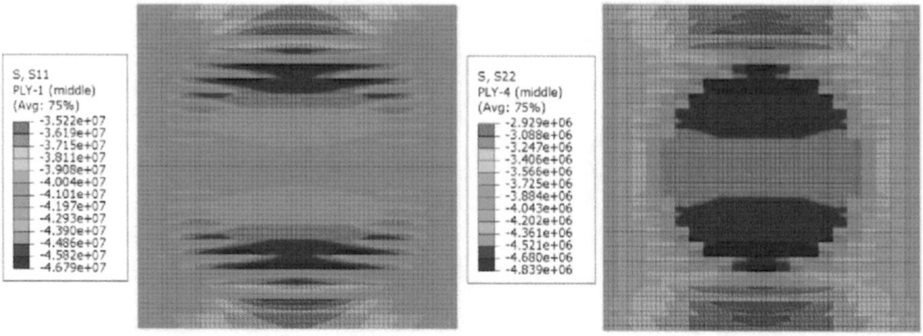

Fig. 2.3 Stresses (Pa) in the load (*horizontal*) direction in the facings of the optimized plate subject to the buckling load (*left*: 0° layers, *right*: 90° layers)

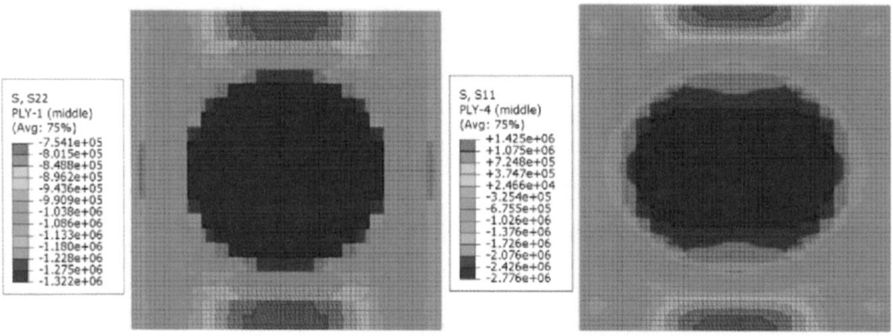

Fig. 2.4 Stresses (Pa) in the direction perpendicular to the load in the facings of the optimized plate subject to the buckling load (*left*: 0° layers, *right*: 90° layers). The load is acting in the horizontal direction

realistic engineering structures (e.g., an ellipsoidal boundary between regions with different fiber volume fractions is unlikely to be endorsed by industry).

In addition to the stability analysis, structural optimization of a compressed plate should ensure that the stresses in the facings and core remain below the allowable limit. The stress check results for the compressed optimized panel shown in Fig. 2.2 are demonstrated in Figs. 2.3 and 2.4. It was found that the stresses in the facings and core do not exceed the allowable level for the respective materials. It should be noted that the issue of strength of facings with variable fiber content involves both the check of local stresses as well as the update of the material strength dependent on the local fiber volume fraction. Such local failure modes as face wrinkling or kinking and core shear failure (e.g., [98]) did not present a problem in the present example. The stresses in the core that remained within the safe range are not shown here for brevity.

It is interesting to compare an optimization of a representative aerospace sandwich plate illustrated in this example with the optimization found in such biological system as the tendon-to-bone insertion site. While the stiffness of the plate varies due to the fiber content, at the insertion site the gradation of the stiffness is achieved through the orientation of collagen fibers and mineral content along the insertion. The final outcome is the structure optimized either for the highest eigenvalues (sandwich plate) or for the highest tensile load carrying capacity (insertion site).

2.6 Conclusions

The current chapter outlined the principles and mathematical backgrounds of FGM in engineering. A review of representative recent studies of such materials was presented. An example of optimization of a sandwich plate with in-surface graded facings resulting in a significant increase in the buckling load and fundamental frequency without a weight penalty was demonstrated.

FGM have found application in numerous engineering areas. The complexity of these material systems requires a comprehensive approach to their design and analysis, incorporating a multiscale formulation from the micromechanical RVE level to macromechanical structural analysis. It is emphasized that a concept like the strength of the material becomes irrelevant in FGM where the strength varies with the position reflecting a distribution of constitutive phases throughout the material. Similar considerations affect the analysis of fracture and such local failure modes as wrinkling in sandwich structures.

In conclusion, we emphasize that numerous natural biological systems are graded. Therefore, a biomimetic approach to design of FGM structures deserves close attention.

References

1. Suresh S, Mortensen A (1998) Fundamentals of functionally graded materials: processing and thermomechanical behaviour of graded metals and metal-ceramic composites. IOM Communications Ltd, London
2. Miyamoto Y (1999) Functionally graded materials: design, processing, and applications. Kluwer Academic Publishers, Boston
3. Birman V, Byrd LW (2007) Modeling and analysis of functionally graded materials and structures. Appl Mech Rev 60:195–216
4. Paulino GH (2008) Multiscale and functionally graded materials. In: Proceedings of the International Conference FGM IX, Oahu Island, Hawaii, 15–18 Oct 2006. AIP conference proceedings, vol 973. American Institute of Physics, Melville
5. Kawasaki A, Niino M, Kumakawa A (2008) Multiscale, multifunctional and functionally graded materials: selected, peer reviewed papers from the 10th International Symposium on MM & FGMs, 22nd–25th Sept 2008, Sendai, Japan. Materials science forum, vol 631–632. Trans Tech, Stafa-Zuriich, Switzerland; United Kingdom; Enfield
6. Mishina H, Inumaru Y, Kaitoku K (2008) Fabrication of ZrO2/AlSl316L functionally graded materials for joint prosthesis. Mater Sci Eng A 475:141–147

7. Qian X, Dutta D (2004) Feature-based design for heterogeneous objects. Comput Aided Design 36(12):1263–1278
8. Kirugulige MS, Kitey R, Tipput HV (2005) Dynamic fracture behavior of model sandwich structures with functionally graded core: a feasibility study. Compos Sci Technol 65:1052–1068
9. Ray A, Mondal S, Das S, Ramachandrarao P (2005) Bamboo—a functionally graded composite-correlation between microstructure and mechanical strength. J Mater Sci 40 (19):5249–5253
10. Willert-Porada M (2010) Design and fabrication strategy in the world of functional gradation. Int J Mater Prod Technol 39(1–2):59–71
11. Genin GM, Kent A, Birman V, Wopenka B, Pasteris JD, Marquez PJ, Thomopoulos S (2009) Functional grading of mineral and collagen in the attachment of tendon to bone. Biophys J 97 (4):976–985
12. Paulino GH, Silva ECN, Le CH (2009) Optimum design of periodic functionally graded composites with prescribed properties. Struct Multidiscip Optim 38(5):469–489
13. Torquato S (2001) Random heterogeneous materials: microstructure and macroscopic properties. Springer, New York
14. Markov K, Preziosi L (2000) Heterogeneous media: micromechanics modeling methods and simulations. Birkhauser, Boston
15. Pindera M-J, Khatam H, Drago AS, Bansal Y (2009) Micromechanics of spatially uniform heterogeneous media: a critical review and emerging approaches. Compos Part B 40:349–378
16. Ostoja-Starzewski M (2008) Microstructural randomness and scaling in mechanics of materials. Chapman & Hall/CRC, Boca Raton, FL
17. Hill R (1965) A self-consistent mechanics of composite materials. J Mech Phys Solids 13:213–222
18. Kanaun SK, Jeulin D (2001) Elastic properties of hybrid composites by the effective field approach. J Mech Phys Solids 49:2339–2367
19. Jones RM (1999) Mechanics of composite materials, 2nd edn. Taylor & Francis, Inc., Philadelphia
20. Fung YC (1994) A first course in continuum mechanics. Prentice-Hall, Englewood Cliffs
21. Silva ECN, Walters MC, Paulino GH (2008) Modeling bamboo as a functionally graded material. In: AIP conference proceedings, pp 754–759 Melville, New York
22. Rahman SCA (2007) A stochastic micromechanical model for elastic properties of functionally graded materials. Mech Mater 39:548–563
23. Cavalcante MAA, Marques SPC, Pindera M-J (2007) Parametric formulation of the finite-volume theory for functionally graded materials—part 1: analysis. J Appl Mech 74 (5):935–945
24. Cavalcante MAA, Marques SPC, Pindera M-J (2007) Parametric formulation of the finite-volume theory for functionally graded materials—part II: numerical results. J Appl Mech 74 (5):946–957
25. Eringen AC, Edelen DGB (1972) On nonlocal elasticity. Int J Eng Sci 10:233–248
26. Gunes R, Reddy JN (2008) Nonlinear analysis of functionally graded circular plates under different loads and boundary conditions. Int J Struct Stab Dyn 8(1):131–159
27. Allahverdizadeh A, Naei MH, Nikkhah Bahrami M (2008) Nonlinear free and forced vibration analysis of thin circular functionally graded plates. J Sound Vib 310(4–5):966–984
28. Li XY, Ding HJ, Chen WQ (2008) Axisymmetric elasticity solutions for a uniformly loaded annular plate of transversely isotropic functionally graded materials. Acta Mech 196 (3–4):139–159
29. Larson RA, Palazotto AN (2009) Property estimation in FGM plates subject to low-velocity impact loading. J Mech Mater Struct 4(7–8):1429–1451
30. Pai PF, Palazotto AN (2007) Two-dimensional sublamination theory for analysis of functionally graded plates. J Sound Vib 308(1–2):164–189

31. Chen H, Yu W (2010) Asymptotical construction of an efficient high-fidelity model for multilayer functionally graded plates. AIAA J 48(6):1171–1183
32. Lu CF, Chen WQ, Xu RQ, Lim CW (2008) Semi-analytical elasticity solutions for bi-directional functionally graded beams. Int J Solids Struct 45(1):258–275
33. Zenkour AM, Allam MNM, Sobhy M (2010) Bending analysis of FG viscoelastic sandwich beams with elastic cores resting on Pasternak's elastic foundation. Acta Mech 212 (3–4):233–252
34. Brischetto S (2009) Classical and mixed advanced models for sandwich plates embedding functionally graded cores. J Mech Mater Struct 4(1):13–33
35. Li Q, Iu VP, Kou KP (2008) Three-dimensional vibration analysis of functionally graded material sandwich plates. J Sound Vib 311(1–2):498–515
36. Ke LL, Wang Y-S (2011) Size effect of dynamic stability of functionally graded microbeams based on a modified couple stress theory. Compos Struct 93:342–350
37. Pradyumna S, Bandyopadhyay JN (2008) Dynamic instability of functionally graded shells using higher-order theory. J Eng Mech 136(5):551–561
38. Asgari M, Akhlaghi M, Hosseini SM (2009) Dynamic analysis of two-dimensional functionally graded thick hollow cylinder with finite length under impact loading. Acta Mech 208 (3–4):163–180
39. Huang H, Han Q (2008) Buckling of imperfect functionally graded cylindrical shells under axial compression. Eur J Mech A-Solid 27(6):1026–1036
40. Li XF, Peng XL, Kang YA (2009) Pressurized hollow spherical vessels with arbitrary radial nonhomogeneity. AIAA J 47(9):2262–2265
41. Batra RC (2008) Optimal design of functionally graded incompressible linear elastic cylinders and spheres. AIAA J 46(8):2050–2057
42. Sofiyev AH, Kuruoglu N, Turkmen M (2009) Buckling of FGM hybrid truncated conical shells subjected to hydrostatic pressure. Thin Wall Struct 47(1):61–72
43. Pradyumna S, Bandyopadhyay JN (2008) Free vibration analysis of functionally graded curved panels using a higher-order finite element formulation. J Sound Vib 318(1–2):176–192
44. Arcininega RA, Reddy JN (2007) Large deformation analysis of functionally graded shells. Int J Solids Struct 44(6):2036–2052
45. Sheng GG, Wang X (2008) Thermomechanical vibration analysis of a functionally graded shell with flowing fluid. Eur J Mech A-Solid 27(6):1075–1087
46. Birman V, Byrd LW (2007) Vibrations of damaged cantilevered beams manufactured from functionally graded materials. AIAA J 45(11):2747–2757
47. Librescu L, Maalawi KY (2007) Material grading for improved aeroelastic stability in composite wings. J Mech Mater Struct 2(7):1381–1394
48. Librescu L, Oh S-Y, Song O (2005) Thin-walled beams made of functionally graded materials and operating in a high temperature environment. J Therm Stress 28(6–7):649–712
49. Ibrahim HH, Yoo HH, Lee KS (2009) Supersonic flutter of functionally graded panels subject to acoustic and thermal loads. J Aircr 46(2):593–600
50. Kashtalyan M, Menshykova M (2008) Three-dimensional analysis of a functionally graded coating/substrate system of finite thickness. Philos Transact R Soc A Math Phys Eng Sci 366 (1871):1821–1826
51. Panda S, Ray MC (2009) Control of nonlinear vibrations of functionally graded plates using 1–3 piezoelectric composite. AIAA J 47(6):1421–1434
52. Ke LL, Wang YS, Yang J, Kitipornchai S (2010) Sliding frictional contact analysis of functionally graded piezoelectric layered half-plane. Acta Mech 209(3–4):249–268
53. Babaei MH, Chen ZT (2008) Analytical solution for the electromechanical behavior of a rotating functionally graded piezoelectric hollow shaft. Arch Appl Mech 78(7):489–500
54. Sladek J, Sladek V, Solek P, Saez A (2008) Dynamic 3D axisymmetric problems in continuously non-homogeneous piezoelectric solids. Int J Solids Struct 45(16):4523–4542
55. Tsai YH, Wu CP (2008) Dynamic responses of functionally graded magneto-electro-elastic shells with open-circuit surface conditions. Int J Eng Sci 46(9):843–857

56. Wu C-P, Tsai Y-H (2007) Static behavior of functionally graded magneto-electro-elastic shells under electric displacement and magnetic flux. Int J Eng Sci 45(9):744–769
57. Birman V (2010) Properties and response of composite material with spheroidal superelastic shape memory alloy inclusions subject to three-dimensional stress state. J Phys D: Appl Phys 43(22)
58. Qian ZH, Jin F, Lu T, Kishimoto K (2009) Transverse surface waves in an FGM layered structure. Acta Mech 207(3–4):183–193
59. Hasheminejad SM, Rajabi M (2007) Acoustic resonance scattering from a submerged functionally graded cylindrical shell. J Sound Vib 302(1–2):208–228
60. Shuvalov AL, Le Clezio E, Feuillard G (2008) The state-vector formalism and the Peano-series solution for modelling guided waves in functionally graded anisotropic piezoelectric plates. Int J Eng Sci 46(9):929–947
61. Du J, Xian K, Yong YK, Wang J (2010) SH-SAW propagation in layered functionally graded piezoelectric material structures loaded with viscous liquid. Acta Mech 212(3–4):271–281
62. Jiangong Y, Bin W, Guoqiang C (2009) Wave characteristics in functionally graded piezoelectric hollow cylinders. Arch Appl Mech 79(9):807–824
63. Cao X, Jin F, Wang Z (2008) On dispersion relations of Rayleigh waves in a functionally graded piezoelectric material (FGPM) half-space. Acta Mech 200(3–4):247–261
64. Liu N, Yang J, Qian ZH, Hirose S (2010) Interface waves in functionally graded piezoelectric materials. Int J Eng Sci 48(2):151–159
65. Li X, Liu J (2009) Scattering of the SH wave from a crack in a piezoelectric substrate bonded to a half-space of functionally graded materials. Acta Mech 208(3–4):299–308
66. Fang XQ (2008) Multiple scattering of electro-elastic waves from a buried cavity in a functionally graded piezoelectric material layer. Int J Solids Struct 45(22–23):5716–5729
67. Bin W, Jiangong Y, Cunfu H (2008) Wave propagation in non-homogeneous magneto-electro-elastic plates. J Sound Vib 317(1–2):250–264
68. Nie GJ, Zhong Z, Batra RC (2011) Material tailoring for functionally graded hollow cylinders and spheres. Compos Sci Technol 71(5):666–673
69. Bobaru F (2007) Designing optimal volume fractions for functionally graded materials with temperature dependent material properties. J Appl Mech 74(5):861–875
70. Zhong Z, Cheng Z (2008) Fracture analysis of a functionally graded strip with arbitrary distributed material properties. Int J Solids Struct 45(13):3711–3725
71. Li YD, Lee KY (2009) Effects of the weak/micro-discontinuity of interface on the fracture behavior of a functionally graded coating with an inclined crack. Arch Appl Mech 79(9):779–791
72. Tohgo K, Iizuka M, Araki H, Shimamura Y (2008) Influence of microstructure on fracture toughness distribution in ceramic-metal functionally graded materials. Eng Fract Mech 75(15):4529–4541
73. Leng SE (2010) Functional graded material with nano-structured coating for protection. Int J Mater Prod Technol 39(1–2):136–147
74. Li YD, Lee KY (2010) Interfacial fracture analysis of a graded piezoelectric layer on a substrate with finite dimension. Arch Appl Mech 80(9):1007–1016
75. Yan Z, Jiang LY (2010) Interaction of parallel dielectric cracks in functionally graded piezoelectric materials. Acta Mech 211(3–4):251–269
76. Chen YJ, Chue CH (2010) Mode III fracture problem of a cracked FGPM surface layer bonded to a cracked FGPM substrate. Arch Appl Mech 80(3):285–303
77. Dag S, Yildirum B, Sarikaya D (2007) Mixed-mode fracture analysis of orthotropic functionally graded materials under mechancial and thermal loads. Int J Solids Struct 44:7816–7840
78. Ueda S, Iogawa T (2010) Two parallel penny-shaped or annular cracks in a functionally graded piezoelectric strip under electric loading. Acta Mech 210(1–2):57–70
79. Ding SH, Li X (2008) Periodic cracks in a functionally graded piezoelectric layer bonded to a piezoelectric half-plane. Theor Appl Fract Mech 49(3):313–320

80. Peng XL, Li XF (2009) Transient response of the crack-tip field in a magnetoelectroelastic half-space with a functionally graded coating under impacts. Arch Appl Mech 79(12):1099–1113
81. Lee KH (2009) Analysis of a transiently propagating crack in functionally graded materials under mode I and II. Int J Eng Sci 47(9):852–865
82. Feng W, Su R (2007) Dynamic fracture behaviors of cracks in a functionally graded magneto-electro-elastic plate. Eur J Mech A-Solid 26(2):363–379
83. Chakraborty A, Rahman S (2008) Stochastic multiscale models for fracture analysis of functionally graded materials. Eng Fract Mech 75(8):2062–2086
84. Kubair DV, Bhanu-Chandar B (2008) Stress concentration factor due to a circular hole in functionally graded panels under uniaxial tension. Int J Mech Sci 50(4):732–742
85. Lee D, Barber JR, Thouless MD (2009) Indentation of an elastic half space with material properties varying with depth. Int J Eng Sci 47(11–12):1274–1283
86. Choi HJ (2009) On the plane contact problem of a functionally graded elastic layer loaded by a frictional sliding flat punch. J Mech Sci Technol 23(10):2703–2713
87. Hu Y, Blouin VY, Fadel GM (2005) Design for manufacturing of 3D heterogeneous objects with processing time consideration. ASME Conf Proc: Design for Manufacturing and Life Cycle Conference, Vol. 4b:523–532
88. Chiu WK, Yu KM (2008) Multi-criteria decision-making determination of material gradient for functionally graded material objects fabrication. Proc IME B J Eng Manufact 222(2):293–307
89. Erisken C, Kalyon DM, Wang H (2010) Viscoelastic and biomechanical properties of osteochondral tissue constructs generated from graded polycaprolactone and beta-tricalcium phosphate composites. J Biomech Eng 132(9):art no. 091013
90. Gorke UJ, Gunther H, Nagel T, Wimmer MA (2010) A large strain material model for soft tissues with functionally graded properties. J Biomech Eng 132(7)
91. Liu Y, Birman V, Chen C, Thomopoulos S, Genin GM (2011) Mechanisms of bimaterial attachment at the interface of tendon to bone. J Eng Mater Technol 133(1):art no. 011006
92. Thomopoulos S, Marquez JP, Weinberger B, Birman V, Genin GM (2006) Collagen fiber orientation at the tendon to bone insertion and its influence on stress concentrations. J Biomech 39(10):1842–1851
93. Hedia HS, Shabara MA, El-Midany TT, Fouda N (2006) Improved design of cementless hip stems using two-dimensional functionally graded materials. J Biomed Mater Res B Appl Biomater 79(1):42–49
94. Hedia HS (2007) Effect of coating thickness and its material on the stress distribution for dental implants. J Med Eng Technol 31(4):280–287
95. Lin D, Li Q, Li W, Swain M (2009) Bone remodeling induced by dental implants of functionally graded materials. J Biomed Mater Res B Appl Biomater 92(2):430–438
96. Abaqus/CAE User's Manual 6.10 (2010) Dassault Systemes Simulia Corp., Providence, RI, USA
97. Eldred MS et al (2008) DAKOTA, A Multilevel Parallel Object-Oriented Framework for Design Optimization, Parameter Estimation, Uncertainty Quantification, and Sensitivity Analysis. vol Version 4.2 User's Manual. Sandia National Laboratories, Livermore, CA 94551
98. Vinson JR (1999) The behavior of sandwich structures of isotropic and composite materials. Technomic, Lancaster, PA

Chapter 3
Models for the Mechanics of Joining Dissimilar Materials

Guy M. Genin and Yanxin Liu

3.1 Introduction

The attachment of dissimilar materials is an age-old problem in mechanics, and a number of clever strategies for bimaterial joining now exist. An aim of this book is to bring out new classes of solutions based upon strategies that can be found in nature and physiology. The aim of this chapter is to present an accessible overview of some of the physical problems that these strategies need to overcome. The approach taken here is to summarize some of the key model problems that can be studied to gain insight into the challenge. The problems presented here fall under the category of small-strain, linear elasticity solutions.

The model attachment system discussed throughout this chapter is the attachment of tendon to bone. Those familiar with mechanics might find this odd, because neither tendon nor bone are particularly linear, and strains in tendon routinely reach the limit of about 10 % that is commonly considered the limit of good taste for the application of small strain theories. A tendon is certainly not a linear spring when deformed significantly, and even for infinitesimal, monotonic deformations, it behaves as a different spring depending upon how quickly it is stretched. Further, an intricate material and structural system can be found at the tendon-to-bone insertion site in a healthy adult [1–5]. However, most of the solutions presented in this chapter have the advantage of simple, closed form expressions that afford better insight into the behavior of bimaterial attachments than would a rigorous numerical solution that accounts for material and geometric nonlinearity. These solutions have relevance in very specific loading cases.

The chapter begins with a concise overview of linear elasticity. The goal of that section is not to teach the subject, but to either alert the expert to the specific

G.M. Genin (✉) • Y. Liu
Department of Mechanical Engineering and Materials Science, Washington University in St. Louis, St. Louis, MO, USA
e-mail: gening@seas.wustl.edu

S. Thomopoulos et al. (eds.), *Structural Interfaces and Attachments in Biology*,
DOI 10.1007/978-1-4614-3317-0_3,

notation that will be used in this chapter, or to provide the initiate with a broad sense of what underlies the boundary value problems presented in this chapter. For a more meaningful discourse on the subject, we suggest Allan Bower's online text [6].

3.2 A Whirlwind Tour of Linear Elasticity

This section presents the basic elements of a boundary value problem in linear elasticity. The goal in each of the model problems discussed in this chapter is to understand how the details of the way two materials are attached and loaded elevate internal forces (stresses) at the attachment site. In each case studied, the boundary value problem involves an idealization of an attachment into a linear elastic "tendon" and a linear elastic "bone," with a sharp interface between them (Fig. 3.1). The inputs to the problem are:

1. The initial shapes of tendon, bone, and their interface, which will often look somewhat less like a potato than Fig. 3.1 but nevertheless be highly idealized.
2. A set of constants that describe the mechanical responses of the tissues, which, in the simplest model problems, consist of two constants for tendon and two constants for bone, which are an elastic modulus E and a Poisson ratio ν.
3. A set of boundary conditions that describe either the displacement or the mechanical tractions applied in each of three orthogonal directions at each point on the outer boundaries of the model.

The outputs are:

1. The internal stress field.
2. The internal displacement field.

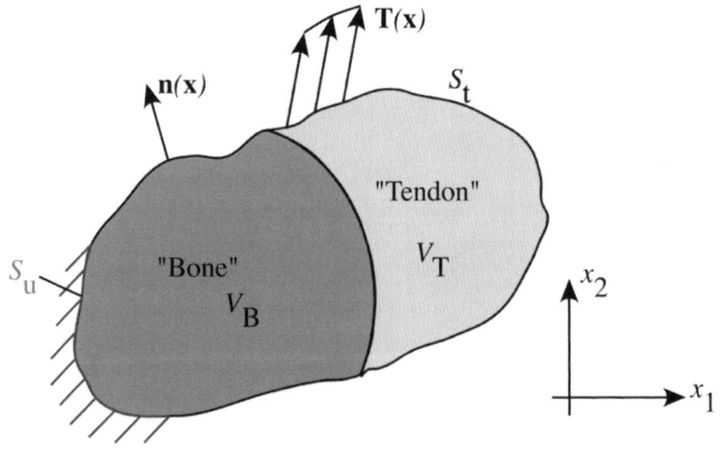

Fig. 3.1 A potato, with some notation useful to the theory of elasticity

3. The displacement at each point and in each direction for which traction was prescribed in the boundary conditions (e.g., the portion S_u of the boundary of V in Fig. 3.1).
4. The traction at each point and in each direction for which displacement was prescribed in the boundary conditions (e.g., the portion S_t of the boundary of V in Fig. 3.1).

These are obtained by solving the following sets of equations at each point within the model:

1. Strain–displacement equations that define the strain tensor field $\boldsymbol{\varepsilon}(\mathbf{x})$ at each point $\mathbf{x}$ within the volume V_{T} of the tendon and V_{B} of the bone in terms of the displacement vector field, $\mathbf{u}(\mathbf{x})$. Here and throughout the chapter, we write these equations using index notation, in which subscripts are understood to represent indices ranging from 1 to 3, commas represent partial differentiation, and repeated indices within a grouping imply summation over the three values of that index. The strain displacement relations are then:

$$\varepsilon_{ij} = \tfrac{1}{2}(u_{i,j} + u_{j,i}) \tag{3.1}$$

where ε_{ij} represents the 3×3 matrix of components of the strain tensor $\boldsymbol{\varepsilon}$ in a particular coordinate system, u_i represents the three components of the displacement vector $\mathbf{u}$ in that coordinate system, and $u_{i,j} = \partial u_i / \partial x_j$.
2. Compatibility relations. Since the nominal strain tensor has six independent components and the displacement vector only three, not every choice of a spatially varying strain field relates to a displacement field. Strain fields that do meet this criterion satisfy the compatibility relations:

$$\varepsilon_{ij,kl} + \varepsilon_{kl,ij} - \varepsilon_{jl,ik} - \varepsilon_{ik,jl} = 0 \tag{3.2}$$

where the additional subscript following the comma represents a second derivative with respect to the components of the coordinate system, so that $\varepsilon_{ij,kl} = \partial^2 \varepsilon_{ij} / \partial x_k \partial x_l$.
3. Constitutive relations that predict the strain tensor at a point in terms of the stress tensor $\boldsymbol{\sigma}$. For the case of linear, isotropic elasticity, these are:

$$\varepsilon_{ij} = \frac{1}{E}[(1+v)\sigma_{ij} - v\delta_{ij}\sigma_{kk}] \tag{3.3}$$

$$\sigma_{ij} = \frac{E}{(1+v)}\varepsilon_{ij} + \frac{E}{(1+v)(1-2v)}\delta_{ij}\varepsilon_{kk} \tag{3.4}$$

where δ_{ij} is Kronecker's delta function that equals 1 when $i = j$ and 0 otherwise, and $\varepsilon_{kk} = \varepsilon_{11} + \varepsilon_{22} + \varepsilon_{33}$.

4. Newton's second law, written for a continuous system that is not accelerating and for which gravitational forces are negligible:

$$\sigma_{ij,j} = 0 \tag{3.5}$$

Traction boundary conditions enter the problem by noting that $T_i = \sigma_{ji}n_j$, where **n** is the outward normal vector of the body's outer boundary at a point at which a traction vector is applied (e.g., the portion S_T of the body in Fig. 3.1). Finding the set of internal vector and tensor fields that uniquely satisfy the above four sets of equations is often not straightforward and is often difficult to do by inspection. Most of the solutions presented in this chapter were derived using planar assumptions (either plane stress, in which out-of-plane stress tensor components are taken as zero or constant, or plane strain, in which out-of-plane strain tensor components are taken as zero or constant), and using a mathematical trick known as a potential function. Although the solution procedures are well beyond the scope of this chapter, we present here a simple example with the hope of preparing a student interested in the subject to follow a derivation in one of the original articles. The example presented here is the stress function of Airy, who defined a function φ such that $\sigma_{xx} = \frac{\partial^2\varphi}{\partial y^2}$, $\sigma_{yy} = \frac{\partial^2\varphi}{\partial x^2}$, and $\sigma_{xy} = \frac{-\partial^2\varphi}{\partial x \partial y}$ or, in cylindrical coordinates, $\sigma_{rr} = \frac{1}{r}\frac{\partial\varphi}{\partial r} + \frac{1}{r^2}\frac{\partial^2\varphi}{\partial^2\theta}$, $\sigma_{\theta\theta} = \frac{\partial^2\varphi}{\partial r^2}$, and $\sigma_{r\theta} = -\frac{\partial}{\partial r}\left(\frac{1}{r}\frac{\partial\varphi}{\partial\theta}\right)$. Substituting this function into Newton's second law results in Newton's second law being identically satisfied within the plane. Substituting these definitions into the constitutive equations, and then substituting the resulting expressions for strain into the compatibility relations results in a single equation for $\varphi : \nabla^4\varphi = 0$. The identification of a solution then involves finding which of the functions φ that satisfy this biharmonic equation meets the boundary conditions for the problem of interest.

One solution presented in this chapter makes use of an energy argument. We note that the average strain energy U per unit volume over a portion of a body, say V_T as in Fig. 3.1, can be written:

$$U = \frac{1}{2}\int_{V_T} \sigma_{ij}\varepsilon_{ij}\, dV \tag{3.6}$$

and the total strain energy in that part of the body is the product of the volume and the strain energy density, $V_T U$.

3.3 An Isotropic Solid Attached to a Rigid Substrate

The simplest possible idealizations of an engineering attachment yield insight into how the morphology of the attachment governs the stress field, and we begin by discussing two such idealizations. We will relate these to the attachment of tendon

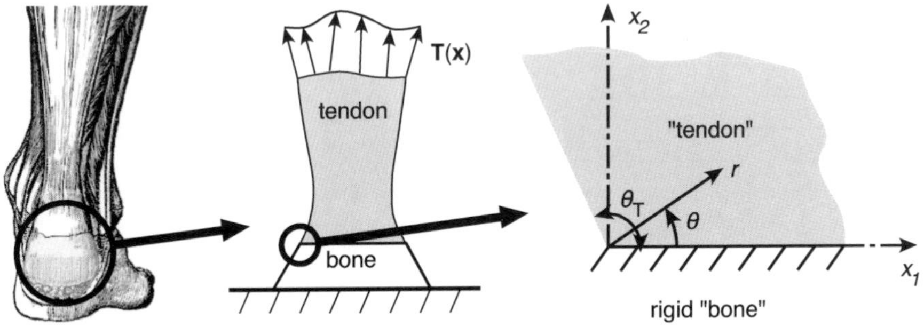

Fig. 3.2 A highly simplified model of a tendon-to-bone attachment, with a schematic of how parameters of the Williams solution relate to this picture. The tendon is linear elastic with elastic modulus E and Poisson ratio v. The insertion angle θ_T of the tendon is shown here as being greater than 90°, although the graphic at the left suggests that nature is in fact smarter than that

to bone. The solutions are for a thin, isotropic material, taken to be a tendon, attached to a rigid substratum, taken to be bone. The tendon is loaded at some position far from the attachment point. The two solutions involve a tendon connected straight to bone in the absence of toughening mechanisms such as a graded interface or tendon/bone interdigitation. However, this particular aspect of the models is not too far distant from the reality of surgical practice, in which all interfacial tissue is resected away and tendon is sutured directly onto bone that has been prepared by drawing blood through abrasion, and little else. We note as well that a tendon is not isotropic. In later sections of this chapter we explore how tendon anisotropy affects stresses, and for now note simply that the isotropic approximations provide superior qualitative insight into the mechanics of attachment, and that the mechanical properties of a healing tendon-to-bone insertion site are believed to be reasonably represented by an isotropic continuum [7].

3.3.1 *The Williams Free Edge Problem*

Williams [8] considered a problem that represents the model shown in Fig. 3.2. The asymptotic stress field in the cylindrical coordinate system shown in Fig. 3.2 can be written:

$$\begin{aligned}\sigma_{rr} &= r^{\lambda-1}(\Phi''(\theta;\lambda) + (\lambda+1)\Phi(\theta;\lambda)) \\ \sigma_{\theta\theta} &= r^{\lambda-1}(\lambda(\lambda+1)\Phi(\theta;\lambda)) \\ \sigma_{r\theta} &= -r^{\lambda-1}\Phi'(\theta;\lambda)\end{aligned} \tag{3.7}$$

where $\Phi(\theta;\lambda)$ is a function whose form is given by Williams [8]. $\Phi(\theta;\lambda)$ contains four unknown constants that must be found along with λ using the boundary conditions. The displacements can be written in terms of these constants using (3.4) and (3.1):

$$\begin{aligned} u_r &= r^{\lambda}\left(\frac{1+v}{E}\right)(-(\lambda+1)\Phi(\theta;\lambda)+(1-n)\Psi'(\theta;\lambda)) \\ u_\theta &= r^{\lambda}\left(\frac{1+v}{E}\right)(-\Phi'(\theta;\lambda)+(1-n)(\lambda-1)\Psi(\theta;\lambda)) \end{aligned} \tag{3.8}$$

where $n = v/(1-v)$, and $\Psi(\theta;\lambda)$, a function whose form is given by Williams [8], contains two of the four unknown constants that are found when determining $\Phi(\theta;\lambda)$.

The key to characterizing the stress field at the point of attachment on the free edge (origin, $r = 0$) is λ: if $\lambda < 1$, the stress at the origin is infinite, and if $\lambda \geq 1$ the leading term of the asymptotic expansion is zero. The four boundary conditions that determine these constants are that (1 and 2) the two displacement components for points on the bone side of the tendon are zero and (3 and 4) the free edge of the tendon is free of tractions in the directions normal and parallel to the surface. This results in a system of equations that has a nontrivial solution only if the following equation is satisfied:

$$\sin^2(\lambda\theta_T) = \left(\frac{1}{3-4n}\right)(4(1-n)^2 - (\lambda\theta_T)^2\sin^2\theta_T) \tag{3.9}$$

Equation (3.9) is transcendental in λ, and an infinite number of λs therefore satisfy it. All of these are valid solutions. The one of interest would seem to be the smallest value, as this suffices to determine whether the stresses at the corner point are unbounded. However, care is usually taken to ensure that the displacement field is bounded even if the stress field is unbounded. Since from (3.8) one can observe that the displacement field scales as r^{λ}, the displacement at $r = 0$ is bounded only if $\lambda > 0$. We therefore look for the smallest $\lambda > 0$ and are interested in identifying whether this smallest value is in the range $0 < \lambda < 1$.

A graph of this minimum λ as a function of the tendon insertion angle θ_T shows that λ decreases monotonically over the range of $0 \leq \theta_T \leq \pi/2$ (Fig. 3.3). At a critical angle, λ drops below 1 and the stress field near the free edge becomes singular. This angle is dependent upon Poisson's ratio. In an isotropic tendon, the threshold tendon insertion angle for the onset of a singularity can be as low as 54°. The exception is $v = 0$, for which the stress is non-infinite even for a 90° insertion angle. Note that in the latter case and in non-singular cases in general, the stresses at the insertion point are not described adequately by considering only the one potentially singular term in the equation.

This problem studied here is far removed from the reality of a tendon, but nevertheless shows the role of tendon morphology in determining the effectiveness of a tendon-to-bone attachment. An outward splay of a tendon at the insertion of tendon to bone can have a profound effect on the stress level on the attachment point.

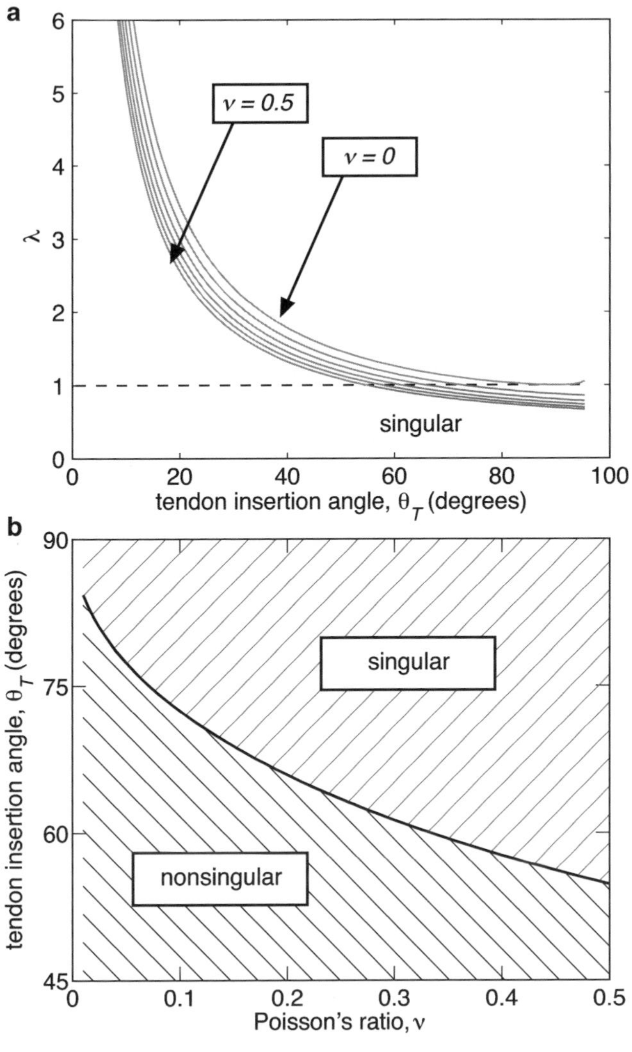

Fig. 3.3 Stresses at $r = 0$ in the Williams solution are unbounded for large tendon insertion angle. (**a**) The exponent on the leading term becomes less than one and the leading term becomes singular for sufficiently high tendon insertion angle. (**b**) The threshold value of tendon insertion angle is a function of Poisson's ratio

3.3.2 Peeling Models

The next model considered involves peeling of a tendon away from a rigid bone as in Fig. 3.4. The tendon is very thin (thickness t much smaller than the width w of the tendon into the page) and is pulled away from the bone with a force f at an angle φ. For the case of a tendon that has no bending resistance and that does not stretch

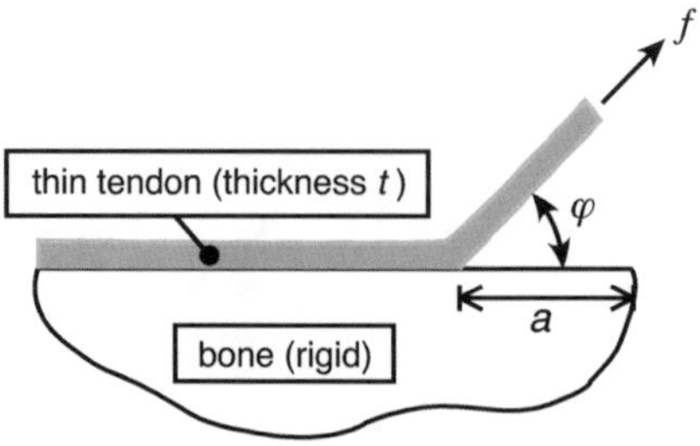

Fig. 3.4 The Kendall peel test model

appreciably when subjected to the critical force f_c needed to debond tendon from bone, the only material parameter that enters the problem is the fracture energy Γ_c. This is the energy per unit area needed to increase the crack length a of the region of tendon that has debonded from the bone. Using energetic arguments, Rivlin [9] calculated the force f_c needed to advance the crack:

$$\frac{f_c}{w} = \frac{\Gamma_c}{1 - \cos\varphi} \tag{3.10}$$

For $\varphi = 90°$, this reproduces a simple Griffith-Irwin type fracture criterion. For φ approaching 0°, the force needed for extension of a crack between the tendon and bone approaches infinity. This model is limited, even from the perspective of elementary linear elastic fracture mechanics. For example, as will be discussed below, one would expect Γ_c to vary with φ. However, even this simple starting point yields some insight into tendon-to-bone attachment mechanics and might explain in part why the bone insertions of, for example, the Achilles tendon are such that there exists a significant overlap region at the heel. The most common site of tears in the Achilles tendon is not where the tendon first contacts bone but rather midsubstance, near this point. This is loosely consistent with expectations from this model: one would not expect a failure at the attachment of tendon to bone with φ so close to 0° unless the force f was sufficient to break the tendon itself or to overwhelm the entire attachment region.

Tendon is compliant compared to bone, so the next appropriate degree of complexity for a peel test model incorporates an elastic tendon. The solution for this case was derived by Kendall [10, 11] and considers a linear elastic tendon of elastic modulus E_T and thickness t in a state of plane strain, which is appropriate for $w \gg t$:

$$\Gamma_c = (1 - \cos\varphi)\frac{f_c}{w} + \frac{f_c^2}{2E_T w^2 t} \tag{3.11}$$

Kendall noted that the elastic term is important only in special cases. The first case is when φ approaches 0°. The second is when the term $f_c/E_T t w$ is large, which corresponds to the case of a relatively large strain being reached at the level of f_c

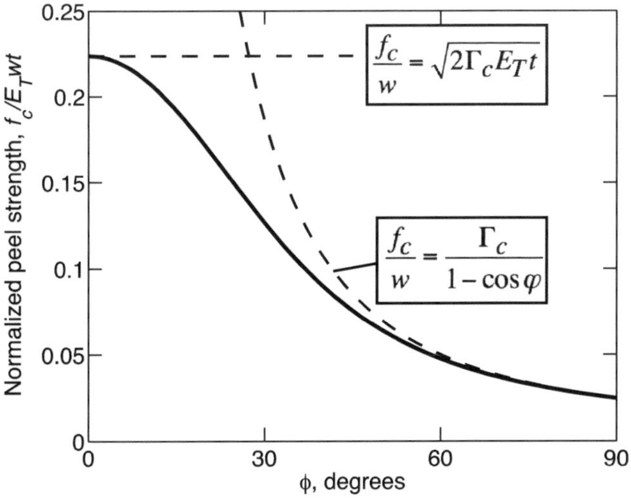

Fig. 3.5 Dependence of peel strength on peeling angle φ in a fictional tendon-to-bone attachment in which the critical energy release rate does not depend upon the peeling angle

that causes pealing. Unlike the case of a rigid tendon, a crack between tendon and bone can advance in this system even if the peel angle is 0°. The crack will advance and the tendon will peel away if the elastic energy released when the crack advances a certain distance exceeds that needed to drive the crack this distance. The elastic term is clearly important for a tendon such as the Achilles tendon, whose functioning is at times like an elastic spring.

The expression (3.11) provides a lower bound on the value of Γ_c needed to ensure that a crudely attached tendon would rupture before becoming detached. We consider the case of an idealized Achilles tendon with $\varphi \approx 0°$. Following Wren et al. [12], we assume a tendon failure strain value of $\varepsilon_u = f_c/E_T wt \approx 0.1$, and a failure stress of $\sigma_u = f_c/wt \approx 80$ MPa. Assuming a thickness t of between 2 mm and 2 cm yields a required $\Gamma_c = (1/2)\, \sigma_u\, \varepsilon_u\, t$ on the order of 8–80 kJ/m^2. This is a fracture toughness range associated with tough engineering materials such as aluminum alloys, high strength steels, and fiberglass [13]. This back-of-the-envelope calculation points to a need for a careful interface design and highlights the difficulty one could expect to encounter in trying to surgically reattach tendon directly to bone: a direct attachment of tendon to bone would not likely ever succeed in gaining the toughness needed to withstand the forces associated with tendon rupture at midsubstance.

Another way that this solution provides insight is through the relative magnitudes of the two terms in (3.11). Even for a highly elastic tendon, the elastic term can be small compared to the crack-opening term (1–cos φ) unless the opening angle is close to 0°. For a tendon, we plotted the two terms in Fig. 3.5; note that Fig. 3.5 is drawn for a fictional attachment in which Γ_c does not vary with φ. The line shown is for the above numbers for tendon, with $E_T = 450$ MPa [14] so that the normalized critical energy release rate $\Gamma_c/2E_Tt \approx 0.05$. In this case, the two terms are approximately equal at $\varphi = 25°$.

The final wrinkle in this solution that we will mention here is that discussed by Williams and Kauzlarich [15] for the case in which the tendon exists in a state of pre-strain. The pre-strain value is given by a uniaxial strain level ε_o, which corresponds to an axial force F required to stretch the portion of the tendon that is adhered to the bone to ε_o:

$$\Gamma_c = (1 - \cos\varphi)\frac{f_c}{w} + \frac{(f_c - F)^2}{2E_T w^2 t} \tag{3.12}$$

The result is that a pretensioning of the attached region actually *increases* the force f needed to cause the tendon to debond. Is this relevant to an idealized tendon-to-bone attachment? This is unclear. Tendons certainly exist in a state of pretensioning, and while this pretensioning is well characterized in the midsubstance, it is not well characterized within the attachment of tendon to bone. We note that pretensioning in the midsubstance adds to f_c and reduces resilience. For pretensioning to be an effective contributor to attachment, the level of pretensioning in the region of tendon adhered to bone would have to exceed that of the tendon at midsubstance.

These solutions have been worked out for arbitrary monotonically increasing nonlinear uniaxial constitutive laws for the tendon and for large strain [16], but these are beyond the scope of the current chapter other than to note that the basic principles remain unchanged.

3.4 Idealized Tendon Attached to Isotropic, Elastic Bone

The next moderate step towards realism is to model the bone with realistic isotropic mechanical properties. This is still a significant approximation. Bone is sufficiently stiff relative to tendon that it is well modeled with the small strain assumptions of linear elasticity, and it is much better modeled as isotropic than tendon is. However, as described later, bone does present anisotropy over the length scale of hundreds of micrometers (osteons), and this length scale is relevant to tendon-to-bone attachment.

The problem of interest was considered by, among others, Bogy [17], Hein and Erdogan [18], and Akisanya and Fleck [19, 20], with important later contributions by many others including Klingbeil and Beuth [21]. Here, an isotropic tendon is attached to an isotropic bone. The insertion angles of the tendon (θ_1) and the bone (θ_2) are both important (Fig. 3.6). The stress at the corner point again has the form:

$$\sigma_{ij}^m = Hr^{\lambda-1}F_{ij}^m(\theta;\lambda) \tag{3.13}$$

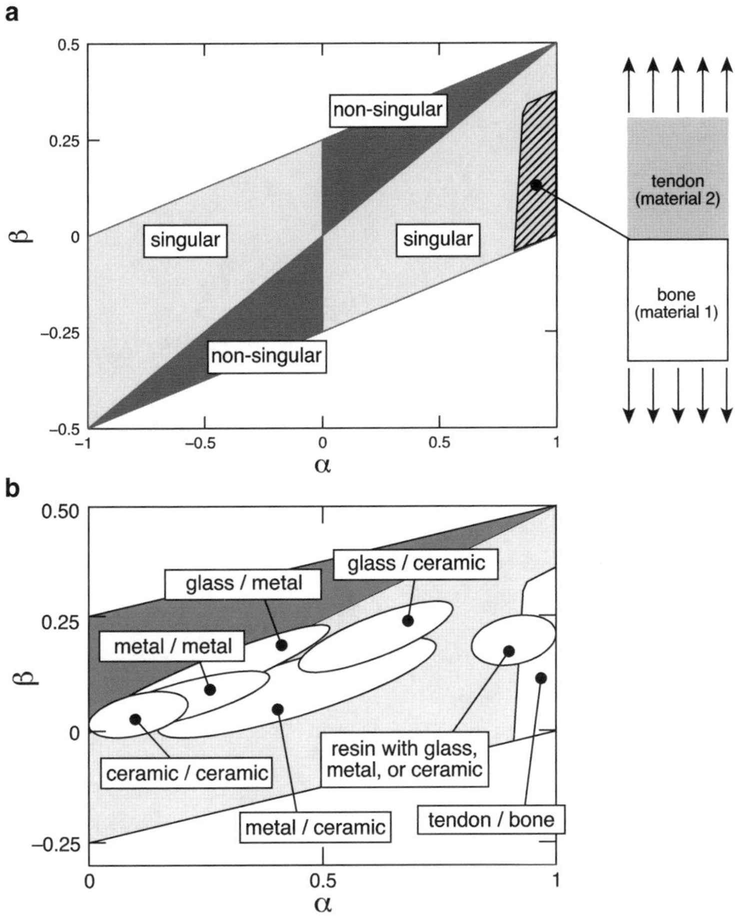

Fig. 3.6 (**a**) All linear, isotropic material mismatches can be represented by the two Dundurs parameters, which range over the shaded region. The lighter regions represent pairs of α and β for which an elastic singularity occurs at the free edge of the interface of a butt joint (inset) between the two materials. Tendon and bone lie within the hatched region. (**b**) Most engineering material pairs congregate in a narrow region of the parameter space, and a few pairs do not result in an elastic singularity for a butt joint and are non-singular. The figure is anti-symmetric about $\alpha = 0$, so data are plotted only for $\alpha > 0$. (**b**) Is based upon data plotted in [23]

and the displacement field has the form:

$$u_i^m = Hr^{\lambda} G_i^m(\theta; \lambda) \tag{3.14}$$

where $m = \{1,2\}$ represents the material number and simple but lengthy expressions for F_{ij} and G_i can be found in [20]. The free edge intensity factor, H, depends upon θ_1 and θ_2 and also upon the material properties of the tendon and bone. The parameter

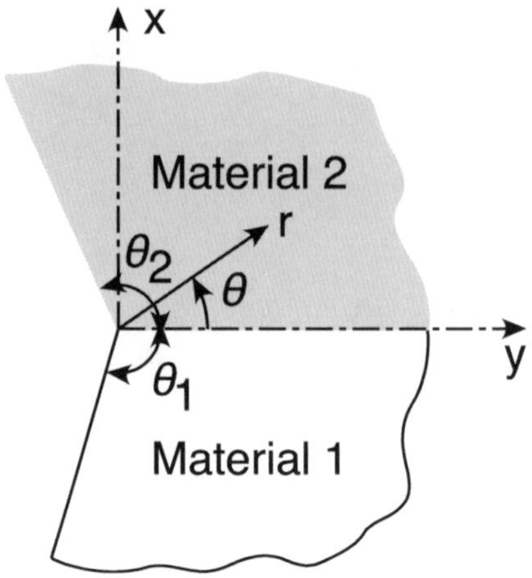

Fig. 3.7 Free edge of a bi-material interface. For a bi-material interface problem, the order of the free edge singularity depends upon the insertion angles and the material properties of the adjoining materials

space is greatly simplified by Dundurs' [22] result that, for a body in plane stress or plane strain loaded by prescribed tractions, the stress distribution depends on only two dimensionless parameters:

$$\alpha = \frac{\mu_1(\kappa_2+1)-\mu_2(\kappa_1+1)}{\mu_1(\kappa_2+1)+\mu_2(\kappa_1+1)}$$
$$\beta = \frac{\mu_1(\kappa_2-1)-\mu_2(\kappa_1-1)}{\mu_1(\kappa_2+1)+\mu_2(\kappa_1+1)}$$

where the subscripts 1 and 2 refer to bone and tendon, respectively; $\mu_i = E_i/2(1+v_i)$, and $\kappa_i = 3-4v_i$ for plane strain. The parameter α can be understood in terms of a dimensionless ratio of the reduced elastic moduli of the two materials: $\alpha = (\bar{E}_1-\bar{E}_2)/(\bar{E}_1+\bar{E}_2)$, where $\bar{E}_i = E_i/(1-\boldsymbol{v}_i^2)$ for plane strain. For attachment of tendon to bone, with bone corresponding to material 1, $\alpha > 0$. All materials must lie within the range $-1 \le \alpha \le 1$, and $\alpha = 1$ corresponds to a tendon attached to a perfectly rigid bone. β also has a specific range of possible values, and these are represented for the case of plane strain in Fig. 3.6 by the shaded region for all materials with positive Poisson ratio. Tendon and bone lie in the hatched region of the plot (elastic modulus for tendon ranging from 50 to 750 MPa; Poisson's ratio for tendon ranging from 0.2 to 0.5; elastic modulus for bone ranging from 10 to 30 GPa; Poisson's ratio for bone ranging from 0.1 to 0.4).

For a "butt joint" in plane strain between tendon and bone, in which a rectangular tendon joins a rectangular bone as pictured in Fig. 3.7 (tendon and bone insertion angles $\theta_1 = \theta_2 = 90°$), the characteristic equation analogous to that of (3.9) can be found in Akisanya and Fleck [20] and can be rewritten in terms of the Dundurs parameters:

$$
\begin{aligned}
0 = &(\alpha - \beta)^2(\lambda^2 - \sin^2(\lambda\pi/2))^2 - \alpha^2(\lambda^2 - \sin^4(\lambda\pi/2)) \\
&+ 2\alpha(\alpha - \beta)(\lambda^2 - \sin^2(\lambda\pi/2))\sin^2(\lambda\pi/2) \\
&+ \sin^2(\lambda\pi/2)(1 - \sin^2(\lambda\pi/2))
\end{aligned}
\tag{3.16}
$$

Following the logic described above for the Williams solution, solutions are sought for which the stresses are singular at $r = 0$ ($\lambda < 1$, cf. (3.13)) but displacements are bounded ($\lambda \geq 0$, cf. (3.14)). In these cases, one concludes that the stress field is singular. One can show from (3.16) that the stress field is for pairs (α, β) in the lighter shaded region of Fig. 3.6, which corresponds to $\alpha(\alpha - 2\beta)>0$. The hatched region corresponding to attachment of tendon and bone lies well within the singular range.

What does this mean for attachment of engineering materials? A broad literature exists that is relevant to relating H and λ to a failure criterion that predicts loads at which the tendon and bone would become debonded. Much of this literature derives from the study of debonding of thin semiconductor films from silicon substrata [21, 24], in addition to the broad literature on structural materials. The overall idea is to first check whether an interface will present a singularity ($\lambda < 1$), and then, if so, whether the value of H, which increases monotonically with the tractions applied to the tendon, is sufficient to cause debonding. We address the first problem in this section and defer the second to the next section.

Suga et al. [25] compiled data for a broad range of engineering material mismatches and found them to be clustered over a fairly narrow range; representative regions are sketched in Fig. 3.6b for several classes of engineering attachments; note that since all data are antisymmetric about $\alpha = 0$, only the region $\alpha > 0$ is shown in Fig. 3.6b. Common engineering material pairs are found predominantly along the lines $\beta = \alpha/4$ and $\beta = 0$, both of which lie well within the singular range. A few metal/metal, metal/glass, and ceramic/ceramic interfaces can be found in the non-singular range, but attachment of tendon to bone is firmly in the singular range.

A singularity between two materials in a butt joint can be eliminated by an interlayer between them. Interlayers are common in protective coatings on turbine blades, where one goal is to provide improved adhesion of layers that provide chemical and thermal protection to the underlying metal blade. In the example we describe here, the goal is to find a material that will not present a singularity when paired in a butt joint with either of the two materials to be joined.

As an example, we explore an interlayer between tendon and bone in Fig. 3.8. The set of all mechanical property pairs ($E_{\text{interlayer}}$, $\nu_{\text{interlayer}}$) that can be paired in a butt joint with tendon without a singular stress field arising is represented by the lightly shaded region; the set of all interlayer properties that can be paired in a butt joint with bone without a singular stress field arising is represented by a darker shaded region. In both cases, the appropriate interlayer material properties are not symmetric about the case of identical material properties, with a broader range of options available for interfaces with a more compliant interface with a lower

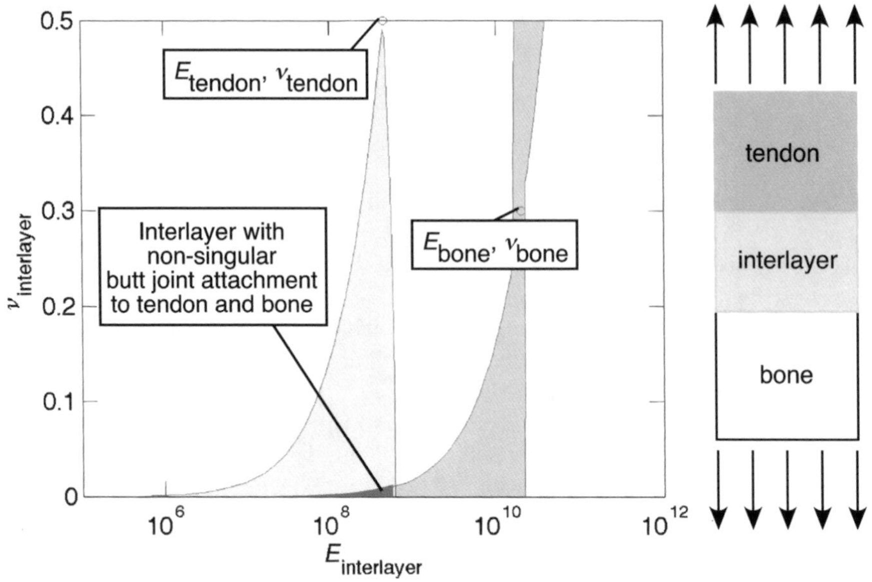

Fig. 3.8 An interlayer can be found that eliminates the singular stress field that would otherwise exist at the connection between two dissimilar materials. The light shaded region shows material constants for material that will not introduce a singular stress field when a butt-jointed to linear elastic "tendon," and the darker shaded region shows a similar set of material properties for attachment to bone. A compliant interlayer with low Poisson ratio can be connected to both tendon and bone without introducing a singular stress field

Poisson ratio. A single material that can provide non-singular butt joints with both tendon and bone is possible, as represented by the black (red in the online version) region in Fig. 3.7. The log scale highlights that a great many of these involve an interlayer that is more compliant than either tendon or bone.

Another interesting aspect of the solution is the effect of the insertion angle. The Xu group has devoted much effort to identifying and evaluating experimentally certain configurations for bimaterial interfaces that reduce singularities [26–28], and we discuss one such case. A configuration that has been tested carefully is one in which both materials exhibit convex outward splays (Fig. 3.9). The example shown involves insertion angles of $\theta_1 = 45°$ and $\theta_2 = 65°$. These insertion angles dramatically reduce the domain of pairs of Dundurs parameters for which a free edge singularity occurs: only for the case of α very close to 1 does a singularity occur. As can be seen by comparing the singular regime to those for engineering attachments in Fig. 3.6, this attachment scheme precludes a singular stress field for nearly all engineering attachments. However, in the case of biological attachment at the tendon-to-bone insertion site, the singular region overlaps with a portion of the possible representative material properties for tendon and bone. This example highlights once more the sensitivity of the stress field to the details of the insertion angles.

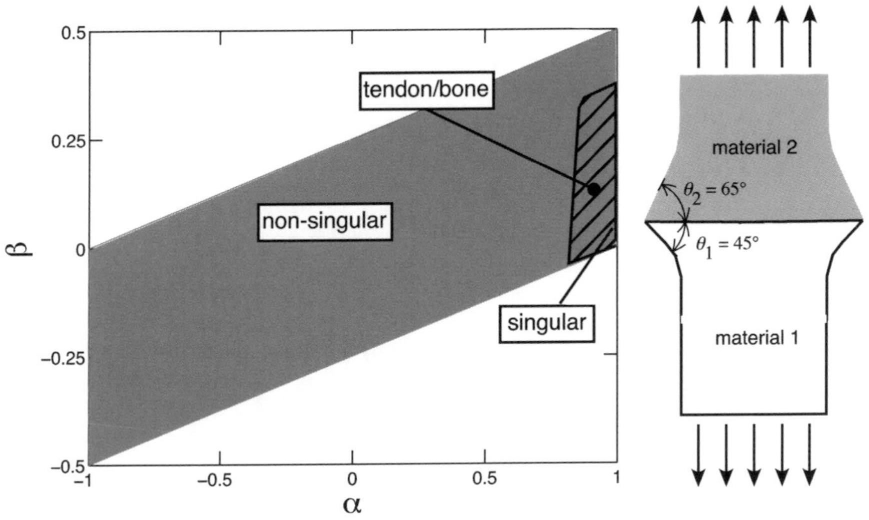

Fig. 3.9 Tailoring of the insertion angle can radically reduce the region in Dundurs parameter space over which a free edge singularity occurs. However, even in this example that precludes a free edge singularity for nearly all engineering material attachments, a singular stress field is possible for attachment of materials within the range of material properties reported for tendon and bone. Data from Wang and Xu [26]

3.5 Free Edge Singularities Between Orthotropic Solids

Section 3.4 focused on attachment of two isotropic materials. Since a focus of this text is biologic attachment and biomaterials are often quite anisotropic, we extend the discussion in this section to the problem of free edge singularities in the attachment of orthotropic materials.

The problem of attachment of general anisotropic materials is much studied, with specialized numerical methodologies well established (e.g., [29–32]), and many published analytical treatments [33–37]. A central challenge is that the number of parameters needed to describe an anisotropic material can be much greater than that needed to describe an isotropic material. Although anisotropic generalizations of Dundurs parameters exist, they have not yet been explored in the context of threshold values for edge singularities. We focus here on a specific case, namely the attachment of an isotropic bone to an orthotropic tendon.

The mechanical properties of a generally anisotropic linear elastic material can include up to 21 constants, but this number can be reduced to five based upon symmetry arguments for a material such as tendon that can be approximated as transversely isotropic. This means that we will consider the case studied in the introductory chapter, in which the idealized tendon has the same stiffness for stressing in any direction perpendicular to that of the dominant direction of the fibers that comprise them. The general anisotropic constitutive law, $\varepsilon_{ij} = S_{ijkl}\sigma_{kl}$, involves a fourth order tensor **S** called the compliance tensor. This tensor is simplified greatly for a transversely isotropic material and can be written in a matrix form:

$$\begin{bmatrix} \varepsilon_{xx} \\ \varepsilon_{yy} \\ \varepsilon_{zz} \\ 2\varepsilon_{yz} \\ 2\varepsilon_{xz} \\ 2\varepsilon_{xy} \end{bmatrix} = \begin{bmatrix} \frac{1}{E_x^{(m)}} & -\frac{v_{xy}^{(m)}}{E_x^{(m)}} & -\frac{v_{xy}^{(m)}}{E_x^{(m)}} & 0 & 0 & 0 \\ -\frac{v_{xy}^{(m)}}{E_x^{(m)}} & \frac{1}{E_y^{(m)}} & -\frac{v_{yz}^{(m)}}{E_y^{(m)}} & 0 & 0 & 0 \\ -\frac{v_{xy}^{(m)}}{E_x^{(m)}} & -\frac{v_{yz}^{(m)}}{E_y^{(m)}} & \frac{1}{E_y^{(m)}} & 0 & 0 & 0 \\ 0 & 0 & 0 & \frac{2(1+v_{yz}^{(m)})}{E_y^{(m)}} & 0 & 0 \\ 0 & 0 & 0 & 0 & \frac{1}{\mu_{xz}^{(m)}} & 0 \\ 0 & 0 & 0 & 0 & 0 & \frac{1}{\mu_{xz}^{(m)}} \end{bmatrix} \begin{bmatrix} \sigma_{xx} \\ \sigma_{yy} \\ \sigma_{zz} \\ \sigma_{yz} \\ \sigma_{xz} \\ \sigma_{xy} \end{bmatrix} \quad (3.17)$$

where the superscript $m = \{1,2\}$ represents material 1 or material 2, and the matrix of elastic constants is called the compliance matrix. The five constants that characterize the constitutive response for each material are: (1) the elastic modulus E_x for stressing in dominant direction of the fibers that comprise the tendon, which we will call the axial direction; (2) the elastic modulus E_y for stressing in any direction perpendicular to the axial direction, which we will call the transverse directions; (3) a shear modulus μ_{xz} that represents the resistance to shear distortion for shearing in the plane normal to the axial direction; (4) a Poisson ratio v_{yz} that describes the contraction in a direction within the plane of transverse isotropy and perpendicular to the direction of a uniaxial straining in a transverse direction; and (5) a Poisson ratio v_{xy} that describes the contraction in the transverse directions associated with uniaxial stretching in an axial direction.

The details of finding an asymptotic solution for the stress field near a free edge at an anisotropic bimaterial interface parallel those of the isotropic problem, with a few exceptions. These are largely due to the existence of ten material constants, with five constants for each of the two adjoining materials. For the case of plane strain, in which the out-of-plane stress components are all set to zero, the material constants that arise in the solution are derived from the compliance matrix in (3.17):

$$\bar{S}_{ij}^{(m)} = S_{ij}^{(m)} - S_{i3}^{(m)} S_{j3}^{(m)} / S_{33}^{(m)} \quad (3.18)$$

where the subscripts i and j range from 1 through 6 to represent the components of the compliance matrix. The solutions all depend upon the four roots M_k of the following characteristic equation (cf. [38]):

$$\bar{S}_{11}^{(m)} (M^{(m)})^4 + (2\bar{S}_{12}^{(m)} + \bar{S}_{66}^{(m)})(M^{(m)})^2 + \bar{S}_{22}^{(m)} = 0 \quad (3.19)$$

The stress field can be written [36, 39]:

$$\begin{aligned}
\sigma_{rr} &= \sum_{k=1}^{4} r^{\lambda-1}(\lambda+1)\lambda A_k^{(m)}\left(-\sin\theta + M_k^{(m)}\cos\theta\right)^2\left(\cos\theta + M_k^{(m)}\sin\theta\right)^{\lambda-1} \\
\sigma_{\theta\theta} &= \sum_{k=1}^{4} r^{\lambda-1}(\lambda+1)\lambda A_k^{(m)}\left(\cos\theta + M_k^{(m)}\sin\theta\right)^{\lambda+1} \\
\sigma_{r\theta} &= -\sum_{k=1}^{4} r^{\lambda-1}(\lambda+1)\lambda A_k^{(m)}\left(-\sin\theta + M_k^{(m)}\cos\theta\right)\left(\cos\theta + M_k^{(m)}\sin\theta\right)^{\lambda}
\end{aligned} \tag{3.20}$$

in which the eight constants $A_k^{(m)}$ (four in each material) are found from the boundary and continuity conditions on stress, and on the displacement field:

$$\begin{aligned}
u_r &= \sum_{k=1}^{4} r^{\lambda}(\lambda+1)A_k^{(m)}\left(p_k^{(m)}\cos\theta + q_k^{(m)}\sin\theta\right)\left(\cos\theta + \mu_k^{(m)}\sin\theta\right)^{\lambda} \\
u_\theta &= \sum_{k=1}^{4} r^{\lambda}(\lambda+1)A_k^{(m)}\left(-p_k^{(m)}\sin\theta + q_k^{(m)}\cos\theta\right)\left(\cos\theta + \mu_k^{(m)}\sin\theta\right)^{\lambda}
\end{aligned} \tag{3.21}$$

where the constants p and q depend on the components of the compliance matrix:

$$p_k^{(m)} = \bar{S}_{11}^{(m)}\left(\mu_k^{(m)}\right)^2 + \bar{S}_{12}^{(m)}, \quad q_k = \bar{S}_{21}^{(m)}\mu_k^{(m)} + \bar{S}_{22}^{(m)}/\mu_k^{(m)} \tag{3.22}$$

As above, the continuity conditions simply require that there be no jump in the displacement or stress when crossing the boundary between the two materials, and the free edge boundary conditions require that the exposed surfaces near the attachment point be traction free. This leads to a set of 32 equations for the eight constants $A_k^{(m)}$, and the existence of a nontrivial solution requires that the determinant of the coefficient matrix vanishes. As above, this leads to an equation that is transcendental in λ. Despite all of this additional complexity, the problem is as simple as the others considered in this chapter: Equation (3.21) shows that the stress field can be singular if the lowest root λ is less than 1, and the tradition is to discard all solutions for which λ is less than 0 as non-physical because (3.21) shows that these lead to unbounded displacements at $r = 0$.

As an example, we repeat here the solution that we described in Liu et al. [39] of a transversely isotropic tendon attaching to an isotropic material. The axis of axisymmetry in the tendon is the y-axis in Fig. 3.7. The properties chosen for the tendon are based upon those reported by [14, 40, 41]: $E_x = 450$ MPa, $E_y = E_z = 45$ MPa, $\mu_{xy} = \mu_{xz} = 0.75E_x/1{,}000$. Following Liu et al. [39], we took for the remaining two independent constants $v_{yz} = 0$ and $v_{xz} = v_{xy} = 2$. The remaining constants needed to populate the compliance matrix S_{ij} can be found from the five constants prescribed: symmetry of the compliance matrix requires that $v_{ij} = v_{ji}$ E_i/E_j (in this relation i and j range from x through z, and no summation occurs over the repeated indices), so that $\nu_{zx} = \nu_{yx} = 0.2$; in the plane of transverse isotropy, $\mu_{yz} = E_y/(2(1 + \nu_{yz}))$.

A word about Poisson's ratio is needed here, because, as seen even for the simplest problems discussed in this chapter, the stress field at the free edge is quite sensitive to the mismatch in Poisson's ratio between the two adjoining materials. Those familiar with linear, isotropic elasticity will recognize the value of 2 for ν_{xz} and ν_{xy} as being outside the thermodynamic bounds for an isotropic material, but they are well within the allowable range for a transversely isotropic material (see, e.g., [42]). The requirement that stressing of any sort must lead to positive stored energy requires that each term on the diagonal of the compliance matrix S_{ij} be positive, and that each term on the diagonal of the inverse of S_{ij} (the stiffness matrix, $C_{ij} \equiv S_{ij}^{-1}$) be positive. The latter requirement yields four criteria for an orthotropic material (e.g., [43]):

$$1 - \nu_{ij}\nu_{ji} > 0 \tag{3.23}$$

and

$$1 - \nu_{xy}\nu_{yx} - \nu_{yz}\nu_{zy} - \nu_{zx}\nu_{xz} - 2\nu_{yx}\nu_{zy}\nu_{xz} > 0 \tag{3.24}$$

For the transversely isotropic material studied here, these can be written:

$$1 - \nu_{yz}\nu_{zy} > 0 \rightarrow \nu_{yz}^2 < 1 \tag{3.25}$$

for the transverse plane, and:

$$2\nu_{yz}\nu_{xy}^2(E_y/E_x) < 1 - \nu_{yz}^2 - 2\nu_{xy}^2(E_y/E_x) \tag{3.26}$$

and

$$\nu_{xy}^2 < E_x/E_y \tag{3.27}$$

for the remaining Poisson ratios. For the numbers chosen to represent tendon, $\nu_{yz} = 0$ satisfies (3.25), and two criteria emerge for ν_{xy} from (3.26) to (3.27). Equation (3.27) requires that $-3.16 < \nu_{xy} < 3.16$, but (3.26) is more restrictive in this case, requiring that $-2.24 < \nu_{xy} < 2.24$. Note that a fully isotropic material in which moduli are the same for all directions of stressing, the above equations require that $-1 < \nu_{\text{isotropic}} < 0.5$.

The order of the free edge stress singularity at the interface between transversely isotropic "tendon" and an isotropic material of elastic modulus $E^{(1)}$ and Poisson ratio $\nu^{(1)} = 0.3$ is shown in Fig. 3.10a. Note that we plotted 0 for all values of $(1–\lambda) > 0$, because the stress field is not singular in such cases. In this example, for two values of $E^{(1)}$ and for an insertion angle $\theta_1 = 90°$, the order of the free edge singularity was studied for a range of tendon insertion angles θ_2. The case of relevance to our theme of tendon attached directly to bone is that of E_2 100 times greater than $E_1^{(x)}$; that is, with the isotropic modulus of bone 100 times greater than

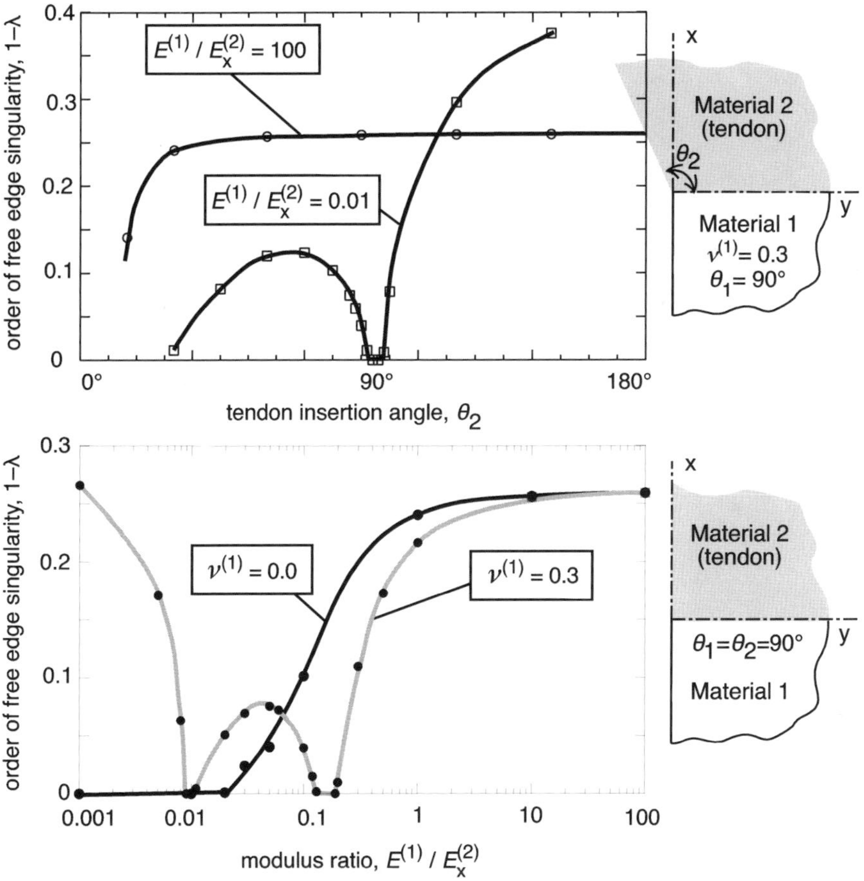

Fig. 3.10 For a biomaterial interface problem, the order of the free edge singularity depends upon the insertion angles and the material orthotropic properties of the adjoining materials

the modulus of the tendon material for stretching in the x-direction, and 1,000 times greater than the modulus of tendon for stretching in the y- or z- directions. The anisotropy of the tendon exacerbates the singularity relative even to the Williams solution: in the William's solution, an isotropic tendon loses the free edge singularity for $\theta_2 < {\sim}60°$, but here even an insertion angle of 15° presents a free edge singularity. The problem is relieved to some degree by attachment through a compliant region. If instead tendon attaches to an isotropic material with E_2 100 times greater than $E_1^{(x)}$, an insertion angle of $\theta_2 < {\sim}30°$ eliminates the free edge singularity. An interesting feature of this is that a second non-singular region arises for $\theta_2 \sim 90°$. One could imagine an effective scheme with a compliant interlayer, in which tendon attaches to a compliant isotropic material at a butt joint ($\theta_1 = \theta_2 = 90°$), which attaches to an isotropic bone. This would eliminate singularities at both interfaces and is loosely related to the scheme that presents at the healthy tendon-to-bone insertion site (cf. [4]).

For the case of a butt joint between tendon and an isotropic material, the order of the singularity is a strong function of both modulus $E^{(1)}$ and Poisson's ratio $\nu^{(1)}$. Two values of $\nu^{(1)}$ were studied over a broad range of modulus $E^{(1)}$ (Fig. 3.10b). For both cases of $\nu^{(1)}$ studied, the order of the singularity approached $(1 - \lambda) \approx 0.26$ for attachment to a relatively stiff isotropic material. The graph shows that this order is relatively constant for $E^{(1)} > \sim 2E_x^{(2)}$, and Fig. 3.10a suggests that this is constant not just for a butt joint but also for any insertion angle $\theta_2 >$ ~30° for the case of tendon attached to a stiff material 1 with $\theta_1 = 90°$. Results suggest that a butt joint between tendon and bone will certainly present a singular stress field, but results again suggest that attachment to a compliant, possibly splayed interlayer, can extinguish the free edge singularity.

Results presented here are somewhat unsatisfying, because they are a smattering of special cases. The literature is full of explorations of special cases because this is an important problem and because no simple way to explore all interfaces exists that is analogous to the Dundurs' parameters (e.g., Fig. 3.6). However, the results do indicate that attaching a material like tendon to an isotropic material that is at least twice as stiff will lead invariably to a singularity over a wide range of insertion angles: as before, an interlayer or careful shaping is needed to avoid a free edge singularity.

3.6 Concluding Remarks

So we found a free edge singularity. Now what? Sections 3.4 and 3.5 focused on situations in which a free edge singularity can arise at the interface between two dissimilar materials. We conclude by describing what one might do to assess whether such a singularity will lead to catastrophic failure of the interface between the two materials, and why researchers who are interested in tendon-to-bone attachment are not much concerned about this.

Several groups have proposed a framework based upon linear elastic fracture mechanics. These concepts follow directly from the problems we have addressed in this chapter: the solution for the stress field around a sharp crack in an infinite solid can be found by considering the case of tendon $\theta_1 = \theta_2 = 180°$ in Fig. 3.7. For the case of materials 1 and 2 being the same linear elastic, isotropic material, and for a remote stress field that is a uniaxial stress σ^{∞} applied in the vertical direction, the asymptotic stress field near the crack has the form:

$$\sigma_{ij} = \frac{K_{\mathrm{I}}}{\sqrt{2\pi r}} \tilde{\sigma}_{ij}(\theta), \tag{3.28}$$

where the stress intensity factor K_{I} is a constant that depends upon geometry and upon σ^{∞}, and the function $\tilde{\sigma}_{ij}(\theta)$ is known (e.g., [44]). Within certain limits, fracture in many materials is well modeled by the criterion $K_{\mathrm{I}} < K_{\mathrm{I}}^{\mathrm{c}}$, where $K_{\mathrm{I}}^{\mathrm{c}}$ is a critical value that can be calibrated experimentally. $K_{\mathrm{I}}^{\mathrm{c}}$ can be related to a more physically intuitive parameter, the fracture energy Γ_{c} that was introduced in Sect. 3.1. For example, for the case of plane strain $\Gamma_{\mathrm{c}} = (1 - v^2)/(K_{\mathrm{I}}^{\mathrm{c}})^2/E$. The available energy $\Gamma = (1 - v^2)(K_{\mathrm{I}})^2/E$ can be compared to the critical fracture energy, Γ_{c}, and fracture can be predicted under certain conditions. Central to these conditions is that the "process zone," which is the region of material just ahead of the crack tip that withstands very high strains without failing, is small compared to the dimensions of the crack and the body in which it is embedded. We will discuss the process zone more in the context of tendon-to-bone attachment.

The free edge intensity factor H in (3.13) can serve the role of a stress intensity factor and serve as an indicator of the likelihood of the onset of fracture. However, fracture need not be catastrophic, and the problem of whether a crack within an interface will advance has been studied by Akisanya and Fleck [20]. The problem studied involves an edge crack embedded within an interface and loaded with the singular stress field of (3.13). The stress field ahead of the crack tip is more complicated (see ref. [45, 46] and the review by Hutchinson and Suo [47]), involving rapid oscillation in the traction between the two materials ahead of the crack tip. However, the concept of a critical fracture energy still holds, with minor extension to account for the sensitivity of fracture toughness to this oscillatory stress field. Klingbeil and Beuth [21, 24] developed an elegant analysis to account for the interactions between free edge and interfacial crack singularities when designing a layered structure, but this is beyond the scope of this chapter.

Why can materials withstand stress singularities, and what does this mean for attachment of biological tissues? In many metals, the mechanisms are fairly well understood and involve the phenomenon of plasticity. Beyond a critical stress level called a yield stress, the stiffness of a metal drops dramatically—this is the end of the linear region of the uniaxial stress vs. strain response shown in Fig. 3.11. This mechanical response results in a reduction of stresses at the crack tip for two reasons. First, the crack tip "blunts," meaning that the metal at the crack tip stretches so as to turn the sharp crack into a blunt crack, thereby eliminating the otherwise infinite stresses locally. Second, the reduction of stiffness of that material at higher strains (the stiffness of relevance is the slope of the tangent to the stress–strain curve) causes stress redistribution away from the crack tip; this occurs even in brittle matrix ceramics [48, 49]. The result is that the material can undergo major irreversible local changes that reduce the severity of the crack without endangering a well-designed structure made of the material.

The situation is different, however, for a living tissue. First, such local injury is undesirable for many tissues. Second, the stress–strain responses of many biological tissues differ fundamentally from those of engineering materials (c.f. the data stress–strain data for a tendon in Fig. 3.11). In addition to withstanding larger strains and reaching lower peak stresses, a typical stress–strain curve is concave up instead of concave down. The consequence is that stiffness ahead of a tear in a tissue can increase, rather than decrease as in a metal. Stress concentrations in a biological tissue can therefore become more rather less severe as stresses increase.

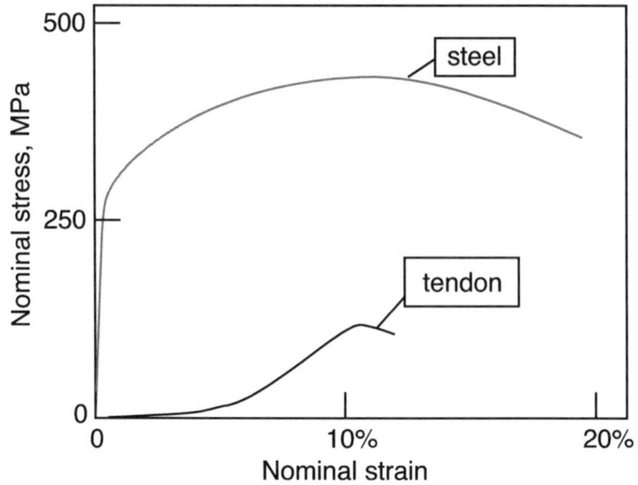

Fig. 3.11 The stress–strain behavior of a metal such as steel involves a characteristic concave down shape, with a drop in stiffness following a yield point corresponding to the onset of permanent "plastic" deformation. The stress–strain behavior of a biological material such as a tendon involves a characteristic concave up shape, with a rise in stiffness over a much larger elastic region

Tissues are nevertheless resilient to tears, with many mechanisms identified within their fibrous protein structures that enhance toughening across length scales [50–52]. However, the body seems to take few chances and uses many schemes for reducing stresses, including tailoring of material and morphological properties of tissues to eliminate free edge singularities, and tailoring of joints to maximize peel resistance.

Acknowledgments This work was supported in part by the National Institutes of Health (HL079165) and by the Johanna D. Bemis trust. Y.L. received a fellowship from the Fannie Stephens Murphy Memorial Fund.

References

1. Genin GM, Kent A, Birman V, Wopenka B, Pasteris JD, Marquez PJ, Thomopoulos S (2009) Functional grading of mineral and collagen in the attachment of tendon to bone. Biophys J 97(4):976–985
2. Silva MJ, Brodt MD, Wopenka B, Thomopoulos S, Williams D, Wassen MH, Ko M, Kusano N, Bank RA (2006) Decreased collagen organization and content are associated with reduced strength of demineralized and intact bone in the SAMP6 mouse. J Bone Miner Res 21(1):78–88
3. Thomopoulos S, Marquez JP, Weinberger B, Birman V, Genin GM (2006) Collagen fiber orientation at the tendon to bone insertion and its influence on stress concentrations. J Biomech 39(10):1842–1851

4. Thomopoulos S, Williams GR, Gimbel JA, Favata M, Soslowsky LJ (2003) Variation of biomechanical, structural, and compositional properties along the tendon to bone insertion site. J Orthop Res 21(3):413–419
5. Wopenka B, Kent A, Pasteris JD, Yoon Y, Thomopoulos S (2008) The tendon-to-bone transition of the rotator cuff: a preliminary Raman spectroscopic study documenting the gradual mineralization across the insertion in rat tissue samples. Appl Spectrosc 62(12):1285–1294
6. Bower AF (2009) Applied mechanics of solids [A free and regularly updated version of this text can be found on http://www.solidmechanics.org]. CRC Press, New York
7. Thomopoulos S, Williams GR, Soslowsky LJ (2003) Tendon to bone healing: differences in biomechanical, structural, and compositional properties due to a range of activity levels. J Biomech Eng 125(1):106–113
8. Williams ML (1952) Stress singularities resulting from various boundary conditions in angular corners of plates in extension. J Appl Mech 19:526–528
9. Rivlin R (1944) The effective work of adhesion. Paint Technol 9:215–216
10. Kendall K (1971) The adhesion and surface energy of elastic solids. J Phys D: Appl Phys 4:1186
11. Kendall K (1975) Thin-film peeling-the elastic term. J Phys D: Appl Phys 8:1449
12. Wren TAL, Yerby SA, Beaupré GS, Carter DR (2001) Mechanical properties of the human achilles tendon. Clin Biomech 16(3):245–251
13. Ashby MF (2005) Materials selection in mechanical design, vol 519. Cambridge University Press, Cambridge, UK
14. Maganaris CN, Paul JP (1999) *In vivo* human tendon mechanical properties. J Physiol 521 (pt 1):307–313
15. Williams JA, Kauzlarich JJ (2004) Peeling shear and cleavage failure due to tape prestrain. J Adhes 80(5):433–458
16. Williams JA, Kauzlarich JJ (2006) The influence of peel angle on the mechanics of peeling flexible adherends with arbitrary load-extension characteristics. Tribol Int 38(11):951–958
17. Bogy D (1971) Two edge-bonded elastic wedges of different materials and wedge angles under surface tractions. J Appl Mech 38:377
18. Hein V, Erdogan F (1971) Stress singularities in a two-material wedge. Int J Fract 7(3):317–330
19. Akisanya A, Fleck N (1992) Brittle fracture of adhesive joints. Int J Fract 58(2):93–114
20. Akisanya A, Fleck N (1997) Interfacial cracking from the freeedge of a long bi-material strip. Int J Solids Struct 34(13):1645–1665
21. Klingbeil N, Beuth J (2000) On the design of debond-resistant bimaterials: part I: free-edge singularity approach. Eng Fract Mech 66(2):93–110
22. Dundurs J (1969) Discussion: edge-bonded dissimilar orthogonal elastic wedges under normal and shear loading. J Appl Mech 36:650
23. Noda NA, Lan X (2012) Stress intensity factors for an edge interface crack in a bonded semi-infinite plate for arbitrary material combination. Int J Solids Struct 49(10):1241–1251
24. Klingbeil N, Beuth J (2000) On the design of debond-resistant bimaterials: part II: a comparison of free-edge and interface crack approaches. Eng Fract Mech 66(2):111–128
25. Suga T, Elssner G, Schmauder S (1988) Composite parameters and mechanical compatibility of material joints. J Compos Mater 22(10):917–934
26. Wang P, Xu LR (2006) Convex interfacial joints with least stress singularities in dissimilar materials. Mech Mater 38(11):1001–1011
27. Xu L, Sengupta S (2004) Dissimilar material joints with and without free-edge stress singularities: part II. an integrated numerical analysis. Exp Mech 44(6):616–621
28. Xu T, Bianco P, Fisher LW, Longenecker G, Smith E, Goldstein S, Bonadio J, Boskey A, Heegaard AM, Sommer B, Satomura K, Dominguez P, Zhao C, Kulkarni AB, Robey PG, Young MF (1998) Targeted disruption of the biglycan gene leads to an osteoporosis-like phenotype in mice. Nat Genet 20(1):78–82

29. Yosibash Z (1997) Computing edge singularities in elastic anisotropic three-dimensional domains. Int J Fract 86(3):221–245
30. Dimitrov A, Andrä H, Schnack E (2002) Singularities near three-dimensional corners in composite laminates. Int J Fract 115(4):361–375
31. Apel T, Mehrmann V, Watkins D (2002) Structured eigenvalue methods for the computation of corner singularities in 3D anisotropic elastic structures. Comput Methods Appl Mech Eng 191(39):4459–4473
32. Yosibash Z, Omer N (2007) Numerical methods for extracting edge stress intensity functions in anisotropic three-dimensional domains. Comput Methods Appl Mech Eng 196(37–40):3624–3649
33. Wang S, Choi I (1982) Boundary-layer effects in composite laminates: part 2: free-edge stress solutions and basic characteristics. J Appl Mech 49:549
34. Wang S, Choi I (1982) Boundary-layer effects in composite laminates: part 1: free-edge stress singularities. J Appl Mech 49:541
35. Ting T (1986) Explicit solution and invariance of the singularities at an interface crack in anisotropic composites. Int J Solids Struct 22(9):965–983
36. Delale F (1984) Stress singularities in bonded anisotropic materials. Int J Solids Struct 20(1):31–40
37. Mittelstedt C, Becker W (2007) Free-edge effects in composite laminates. Appl Mech Rev 60:217
38. Lekhnitskii SG (1968) Anisotropic plates. Gordon and Breach, New York
39. Liu Y, Birman V, Chen C, Thomopoulos S, Genin GM (2011) Mechanisms of bimaterial attachment at the interface of tendon to bone. J Eng Mater Technol 133:011006
40. Weiss JA, Gardiner JC, Bonifasi-Lista C (2002) Ligament material behavior is nonlinear, viscoelastic and rate-independent under shear loading. J Biomech 35(7):943–950
41. Yin L, Elliott DM (2004) A biphasic and transversely isotropic mechanical model for tendon: application to mouse tail fascicles in uniaxial tension. J Biomech 37(6):907–916
42. Ting T, Chen T (2005) Poisson's ratio for anisotropic elastic materials can have no bounds. Q J Mech Appl Math 58(1):73–82
43. Jones RM (1999) Mechanics of composite materials, 2nd edn. Taylor & Francis, Inc., Philadelphia
44. Tada H, Paris PC, Irwin GR, Engineers ASoM (2000) The stress analysis of cracks handbook, vol 130. ASME press, New York
45. Williams M (1959) The stresses around a fault or crack in dissimilar media. Bull Seismol Soc Am 49(2):199–204
46. Rice JR (1988) Elastic fracture mechanics concepts for interfacial cracks. J Appl Mech-Trans ASME 55(1):98–103
47. Hutchinson JW, Suo Z (1992) Mixed mode cracking in layered materials. Adv Appl Mech 29:63–191
48. Genin GM, Hutchinson JW (1997) Composite laminates in plane stress: constitutive modeling, and stress redistribution due to matrix cracking. J Am Ceram Soc 80(5):1245–1255
49. Genin GM, Hutchinson JW (1999) Failures at attachment holes in brittle matrix laminates. J Compos Mater 33(17):1600–1619
50. Gao H, Ji B, Buehler MJ, Yao H (2005) Flaw tolerant nanostructures of biological materials. Mechanics of the 21st Century, pp 131–138, New York: Springer
51. Buehler MJ, Keten S, Ackbarow T (2008) Theoretical and computational hierarchical nanomechanics of protein materials: deformation and fracture. Prog Mater Sci 53(8):1101–1241
52. Liu Y, Thomopoulos S, Birman V, Li JS, Genin G (2011) Bi-material attachment through a compliant interfacial system at the tendon-to-bone insertion site. Mech Mater 44:83–92

Part II
Natural Examples of Transitions from Stiff to Compliant Materials

Chapter 4
Ligament and Tendon Enthesis: Anatomy and Mechanics

Matteo M. Tei, Kathryn F. Farraro, and Savio L.-Y. Woo

4.1 Introduction

The insertions of ligaments and tendons to bone are morphologically and biomechanically complex. Within the length of 1 mm, the insertion is transformed from soft connective tissue to hard bone. In general, this transformation consists of four zones; i.e., collagen fibers, non-mineralized fibrocartilage, mineralized fibrocartilage, and bone, making it suitable to transmit loads with minimal stress concentration. However, the morphology of ligament and tendon insertions can vary greatly from one ligament or tendon to another as well as between the two ends of the same ligament. Adding to this complexity, factors such as age, skeletal maturation, and physical activity have also been shown to affect the morphological and biomechanical properties of these entheses, which could, in turn, have a significant influence on their modes of failure caused by daily or sports activities.

In this chapter, we will begin by discussing the anatomy of the enthesis, including a review of the gross morphology as well as histology and appearance of two distinct types of insertions: the direct and indirect insertions to bone. We will also touch upon the vascular and nerve supply, including associated blood vessels and neuroreceptors. This will be followed by details on the biomechanical function of insertion sites, including some challenges with methods involved in determining their properties.

We will then review the changes that occur across the insertion site during growth and skeletal maturity. Specific structural changes of insertion sites during skeletal maturation and the asynchronous change between the properties of the ligament insertion and substance will be explained using the femur-MCL-tibia complex (FMTC) as an example. This will be followed by a description of

M.M. Tei • K.F. Farraro • S.L.-Y.Woo (✉)
Musculoskeletal Research Center, Department of Bioengineering, Swanson School of Engineering, University of Pittsburgh, Pittsburgh, PA, USA
e-mail: mmt44@pitt.edu; kff7@pitt.edu; ddecenzo@pitt.edu

S. Thomopoulos et al. (eds.), *Structural Interfaces and Attachments in Biology*,
DOI 10.1007/978-1-4614-3317-0_4, © Springer Science+Business Media New York 2013

age-related changes in ligaments and tendons and their insertions. Finally, the negative effects of immobilization on the insertion and its slow recovery following remobilization, together with positive effects of exercise, will be presented with an illustration of how activity level can be related to biomechanical properties by a highly nonlinear curve.

One of the greatest challenges in studying ligament and tendon entheses is accurate determination of their biomechanical properties, due to their complexity and irregular geometry. With the development of the video dimensional analyzer (VDA) system, the nonuniform elongation between the insertion site and along the ligament could be measured. As a result, it has been shown that the percent elongation at or near the insertion is always higher than that in the ligament or tendon substance. We will also review other technologies, such as the use of a laser micrometer, to determine the cross-sectional area of ligaments and tendons so that their tensile stress could be properly determined. With the knowledge of a stress–strain relationship, the mechanical properties of the ligament substance could be determined and separated from the structural properties of the bone-ligament-bone complex.

To conclude, we will discuss repair of the insertion sites of ligaments and tendons after injury, including surgical reconstruction using a tissue autograft or allograft. As graft-bone healing has not been able to replicate the normal soft tissue-to-bone enthesis, new biomimetic technologies, including the use of bioscaffolds aiming to reproduce the zones of transition across the insertion, are being explored. Although the availability of new biomaterials that could assist the body in recreating the complex insertion site indeed offers many exciting possibilities, many challenges still remain, as in-depth knowledge of the composition and properties of ligament and tendon insertion sites is still lacking. It is our belief that fundamental studies to improve our understanding of enthesis structure, function, and their relationship are needed before one can be in a position to move forward with regeneration of an enthesis on a scientific basis.

4.2 Anatomy

4.2.1 Morphology

The morphology of ligament and tendon insertions to bone is among the most complex of all biological tissues. The transformation of soft to hard tissue requires a gradual transition of collagen fibers to non-mineralized fibrocartilage, then to mineralized fibrocartilage, and finally to bone. In addition, the structure of the insertion site is different from ligament to ligament, as well as between the two ends of the same ligament. Nevertheless, researchers have been able to categorize ligament and tendon insertions into two general types: direct insertions and indirect insertions.

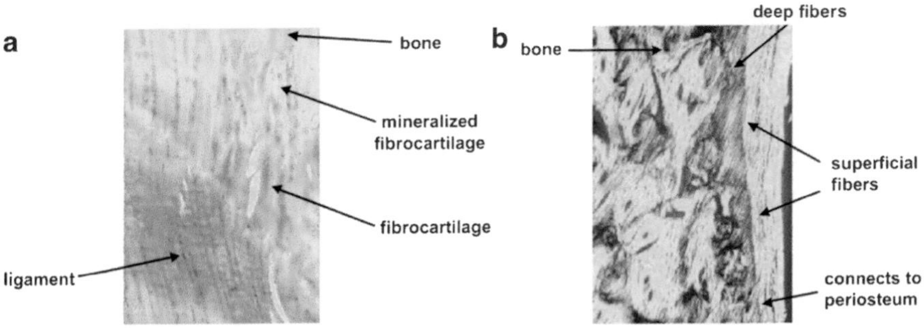

Fig. 4.1 Photomicrograph demonstrating a direct insertion: the femoral insertion of rabbit medial collateral ligament (**a**), and an indirect insertion: the tibial attachment of the MCL (**b**) (reproduced, with permission, from [11])

4.2.1.1 Direct Insertions

Microscopically, superficial and deep fibers of the ligaments and tendons are inserted into bone with the deep fibers meeting the bone at right angles with four distinct zones. *Zone 1* consists of type I collagen as the extracellular matrix with fibroblasts. There are also capillaries, arterioles, and venules running parallel to the collagen fibers, and this zone is free of nerves and nerve endings. In *Zone 2*, the cells become larger and more rounded and chondrocyte-like. Cells in this zone are arranged in rows between the parallel collagen fibers. The Golgi organelles become prominent, and the cell processes are short, with most appearing to remain in a lacunar region that extends 1–2 μm around the cells. Microscopically, this zone has an appearance similar to fibrocartilagenous tissues. In *Zone 3*, the tissue becomes mineralized fibrocartilage. Light microscopy shows a clear line of calcification, called the "tidemark." The tidemark is usually smooth in contour, but is sometimes irregularly shaped. About 12 μm away, the mineral crystals increase in number and aggregate into masses so that individual crystals become less obvious. The deeper part of zone 3 is also characterized by dense mineral deposits both within and between the collagen fibers. Finally, in *Zone 4*, it becomes bone, as the inserting tissue merges with the bone matrix collagen fibrils. The bone matrix proteoglycans are represented by chondroitin sulfate, similar to the small proteoglycans of cartilage, whereas the proteoglycans of ligaments and tendons are represented by dermatan sulfate.

The femoral attachment of the MCL to the femur is a good example of a direct insertion. The MCL inserts in the femoral epiphyseal area by passing acutely into the cortex through a well-defined zone of fibrocartilage and with minimal contribution into the overlying periosteum (Fig. 4.1a).

4.2.1.2 Indirect Insertions

Unlike direct insertions, the superficial components of an indirect insertion blend into the periosteum, while the deep components of fibers of indirect insertions attach to the bone with little or none of the transitional zone of the fibrocartilage seen in direct insertions. Here, the collagen fibers meet the bone at an acute angle, and there is a tidemark separating the mineralized and non-mineralized tissue.

The distal (tibial) attachment of the MCL to the tibia is a good example of an indirect insertion (Fig. 4.1b). Here, superficial fibers are attached to the periosteum while deeper fibers are directly attached to the bone at acute angles [1].

4.2.1.3 Vascular and Nerve Supply

The insertion sites of ligaments and tendons are relatively avascular, as the blood supply to the soft tissues comes from the joint capsules. Commonly, the vessels in the marginal part of the insertion area of the ligament or tendon connect with those of the periosteum. Therefore, the vessels of the external peritendineum and of the periosteum are the major vessels disrupted in avulsion injuries at the bone surface. Superficial blood vessels in the anastomase merge with vessels of the periosteum in most tendon-bone junctions, but intratendinous vessels remain separated from the vasculature of bone except in circumscribed diphysoperiosteal insertions, characterized by those to spinae, trabeculae, or tuberosities of bone.

The nerve supply has a pattern similar to that of the blood supply in that there are no nerves that cross the zone of fibrocartilage to innervate both sides of the insertion site. However, bones, tendons, and ligaments all have abundant neural elements that may transmit important information in the analysis of joint motion, position, and acceleration. Nerve endings and Pacini and Ruffini receptors have been found in the interfascicular connective tissue. These receptors seem to possess a "limit-detection function" of the physiological tolerable limit of movement or may control small movements via the perception of acceleration [2]. Pacini and Ruffini receptors, Golgi tendon organ-like receptors, and free nerve endings were found in proximity to the insertions of the anterior cruciate ligament (ACL) [3]. Furthermore, Grigg and associates described that the afferents in the posterior articular nerve (PAN) from the posterior capsule of the knee joint were sensitive to linear stress, and that their role is to signal the limit of the joint motion in extension, in addition to the afferents coming from the knee ligaments [4–6].

4.2.2 Biomechanical Function

The insertion site functions to transmit a load between the flexible yet strong tension-bearing ligament or tendon into rigid, less compliant bone without damaging the soft tissue [7]. However, the load magnitude varies greatly between tendons and ligaments as well as between different joints. Typically, *in vivo* forces on tendon insertions are large because of muscular contractions, while forces in ligaments tend to be relatively small. To facilitate this load transfer and prevent tearing at the attachment site, a gradual change in tissue composition across the insertion site between soft tissue and bone is needed [8, 9].

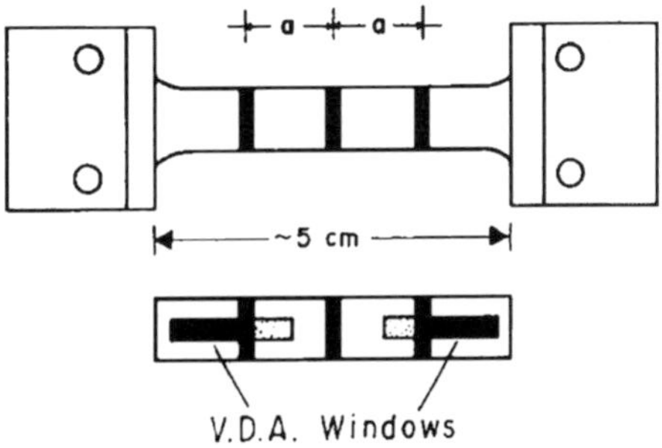

Fig. 4.2 Stained gauge lines on test specimen and video dimensional analyzer (VDA) windows for tensile strain determination (reproduced, with permission, from [18])

Determining the biomechanical properties of ligaments and tendons as well as their insertions is crucial to understanding the structure-function relationship for purposes of homeostasis for injury prevention, repair, and healing. However, the complex nature of insertion sites presents significant challenges when the properties of the insertion site are separated from that of the tissue substance. Variation in insertion type (direct or indirect), tissue geometry, matrix composition and distribution, and orientation of collagen fibers makes it even more difficult to make generalizations about properties of ligament and tendon entheses. For example, in the supraspinous tendon, Thomopoulos and associates [10] found that collagen fibers were significantly less organized at the bony insertion compared to the muscle insertion.

An additional challenge in determining the biomechanical properties of the ligament or tendon insertion site is the size of the test specimen. For ligaments such as the MCL, it is necessary to prepare the test specimen with the femoral and tibial bony attachments because the ligament substance is relatively short, so the test specimen is that of a bone-ligament-bone complex [8]. An apparatus was developed for uniaxial tensile testing using a VDA system to determine nonuniform properties of the rabbit FMTC. The MCL is stained with several gauge lines for tensile strain determination of the ligament midsubstance and insertion sites (Fig. 4.2). This data and the output from a tensile load cell on a materials testing machine produce a load-elongation diagram and stress–strain curve.

A typical load-elongation curve for the FMTC is shown in Fig. 4.3, characterized by a toe region, a linear region, and a failure region [11, 12]. The nonlinearity of this curve illustrates the ligament's function in guiding joint motion under low loading conditions, while limiting excess motion and protecting the cartilage at higher loads.

Using strain data obtained with the VDA system in the MCL, it was found that the strain of the ligament substance is consistently smaller than the specific deformations calculated for the bone-ligament-bone complex [8]. These results suggest that the deformations near or at the ligament insertion sites to bone are larger than in the midsubstance. This large variation of regional strain values along the ligament substance highlights the possibility that larger deformations near insertions may predispose these areas to higher incidence of tensile failure at low stretch rates and stresses the need to characterize and understand the differences in biomechanical properties between the ligament substance and insertion.

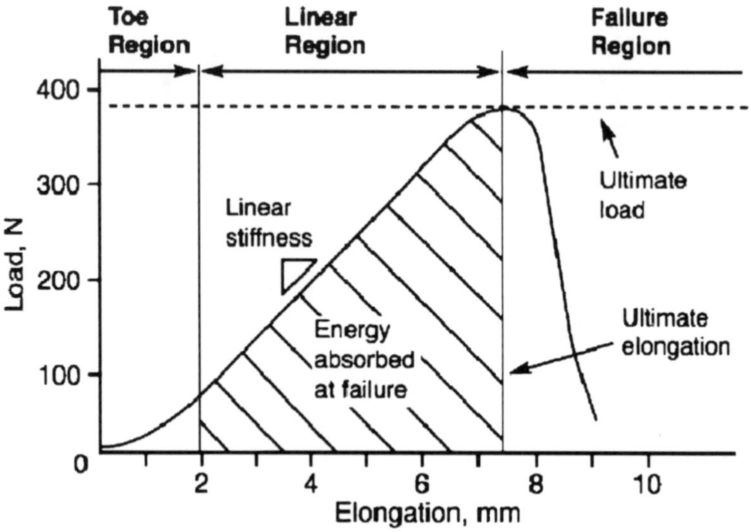

Fig. 4.3 Typical load-elongation curve of the femur-MCL-tibia complex

4.3 Development, Growth, and Aging

4.3.1 Changes with Skeletal Maturity

4.3.1.1 Embryology

The development of ligaments and tendons to bone is unique and it is important to better understand the structure-function relationships in these tissues. Between 7 and 8 weeks of embryonic life, the ligaments, tendons, and joint capsules begin development by cellular condensations, forming in situ as a unit without migration. The overall development of the insertion site proceeds along with that of the bone.

4.3.1.2 Skeletally Immature

Before skeletal maturation, bone growth is longitudinal and coincides with the lengthening of the insertion site, so that a constant position relative to the growth plate and adjacent joint can be maintained. This is why the indirect insertion is needed. Dörlf [62] sought to explain the cause and method of migration of tendon insertions in immature rabbits by using Tetracycline as a marker of osteogenesis at the insertion sites. He found that insertion site migration is caused by dragging of the insertion by the periosteum, which is itself pulled by the epiphyses as they grow away from the diaphyses of the bone. In our studies of the rabbit MCL, we have

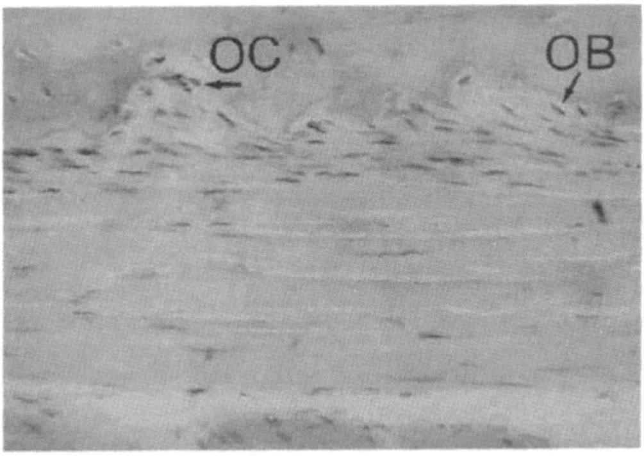

Fig. 4.4 A photomicrograph showing the distal (tibial) insertion of the MCL from a skeletally immature rabbit. Note that the osteoclasts (OC) and osteoblast (OB) and the oblique deeper fibers' insertion to bone have not yet been well established (reproduced, with permission, from [14])

found that the insertion site on the tibial side is affected by its proximity to the growth plate where (1) osteoclastic activity in this region weakens the subperiosteal attachment and (2) part of the ligament insertion is at the area of the metaphysis.

The examination of the tibial insertions of skeletally immature rabbit specimens revealed several differences when compared to mature samples. The metaphysis of the proximal tibia in the skeletally immature rabbit was composed of bars containing calcified cartilage, and the primary spongy bone was undergoing reorganization as exemplified by the increased presence of osteoclasts and osteoblasts (Fig. 4.4). The delayed maturation of the MCL-tibia junction may be due to this increased complexity compared to that of the MCL substance. Therefore, this junction was an area of weakness in the FMTC and the skeletally immature specimens failed by tibial avulsion. This finding was well-illustrated by histological evaluation of the components of the FMTC, which showed that the weakest link in skeletally immature rabbits was the tibial insertion, a result of the maturation process that included bone remodeling activities in the subperiosteal region of this attachment. Thus, some of the deep oblique fibers had not yet attached to bone and the ligament attachment became more dependent on the periosteal component. In contrast, the femoral insertion had a direct penetration of fibers into the metaphyseal cortex. There were no histological differences noted at the femoral insertion of the MCL as a function of skeletal maturity.

4.3.1.3 Skeletally Mature

As the insertion site changes structurally and compositionally with skeletal maturation, there are also significant changes in the structural properties of the femur-MCL-tibia complex during maturation of the rat and rabbit. At this indirect insertion, skeletal maturity is characterized by the deep fibers anchoring solidly into the bone. Tipton and associates [13] and our research center [14, 15] found that in the rabbit, the strength of the FMTC did not plateau until closure of the epiphyses at about 7 months of age, and tensile failure of skeletally immature animals occurred by tibial avulsion in all cases [14]. In contrast, older rabbit specimens exhibited

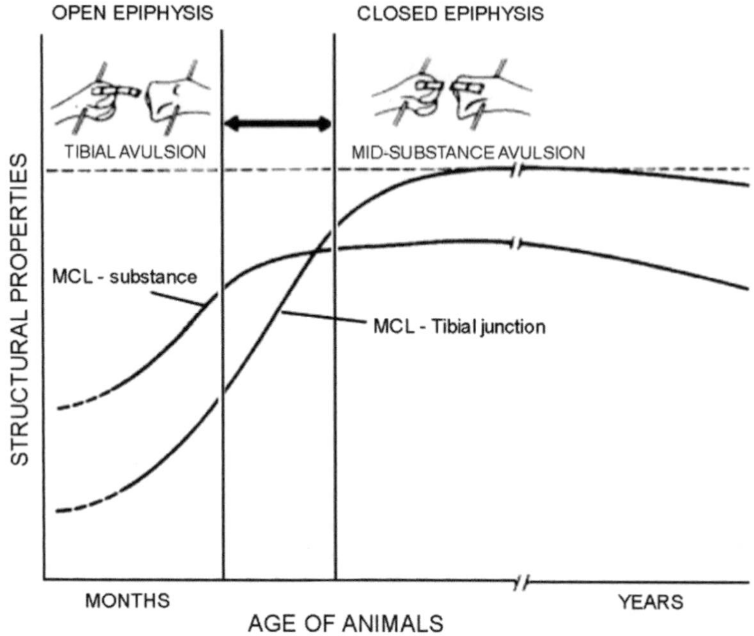

Fig. 4.5 Schematic description of the changes in the tensile properties and failure modes of the rabbit femur-MCL-tibia complex (FMTC) with age

tensile failure of the FMTC by midsubstance failure, as the strength of the MCL-tibia insertion increased with skeletal maturity.

A schematic representation of the effects of maturation on the biomechanical properties of the FMTC is shown in Fig. 4.5. Prior to skeletal maturity, the strength of the MCL substance reached its peak value, while the bone-ligament junction, especially at the proximal tibial insertion site, was being established. Therefore, the MCL substance was stronger, and the FMTC failed by tibial avulsion. Once skeletal maturity was reached, the proximal tibial insertion site became solidly established, while the tensile strength of the MCL substance changed minimally.

4.3.2 Aging

With aging, there are significant changes in the periosteum, as the superficial fibrous layer becomes comprised of fibroblasts and fibrocytes interposed between multidirectional collagen layers permeated by elastic tissue. The deeper osteogenic layer now contains precursor osteogenic cells and mature osteoblasts, changes that are coupled with a loss of organelles. Aging is also characterized by a loss of cells and organelles associated with normal functional activities. Lipofuscin also appears in all of aged cells, including osteocytes. Despite these severe ultrastructural

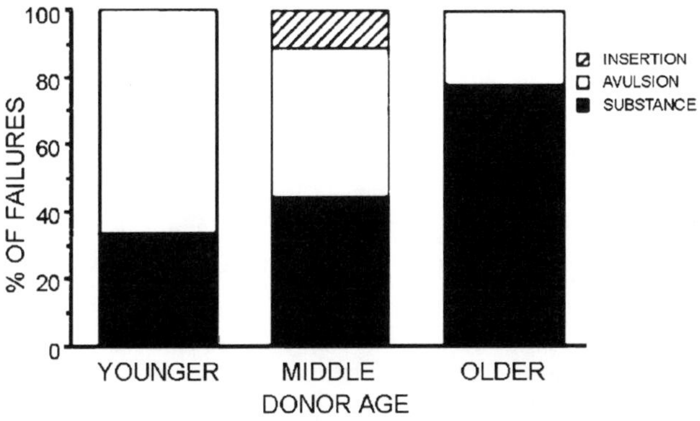

Fig. 4.6 Histogram of modes of failure of human femur-ACL-tibia complex (FATC) tested from the younger, middle, and older donors studied (reproduced, with permission, from [9])

alterations with age, it appears that sufficient organelles remain in a few cells of each layer to maintain viability.

Biomechanical studies of soft tissue-bone junctions in cadaver specimens from donors over than 50 years of age have shown significant reductions in the structural properties of the femur-ACL-tibia complex (FATC). In our research center, we have found that the failure mode changed with age. In younger donors, tibial avulsion was much more common, whereas in older donors, there were more midsubstance failures (Fig. 4.6). This shift in failure mode was accompanied with a decrease in linear stiffness, ultimate load, and energy absorbed at failure for the older group, suggesting that there is a more rapid deterioration of the ACL substance with increasing age [9].

It should be noted that this unusually fast degradation of the ACL is unique to this ligament, as the FMTC showed insignificant change in stiffness or ultimate load with age in the rabbit model [14]. This illustrates the uniqueness of each ligament in its growth, development, and aging. Investigators should thus be cautious when extrapolating age-related changes from one ligament to another.

4.4 Stress and Motion-Dependent Homeostasis

4.4.1 Immobilization

Even short periods of immobilization have deleterious effects on tendons, ligaments, and bone, as well as the insertion sites. Osteoclasts at the bony insertion have been found to resorb bone and sever the deep fibrous attachment, severely weakening the insertion and rendering it susceptible to failure by avulsion, as it is now limited to the superficial attachment where the collagen fibers become confluent with the periosteum [16].

Mechanical and biochemical changes also occur in these soft tissues following immobilization. There are significant increases in joint stiffness with alterations of articular cartilage. With longer periods of immobilization, areas of necrosis in cartilage are seen in underlying contacting areas. Ulcerations could also occur even in non-contact areas. The significance of these findings is escalated when one considers the dependency of the insertion site on maintaining structural integrity. This is especially important for the collateral ligaments of the knee, where the collagen fibrils of the distal attachments become confluent with the periosteum, with some fibrils passing directly into the bone. There are also profound changes in the substance of the ligament, as fibrils morphologically alter their normal arrangement and cellular organization. Concomitant biochemical changes include reduction of glycosaminoglycans and water as well as significant changes in the mass, rate of turnover, and cross-linking of collagen. It was noted that, after immobilization, disruption of the MCL-tibia junction was great, with a time-dependent decrease in ultimate load and an increase in tibial avulsions, indicating that a longer period of immobilization resulted in greater resorption of bone [1]. In the ACL insertion, however, the effects of immobilization were more modest, with no appreciable change observed in either attachment under light microscopy and no incidence of increased avulsion failure [17].

4.4.2 Remobilization

Despite the deleterious effects of immobilization on ligaments and tendons and their insertion sites, a reversal of these effects has been demonstrated, although it takes much more time. In our research center, we found that the mechanical properties of the MCL returned to control values relatively quickly following remobilization. However, the structural properties of the FMTC remained inferior because of incomplete recovery at the insertion site, as shown by areas of resorbed bone and the presence of osteoclasts, as well as regions where disorganized tissue was undergoing reossification. Failures therefore continued to occur at bone insertion sites.

Thus, there is an asynchronous recovery rate between the insertion site and the ligament substance following immobilization and remobilization. The recovery of the MCL substance is much faster than that of the insertion, and 52 weeks of remobilization after immobilization may be required in order to restore the MCL insertion [1].

Based on these findings, we proposed a set of hypothetical curves to represent the biomechanical properties in response to immobilization, remobilization, and exercise. These curves illustrate the reduction in biomechanical performance with immobilization, improvement with remobilization, and the asynchronous recovery rate between the ligament substance and insertion site (Fig. 4.7).

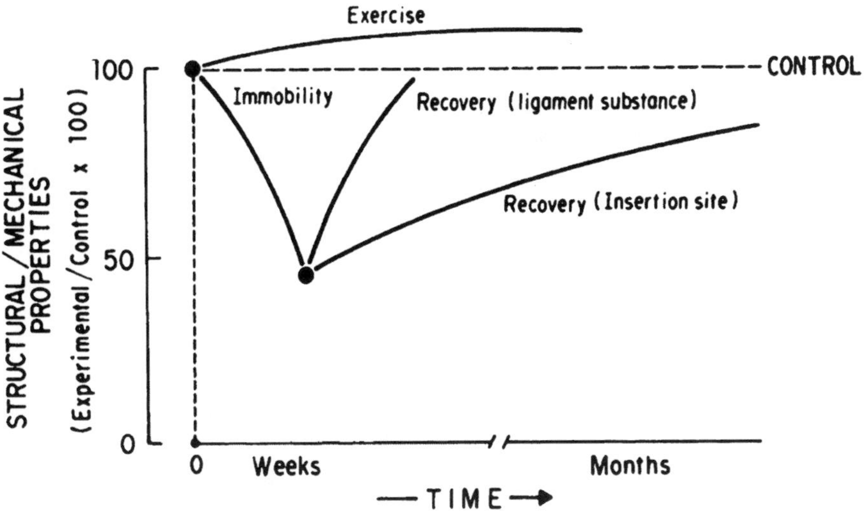

Fig. 4.7 Curves summarizing the homeostatic responses of the components of the bone-ligament-bone complex when it was subjected to different levels of physical activity (reproduced, with permission, from [1])

4.4.3 *Effects of Exercise*

The relationship between physical activity and soft tissue and insertion site properties has also been shown to have an effect on ligament and tendon entheses. Laboratory studies have directly addressed the effect of exercise on these tissues, including some reports on the effects of exercise on tissue biomechanical properties [18–20].

Our research center has performed studies of the biochemical and biomechanical properties of the isolated swine extensor tendon using 1-year-old swine following a 1-year exercise regime [18]. A second, sedentary group was used as a control. Load-deformation curves were produced typical of the characteristic nonlinear tensile behavior of tendons, beginning with an initial toe region of low stiffness, where the ligament has not been fully extended, followed by an intermediate linear region, and finally a yield region as fibers begin to fail and the tendon ruptures. Exercised medial and lateral tendons were found to have a significantly higher ultimate strength (σ_{max}) and lower ultimate strain (ε_{max}). Contrary to several previous studies, size and composition of the tendons were shown to be affected by exercise, as cross-sectional area of exercised tendon was found to be 22% greater than the sedentary control, tendon weights were significantly higher, and collagen content was found to be significantly greater in the lateral extensor. Thus, this study demonstrated a clear increase in mechanical properties in addition to hypertrophy and increased collagen content of the tendon.

A parallel study using the swine flexor tendon was also done [20]. Exercise was found to improve the strength of the flexor tendon, as exercised tendons displayed an ultimate load and linear load-deformation slope 19 and 26% higher than control

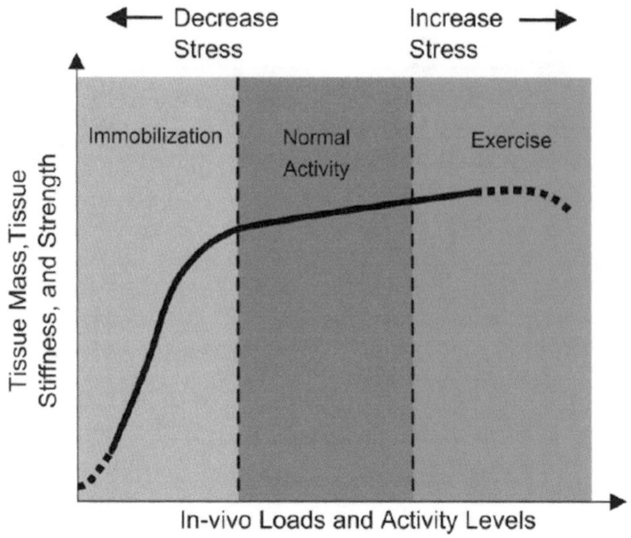

Fig. 4.8 Homeostatic response of ligaments and tendons to physical activity and *in vivo* loading (reproduced, with permission, from [61])

specimens; however, ultimate elongation was not found to be significantly different between groups. No significant difference was found in the cross-sectional area or wet or dry weight between groups. Similarly, no statistically significant difference was found between the stress–strain relationships of exercised and control specimens. However, despite the lack of change in the stress–strain curve, a large increase in the ultimate load was found, while tensile failure at the tendon insertion to bone occurred. These data suggest that exercise has a positive effect on the strength of bony insertions.

The differences in the effects of exercise on the extensor compared to flexor tendons is likely due to their anatomical location and function. The flexor tendon has an inherent high strength and resiliency, and thus is unlikely to hypertrophy. Additionally, it is constrained by and must glide within a sheath, so there is little room for additional growth. In contrast, the extensor tendon does not experience spatial limitations and has a different biochemical composition that may be favorable for increased collagen production in response to stress [20].

Based on the results of studies of joint immobilization and exercise, a highly nonlinear curve describes the relationship between load and activity level and the biomechanical properties of ligaments and tendons (Fig. 4.8). The left region of the curve represents a rapid reduction in tissue properties and mass caused by immobilization; in contrast, the right region of the curve shows only a slight increase in mechanical properties following exercise. Thus, despite the striking penalty found by immobilization after injury, long-term exercise regimens seem to provide only moderate improvement in tendon properties [11]. Further, this concept has led to the approach of using controlled passive joint motion as a therapy for ligament injuries [21].

4.5 Nonuniform Biomechanical Properties Between Ligament/Tendon Substance and Its Enthesis

The complexity and geometric irregularity of insertion sites makes it very difficult to separate the biomechanical properties of the insertion sites and the ligament or tendon midsubstance. Nevertheless, efforts have been made in the development of testing devices and procedures such that a better understanding of the variation in these properties can be made and quantitative data can be obtained.

4.5.1 Cross-Sectional Area Measurement

Accurate measurements of the cross-sectional area of the ligament or tendon substance are necessary in the determination of stresses in these tissues during uniaxial tensile tests. In the early days, devices and techniques included dial calipers, constant pressure area micrometers, and thickness micrometers, but these devices all required physical contact with the specimen, causing deformation and thus affecting the cross-sectional area measurements. In our laboratory, we developed a laser micrometer to determine the cross-sectional shape and area of soft tissue without needing to make contact with the specimen [22, 23]. Recently, we have used a laser micrometer system with charge-coupled device (CCD) laser displacement sensors to rapidly measure the cross-sectional area of soft tissues, including those containing concavities [24]. This system has proven able to determine cross-sectional area of soft tissues in an accurate, repeatable, and rapid manner.

A schematic of the system and frame is shown in Fig. 4.9a. The device is composed of two main components: a CCD laser displacement sensor and a rotary

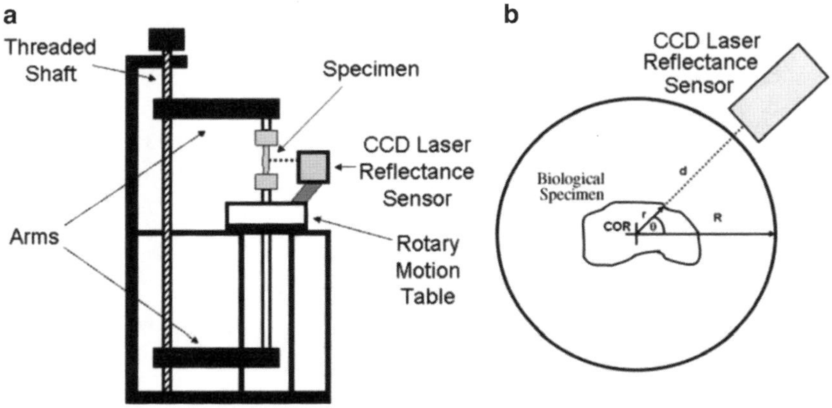

Fig. 4.9 (**a**) A simplified schematic of the charge-coupled device (CCD) laser reflectance system and frame. (**b**) A diagram depicting an overhead view of the CCD laser reflectance system with a biological specimen over the center of rotation (COR) of the system (reproduced, with permission, from [24])

motion table. The laser sensor is attached to the rotary motion table and moves in a circle as the table rotates around the stationary specimen, which is longitudinally mounted along the table's center of rotation. Figure 4.9b shows an overhead view of the path of the laser. As it moves, the sensor measures the distance to the specimen surface and calculates values of a radius, r, the difference between the total and measured radii of the system.

By plotting r along with the angular position of the laser system in polar coordinates, an algorithm using Simpson's rule can be used to calculate the cross-sectional area:

$$\text{Area} = \sum_{\phi=0.05}^{360} \frac{0.05\pi(r(\phi) + r(\phi + 0.05))^2}{1440}. \qquad (4.1)$$

4.5.2 Measurement of Mechanical Properties of Tissue

The early development of a VDA system to determine ligament strain of the rabbit FMTC during uniaxial tensile testing has yielded accurate, reproducible, and automatic measurements [8]. With proper measurement of the cross-sectional area of the ligament, the stress in the ligament could also be determined, and the stress–strain relationship would represent the mechanical properties of the ligament substance. A typical stress–strain curve is shown in Fig. 4.10, illustrating a characteristic shape and associated mechanical properties.

However, it should be noted that the tissue specimen must have uniform cross-sectional area, an appropriate aspect ratio, proper alignment, and uniform stress in order to obtain accurate stress–strain values. In the case of the MCL, obtaining a uniform stress distribution is rather straightforward, as it has a relatively uniform cross section. On the other hand, the complex anatomy of the ACL presents difficulties which make simultaneous loading of all the collagen fibers of the entire ligament nearly impossible [25]. Thus, for mechanical testing, it is usually separated into medial and lateral bundles, and one bundle is chosen to be transected and removed. The other bundle is then rotated for longitudinal alignment for tensile testing.

4.5.3 Tissue Strain vs. Percent Elongation

To describe the change in length of ligaments and tendons in response to tensile loading, both strain and percent elongation have been reported in the literature. The difference in these parameters is that strain refers to the tissue substance, while

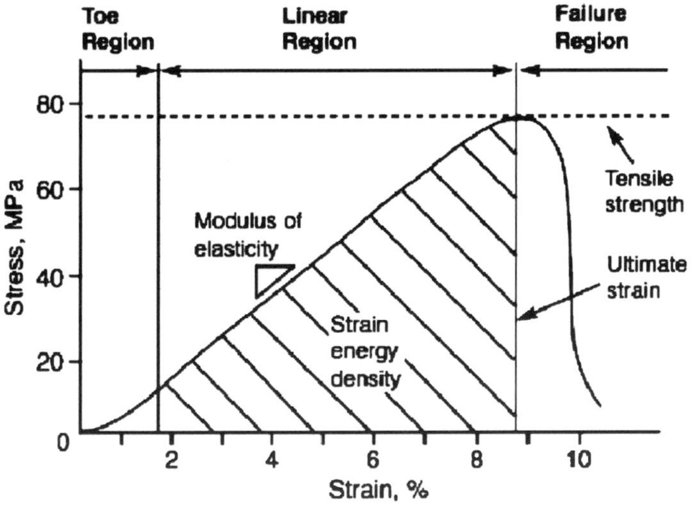

Fig. 4.10 Typical stress–strain curve showing the mechanical properties of the MCL

percent elongation describes the entire bone-ligament-bone complex. Strain is defined as:

$$\varepsilon = \frac{l - l_0}{l_0} \tag{4.2}$$

where l_o represents the initial distance between gauge markers on the tissue substance and l represents the final distance. In contrast, percent elongation is equal to the crosshead displacement of the material testing machine divided by the estimated original length of the tissue specimen [8]. Previously, researchers did not distinguish between these two values, often reporting percent elongation as strain with values well outside the true limits of ligaments and tendons. For example, Noyes and associates erroneously reported the average strains of the ACL at failure to be 50–60% [26, 27].

Using the previously described methods and technology for biomechanical testing, large percent elongation values based on clamp-to-clamp measurements of ligaments and tendons (on the order of 20–50% at failure) with much smaller strains (less than 20%) could be demonstrated. Noyes et al. [28] studied the strain distribution of human ACL subbundles using load-to-failure testing, finding the percent elongation to be 25–30%. However, in measuring local surface strain, they found a large spatial variation in strain, with the highest strain at the insertion sites and strain as low as 7% in the midsubstance tissue. Studies in our research center have produced analogous results, as the strains at failure for the MCL substance in dogs, swine, and rabbit were found to be 14, 12, and 7%, while percent elongation of the FMTC was 21, 30, and 16% [8]. Lam et al. [29] also achieved similar results in the rabbit MCL, finding the largest strain rates at the femoral insertion of the ligament and decreasing into the midsubstance tissue. In other words, the findings suggest that insertion sites can undergo greater elongation before failure.

The reason for differences in the elongation of the ligament substance and the ligament strain may be due to the changes in tissue composition that occur across the insertion. The tissue changes from the ligament or tendon substance (primarily collagen type I with some proteoglycans), to fibrocartilage (collagen types I, II, III, and aggregan), and finally to bone (collagen type I). Histologically, a change in cell shape and decrease in collagen orientation has been observed nearing the bony insertion [10]. Particularly in ligaments such as the ACL, the insertion site is often much wider than the midsubstance tissue [30], and thus collagen fibers are not able to fully align under tension and achieve the stiffness found in the ligament substance.

Recently, new techniques have been developed to better characterize the strain distributions across ligaments and tendons. Spalazzi et al. [31] used ultrasound elastography to examine the response of the ACL substance and insertion site under tension, finding only tensile strain in the ligament substance, but both tensile and compressive strain in the insertion. A nonuniform strain distribution was also observed from the tissue substance to the bone, and strain was found to be highest at the insertion site.

4.6 Repair of Ligament and Tendon Insertion Sites After Injury

Repair of the soft tissue-bone junction following avulsion injuries depends on the location and severity of the injury. Some investigators advocate nonsurgical therapy for nondisplaced or minimally displaced avulsion injuries [32–34]. Others prefer reattaching the soft tissue end (tendon, ligament, or joint capsule) to the denuded bone with transosseous nonabsorbable sutures, screws with toothed or spiked washers, and staples [35–37]. Results of these procedures can vary greatly and are dependent on the method used as well as the tissue type. For example, Robertson and associates [38] showed that screw fixation with a plastic spiked washer or soft tissue plate had initial loading capabilities superior to those with staple and suture fixation. In terms of the ultimate load at failure during tensile test, the screw with the spiked washer proved to be optimal for capsular tissue or thicker tendons, while the screw with the soft tissue plate was best for thinner tendinous tissue. In the past several years, improvement of the arthroscopic technique has led to the development of different types of suture anchors, which have become one of the most commonly used tools for arthroscopic repair of the rotator cuff and glenoid labrum in the shoulder [39, 40]. Suture anchors consist of metallic or bioabsorbable anchors that are inserted into bone with attached eyelets to pass sutures through. These devices provide firm fixation of soft tissue to bone, which is required for tendon-bone healing. Recently, suture anchors have also been used for hip arthroscopy, especially for tears of the acetabular labrum [41].

For some injuries, such as that of the ACL, the aforementioned treatment strategies have not worked well, and surgical reconstructive procedures using replacement grafts (tissue or synthetic materials) are performed to restore joint stability. In the case of tissue grafts, secure fixation to bone is needed to facilitate graft-bone healing [42–44]. Synthetic grafts made out of carbon and Dacron fibers have resulted in bony ingrowths to the most peripheral fibers of the grafts [45, 46]. Still others have used porous-coated plugs on the ends of the grafts to help bone fixation and have produced improved results [47].

Nevertheless, the re-establishment of the soft tissue insertion to bone remains to this day as one of the greatest challenges in orthopaedics [47]. In the case of ACL reconstruction, fixation of the graft to bone remains the weakest link, as more than half of failures occur there [48]. It is therefore clear that these surgical procedures have not been able to recreate the composition, geometry, and biomechanical properties to the level of complexity that exists within and between the insertion sites [10].

New strategies in functional tissue engineering that combine cells, growth factors, and/or bioscaffolds as implants that could mimic the natural enthesis are being explored [11, 49–53]. These implants can be designed for the body to promote the growth and differentiation of appropriate cell types, regulate matrix composition, and exhibit appropriate biomechanical properties of the interface; therefore, this is a huge step in the right direction. Lu and Jiang have designed biomimetric scaffolds for ligament and tendon attachments to bone that have the heterogenous composition and biomechanical properties found across an enthesis [54]. These authors have advocated the use of the triphasic scaffold by engineering three separate yet continuous regions [54–56]: Phase A, which corresponded to the ligament substance and contains PLGA (10:90) mesh and seeded fibroblasts to promote soft tissue growth; Phase B, which corresponds to the region of fibrocartilage; and Phase C, which contains seeded osteocytes, sintered PLGA (85:15), and 45S5 glass composite microspheres to promote the formation of bone in the bony region. At 2 months after implantation, developing tissue was found that contained the continuous gradient of tissue types, including both the ligament and bony regions as well as the intermediate region of fibrocartilage, which are similar to that of the neonatal ACL-bone junction. As all insertions to bone are multifaceted, with regions of ligament, non-mineralized, mineralized fibrocartilage, and bone, replicating the properties with a gradient of tissue types is the first step to produce a longer-lasting and successful biomimetric graft [57].

In spite of these encouraging early results, much work remains so that tissue growth and maturation occurs in each distinct region of the insertion site. The readers are encouraged to read the recent work of Helen H. Lu (Columbia University) and Stavros Thomopoulos (Washington University in St. Louis) and their coworkers to gain a better perspective on challenges and opportunities in this area of research. For appropriate technology to be applied in the laboratory and eventually to the clinical settings, one must continue to gain knowledge on the molecular, cellular, and tissue biology and biomechanics of each component of the insertion site. Furthermore, one will also need to develop other novel biomaterials such as nanofibers [55, 58], biodegradable and bioresorbable magnesium alloys [59, 60], and so on, to be used as scaffolds. With functional tissue engineering, we can be hopeful that multiphasic scaffolds with unique and desired characteristics can be made and implanted for rapid integration with native tissues to take place and eventually remodel into a native-like insertion site.

Acknowledgements This work was supported in part by the Commonwealth of Pennsylvania, McGowan Institute for Regenerative Medicine, NIH (MCL Grant 14918), and an NSF ERC Grant (#0812348).

References

1. Woo SLY, Gomez MA, Sites TJ, Newton PO, Orlando CA, Akeson WH (1987) The biomechanical and morphological-changes in the medial collateral ligament of the rabbit after immobilization and remobilization. J Bone Joint Surg Am 69A(8):1200–1211
2. Haus J, Halata Z (1990) Innervation of the anterior cruciate ligament. Int Orthop 14 (3):293–296
3. Aydog ST, Korkusuz P, Doral MN, Tetik O, Demirel HA (2006) Decrease in the numbers of mechanoreceptors in rabbit ACL: the effects of ageing. Knee Surg Sports Traumatol Arthrosc 14(4):325–329
4. Grigg P (1975) Mechanical factors influencing response of joint afferent neurons from cat knee. J Neurophysiol 38(6):1473–1484
5. Grigg P, Harrigan EP, Fogarty KE (1978) Segmental reflexes mediated by joint afferent neurons in cat knee. J Neurophysiol 41(1):9–14
6. Grigg P, Hoffman AH (1982) Properties of Ruffini afferents revealed by stress-analysis of isolated sections of cat knee capsule. J Neurophysiol 47(1):41–54
7. Buckwalter JA, Woo SL-Y (1996) Age-related changes in ligaments and joint capsules: implications for participation in sports. Sports Med Arthrosc 4:250–262
8. Woo SLY, Gomez MA, Seguchi Y, Endo CM, Akeson WH (1983) Measurement of mechanical properties of ligament substance from a bone ligament bone preparation. J Orthop Res 1(1):22–29
9. Woo SLY, Hollis JM, Adams DJ, Lyon RM, Takai S (1991) Tensile properties of the human femur-anterior cruciate ligament-tibia complex—the effects of specimen age and orientation. Am J Sports Med 19(3):217–225
10. Thomopoulos S, Williams GR, Gimbel JA, Favata M, Soslowsky LJ (2003) Variation of biomechanical, structural, and compositional properties along the tendon to bone insertion site. J Orthop Res 21(3):413–419
11. Woo SLY, Abramowitch SD, Kilger R, Liang R (2006) Biomechanics of knee ligaments: injury, healing, and repair. J Biomech 39(1):1–20
12. Woo SLY, Thomas M, Saw SSC (2004) Contribution of biomechanics, orthopaedics and rehabilitation: the past, present and future. Surgeon 2(3):125–136
13. Tipton CM, Matthes RD, Martin RK (1978) Influence of age and sex on strength of bone-ligament junctions in knee joints of rats. J Bone Joint Surg Am 60(2):230–234
14. Woo SLY, Peterson RH, Ohland KJ, Sites TJ, Danto MI (1990) The effects of strain rate on the properties of the medial collateral ligament in skeletally immature and mature rabbits—a biomechanical and histological study. J Orthop Res 8(5):712–721
15. Woo SLY, Orlando CA, Gomez MA, Frank CB, Akeson WH (1986) Tensile properties of the medial collateral ligament as a function of age. J Orthop Res 4(2):133–141

16. Woo SLY, Buckwalter JA (1988) Injury and repair of the musculoskeletal soft tissues. J Orthop Res 6(6):907–931
17. Newton PO, Woo SLY, Mackenna DA, Akeson WH (1995) Immobilization of the knee joint alters the mechanical and ultrastructural properties of the rabbit anterior cruciate ligament. J Orthop Res 13(2):191–200
18. Woo SLY, Ritter MA, Amiel D, Sanders TM, Gomez MA, Kuel SC, Garfin SR, Akeson WH (1980) The biomechanical and biochemical properties of swine tendons—long-term effects of exercise on the digital extensors. Connect Tissue Res 7(3):177–183
19. Woo SLY, Amiel D, Akeson WH, Kuei SC, Tipton CM (1979) Effect of long-term exercise on ligaments, tendons, and bones of swine. Med Sci Sports Exerc 11(1):105
20. Woo SLY, Gomez MA, Amiel D, Ritter MA, Gelberman RH, Akeson WH (1981) The effects of exercise on the biomechanical and biochemical properties of swine digital flexor tendons. J Biomech Eng-T ASME 103(1):51–56
21. Frank C, Akeson WH, Woo SLY, Amiel D, Coutts RD (1984) Physiology and therapeutic value of passive joint motion. Clin Orthop Relat Res 185:113–125
22. Lee TQ, Woo SLY (1988) A new method for determining cross-sectional shape and area of soft-tissues. J Biomech Eng-T ASME 110(2):110–114
23. Woo SLY, Danto MI, Ohland KJ, Lee TQ, Newton PO (1990) The use of a laser micrometer system to determine the cross-sectional shape and area of ligaments—a comparative-study with 2 existing methods. J Biomech Eng-T ASME 112(4):426–431
24. Moon DK, Abramowitch SD, Woo SLY (2006) The development and validation of a charge-coupled device laser reflectance system to measure the complex cross-sectional shape and area of soft tissues. J Biomech 39(16):3071–3075. doi:10.1016/j.jbiomech.2005.10.029
25. Danto MI, Woo SLY (1993) The mechanical-properties of skeletally mature rabbit anterior cruciate ligament and patellar tendon over a range of strain rates. J Orthop Res 11(1):58–67
26. Noyes FR, Delucas JL, Torvik PJ (1974) Biomechanics of anterior cruciate ligament failure—analysis of strain-rate sensitivity and mechanisms of failure in primates. J Bone Joint Surg Am 56(2):236–253
27. Noyes FR, Grood ES (1976) Strength of anterior cruciate ligament in humans and Rhesus-monkeys. J Bone Joint Surg Am 58(8):1074–1082
28. Noyes FR, Butler DL, Grood ES, Zernicke RF, Hefzy MS (1984) Biomechanical analysis of human ligament grafts used in knee-ligament repairs and reconstructions. J Bone Joint Surg Am 66A(3):344–352
29. Lam TC, Shrive NG, Frank CB (1995) Variations in rupture site and surface strains at failure in the maturing rabbit medial collateral ligament. J Biomech Eng-T ASME 117(4):455–461
30. Harner CD, Baek GH, Vogrin TM, Carlin GJ, Kashiwaguchi S, Woo SLY (1999) Quantitative analysis of human cruciate ligament insertions. Arthroscopy 15(7):741–749
31. Spalazzi JP, Gallina J, Fung-Kee-Fung SD, Konofagou EE, Lu HH (2006) Elastographic imaging of strain distribution in the anterior cruciate ligament and at the ligament-bone insertions. J Orthop Res 24(10):2001–2010. doi:10.1002/jor.20260
32. Hastings DE (1980) The non-operative management of collateral ligament injuries of the knee-joint. Clin Orthop Relat Res 147:22–28
33. Weiss JA, Woo SLY, Ohland KJ, Horibe S, Newton PO (1991) Evaluation of a new injury model to study medial collateral ligament healing—primary repair versus nonoperative treatment. J Orthop Res 9(4):516–528
34. Edson CJ (2006) Conservative and postoperative rehabilitation of isolated and combined injuries of the medial collateral ligament. Sports Med Arthrosc 14(2):105–110
35. Firoozbakhsh KK, DeCoster TA, Moneim MS, McGuire MS, Naraghi FF (1996) Staple leg profile influence on pullout strength—a biomechanical study. Clin Orthop Relat Res 331:300–307
36. Beynnon BD, Meriam CM, Ryder SH, Fleming BC, Johnson RJ (1998) The effect of screw insertion torque on tendons fixed with spiked washers. Am J Sports Med 26(4):536–539

37. Fealy S, Rodeo SA, MacGillivray JD, Nixon AJ, Adler RS, Warren RF (2006) Biomechanical evaluation of the relation between number of suture anchors and strength of the bone-tendon interface in a goat rotator cuff model. Arthroscopy 22(6):595–602
38. Robertson DB, Daniel DM, Biden E (1986) Soft-tissue fixation to bone. Am J Sports Med 14 (5):398–403
39. Koh KH, Kang KC, Lim TK, Shon MS, Yoo JC (2011) Prospective randomized clinical trial of single- versus double-row suture anchor repair in 2-to 4-cm rotator cuff tears: clinical and magnetic resonance imaging results. Arthroscopy 27(4):453–462
40. Philippon MJ, Souza BGSE, Briggs KK (2010) Labrum: resection, repair, and reconstruction. Sports Med Arthrosc 18(2):76–82
41. Ozbaydar M, Elhassan B, Warner JJP (2007) The use of anchors in shoulder surgery: a shift from metallic to bioabsorbable anchors. Arthroscopy 23(10):1124–1126
42. Drogset JO, Straume LG, Bjorkmo I, Myhr G (2011) A prospective randomized study of ACL-reconstructions using bone-patellar-tendon-bone grafts fixed with bioabsorbable or metal interference screws. Knee Surg Sports Traumatol Arthrosc 19(5):753–759
43. Cerulli G, Zamarra G, Vercillo F, Pelosi F (2011) ACL reconstruction with "the original all-inside technique". Knee Surg Sports Traumatol Arthrosc 19(5):829–831
44. Emond CE, Woelber EB, Kurd SK, Ciccotti MG, Cohen SB (2011) A comparison of the results of anterior cruciate ligament reconstruction using bioabsorbable versus metal interference screws a meta-analysis. J Bone Joint Surg Br 93A(6):572–580
45. Weiss AB, Blazina ME, Goldstein AR, Alexander H (1985) Ligament replacement with an absorbable copolymer carbon-fiber scaffold—early clinical-experience. Clin Orthop Relat Res 196:77–85
46. Richmond JC, Manseau CJ, Patz R, McConville O (1992) Anterior cruciate reconstruction using a Dacron ligament prosthesis—a long-term study. Am J Sports Med 20(1):24–28
47. Dunn MG, Tria AJ, Kato YP, Bechler JR, Ochner RS, Zawadsky JP, Silver FH (1992) Anterior cruciate ligament reconstruction using a composite collagenous prosthesis—a biomechanical and histologic-study in rabbits. Am J Sports Med 20(5):507–575
48. Paxton JZ, Donnelly K, Keatch RP, Baar K, Grover LM (2010) Factors affecting the longevity and strength in an *in vitro* model of the bone-ligament interface. Ann Biomed Eng 38 (6):2155–2166
49. Scherping SC Jr, Schmidt CC, Georgescu HI, Kwoh CK, Evans CH, Woo SL-Y (1997) Effect of growth factors on the proliferation of ligament fibroblasts from skeletally mature rabbits. Connect Tissue Res 36(1):1–8
50. Hildebrand KA, Woo SL-Y, Smith DW, Allen CR, Deie M, Taylor BJ, Schmidt CC (1998) The effects of platelet-derived growth factor-BB on healing of the rabbit medial collateral ligament: an *in vivo* study. Am. Orthopaedic Society for Sports Medicine 1997 O'Donoghue Sports Injury Research Award paper. Am J Sports Med 26(4):549–554
51. Martinek V, Latterman C, Usas A, Abramowitch S, Pelinkovic D, Seil R, Lee J, Robbins P, Woo SL-Y, Fu FH, Huard J (2002) Enhancement of the tendon-bone integration of ACL tendon grafts with BMP-2 gene transfer: a histological and biomechanical study. J Bone Joint Surgery 84A(7):1123–1131
52. Karaoglu S, Fisher M, Woo SL-Y, Fu Y-C, Liang R, Abramowitch SD (2008) Use of a bioscaffold to improve healing of a patellar tendon defect after graft harvest for ACL reconstruction: a study in rabbits. J Orthop Res 26(2):255–263
53. Liang R, Woo SL-Y, Nguyen TD, Liu P-C, Almarza A (2008) A bioscaffold to enhance collagen fibrillogenesis in healing medial collateral ligament in rabbits. J Orthopaedic Research 26(8):1098–1104
54. Lu HH, Jiang J (2006) Interface tissue engineering and the formulation of multiple-tissue systems. Adv Biochem Eng Biotechnol 102:91–111
55. Spalazzi JP, Dagher E, Doty SB, Guo XE, Rodeo SA, Lu HH (2008) *In vivo* evaluation of a multiphased scaffold designed for orthopaedic interface tissue engineering and soft tissue-to-bone integration. J Biomed Mater Res A 86A(1):1–12

56. Spalazzi JP, Doty SB, Moffat KL, Levine WN, Lu HH (2006) Development of controlled matrix heterogeneity on a triphasic scaffold for orthopedic interface tissue engineering. Tissue Eng 12(12):3497–3508
57. Lu HH, Subramony SD, Boushell MK, Zhang XZ (2010) Tissue engineering strategies for the regeneration of orthopedic interfaces. Ann Biomed Eng 38(6):2142–2154
58. Moffat KL, Kwei ASP, Spalazzi JP, Doty SB, Levine WN, Lu HH (2009) Novel nanofiber-based scaffold for rotator cuff repair and augmentation. Tissue Eng Part A 15(1):115–126
59. Staiger MP, Pietak AM, Huadmai J, Dias G (2006) Magnesium and its alloys as orthopedic biomaterials: a review. Biomaterials 27(9):1728–1734
60. Witte F, Feyerabend F, Maier P, Fischer J, Stormer M, Blawert C, Dietzel W, Hort N (2007) Biodegradable magnesium-hydroxyapatite metal matrix composites. Biomaterials 28 (13):2163–2174
61. Woo SLY, Hollis JM, Adams DJ, Lyon RM, Takai S (1987) Treatment of the medial collateral ligament injury, II: structure and function of canine knees in response to differing treatment regimes. Am J Sports Med 15(1):22–29
62. Dörlf J (1980) Migration of tendinous insertions. I. Cause and mechanism. J Anat 131 (Pt 1):179–95

Chapter 5
The Bone–Cartilage Interface

Virginia L. Ferguson and Rachel C. Paietta

5.1 Introduction

Bone–cartilage interfaces in the body anchor together stiff bone and compliant cartilage in a thin ($\leq$100's of microns) [1] region that progressively calcifies with aging. This bone–cartilage, or osteochondral, interface is of critical importance in articular joints and the spine due to the significant occurrence and health detriments of osteoarthritis and intervertebral disc (IVD) degeneration [2]. In 2008, 27 million individuals in the U.S. suffered from clinical osteoarthritis [3]. A separate analysis showed that as many as 40% of adults experience herniated discs in the lumbar spine which require surgical repairs [4]. One potential solution for repair of damaged cartilage or IVD is to replace the soft tissue with a synthetic replacement, yet engineered cartilage implants often fail due to a lack of mechanical anchoring [5]. Another solution, total joint replacement, is destructive to the surrounding tissue [6, 7], has a limited lifetime (~15 years for femoral head replacements), and is not a viable option for young patients needing successive replacements. Instead, recent efforts have focused on integrating engineered tissues and devices into the osteochondral interface or underlying bone [5, 8–14]. Synthetic grafts are improving in functionality for repair of joints and entheses (i.e., the bone–tendon attachment); however, such engineered solutions have yet to succeed, possibly because they lack equivalent material properties and functionality as compared to the native, healthy tissue.

One common approach to designing artificial osteochondral interfaces is to adhere or form a continuum between stiff, bone-like and soft, cartilage-like materials [5, 14, 15]; however, such solutions have not yet shown efficacy in the harsh loading environment of the osteochondral region [14]. The natural mechanisms for functional grading of hard–soft tissue interfaces are considered

V.L. Ferguson (✉) • R.C. Paietta
Department of Mechanical Engineering, University of Colorado, Boulder, CO, USA
e-mail: virginia.ferguson@colorado.edu; Rachel.Paietta@Colorado.edu

S. Thomopoulos et al. (eds.), *Structural Interfaces and Attachments in Biology*,
DOI 10.1007/978-1-4614-3317-0_5,

Table 5.1 Scales of hierarchical organization within bone and cartilage

	Unit (m)	Bone [36]	Cartilage [37]
Nano-scale	10^{-10}–10^{-9}	Ca^{2+},PO_4^{3-}, H_2O	Na+, Ca^2+, SO-, COO^-, H_2O
Ultra-scale	10^{-8}–0^{-6}	Collagen	Collagen
		Hydroxyapatite	Proteoglycans
Micro-scale	10^{-7}–10^{-4}	Lamella	Cells
		Cells	Collagen fibril organization
Tissue-scale	10^{-4}–10^{-2}	Osteons	Articular cartilage
		Trabeculae	Disc regions
Macro-scale	10^{-2}–1	Whole bones	Joints

by only a few researchers. Attempts to mimic functionality or specific features of the natural tissue in tissue engineered constructs have met with limited success [11, 16–19]. Perhaps the greatest shortcoming in our ability to design improved materials for osteochondral replacement lies in our current, narrow understanding of how the biologic osteochondral interface is engineered *in vivo* to facilitate stress transfer.

Structurally, the osteochondral interface possesses a hierarchical organization (Table 5.1) that is functionally graded, where collagen fibers extend from the deep zones of soft cartilage into a calcified region (termed "the zone of calcified cartilage," or ZCC) through a series of wavy tidemarks (Fig. 5.1). However, the mechanisms of efficient load transfer through this region are not well understood. Quantitative backscattered electron (qBSE) imaging of the human femoral head sometimes shows a stepwise decrease in mineral density from bone to soft, hyaline cartilage [20]. Yet qBSE and other techniques have also shown that many healthy osteochondral regions include a ZCC that increases in mineral density immediately adjacent to hyaline cartilage. A relatively sharp interface exists where the ZCC meets the hyaline cartilage (Fig. 5.2) [20–23]; however, such a sharp interface is counterintuitive. While abrupt junctions between materials create a high localization of stress and failure [24–27], the osteochondral region in healthy human tissues rarely fails. Functional grading in natural [28–31] and engineered materials [32–35] minimizes stresses at the interfaces of dissimilar materials, yet the mineral content in the osteochondral region is not uniformly graded. This chapter will review the biomechanical implications of the compositional and microstructural makeup of the native osteochondral tissues and how these tissues are structured to effectively transmit loads without failing.

Further, preparing undecalcified tissue sections across such a dissimilar bimaterial interface is difficult and limits the range of possible analyses. Many routine assays also require significant processing that alters tissue morphology or properties. As such, the *in vivo*, micro- to nano-meter length scale histology and mechanical properties that are relevant to the interface's function remain understudied. The tissue organization has been well characterized via decalcified tissue histology and other assays that require decalcification. However, removal of the mineral phase eliminates the ability to study the role of the highest modulus component. This chapter will describe existing knowledge gaps and explore what is

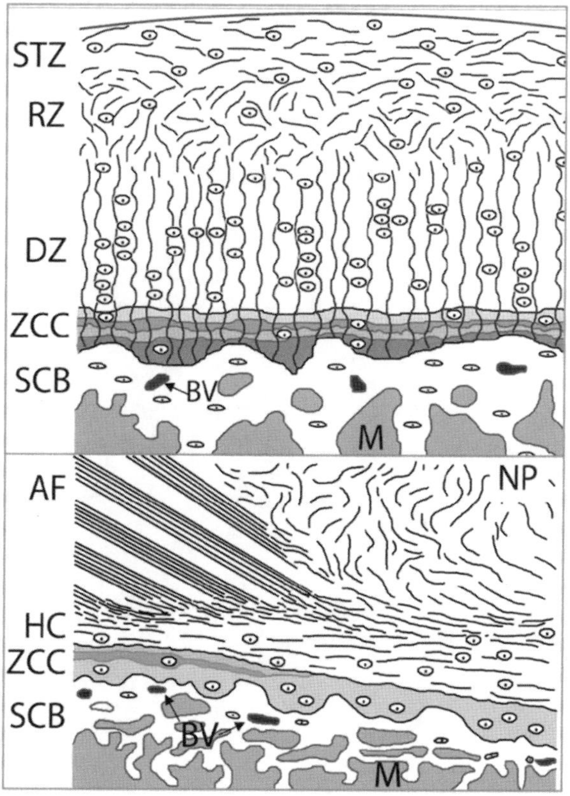

Fig. 5.1 Schematic representation of normal histology for the osteochondral interface region of synovial (*top panel*) and cartilaginous (*bottom panel*) joints (adapted, with permission, from [37] and [42], respectively). In both joint types, collagen fibrils in the hyaline cartilage (HC) become mineralized and anchor the soft tissue to the underlying bone. This ZCC (zone of calcified cartilage) is demarcated by wavy tidemarks and contains chondrocytes that may regulate mineralization. The ZCC is interlocked with the underlying SCB (subchondral bone) (*white*), where the border is marked by a tortuous cement line (*black*). *DZ* deep, *RZ* radial, and *STZ* superficial tangential zones of HC, *AF* annulus fibrosus, *NP* nucleus pulposis, *BV* blood vessel, and *M* marrow space

known regarding how bone and cartilage are integrated in order to facilitate the normal mechanical function of the ostechondral interface. This chapter also considers how functionality is disrupted with aging, altered mechanical loading, and disease. Improvements in our understanding, through a review of the existing literature and identification of lingering questions, will enable better design of tissue engineered osteochondral materials and improve our ability to robustly integrate hard and soft engineered materials.

5.2 Morphological Foundations of the Bone–Cartilage Interface

The osteochondral unit forms an interface between the highly dissimilar materials of soft, non-mineralized cartilage and the underlying stiff bone. This region forms a layered structure that includes three distinct entities (Fig. 5.1): subchondral bone (SCB), calcified cartilage, and soft hyaline cartilage. In the osteochondral interface within the spinal tissues, the hyaline cartilage further joins the underlying bone with an additional layer of fibrocartilage (i.e., the annulus fibrosus). The physical

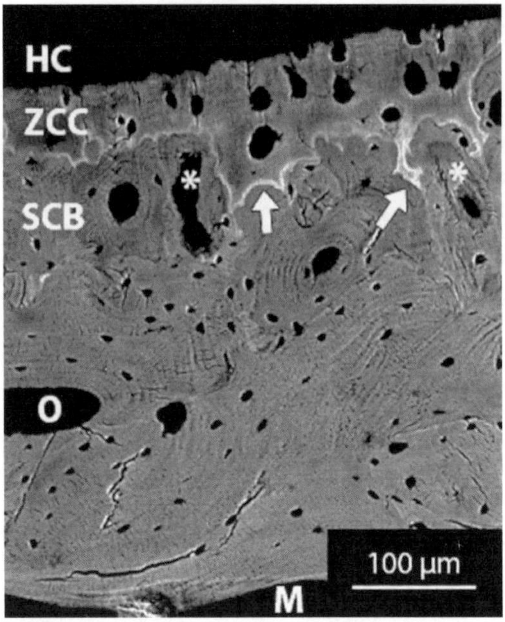

Fig. 5.2 Calibrated backscattered electron image of the osteochondral region in rabbit tissue showing the HC = hyaline articular cartilage, ZCC, and SCB, where the absence of mineral density in the HC is shown as *black* (*gray* level = 0) and mineralized regions in shades of *gray* to *white* (up to *gray* level = 255). *Wavy tidemarks* indicate regions of HC that are permeated with mineral; a white tortuous cement line (*arrows*) marks the boundary where the ZCC is anchored to the underlying SCB. *Asterisks* denote regions where ZCC and/or SCB has been removed by osteoclasts and infilled with newly formed bone by osteoblasts. O = example of an osteon that surround a central Haversian canal where blood vessels reside. M = marrow space within subchondral trabecular bone structure. The mineralized ZCC shows a smooth appearance as compared to the greater texture of mineral within the SCB

interaction between the osteochondral components creates a robust, continuous connection between materials possessing dissimilar properties. This section explores how this region both facilitates and presents challenges for the anchoring of cartilage to bone and synthesizing biomimetic biomaterial systems.

Like most biological tissues [36], the bone–cartilage interface possesses a hierarchy that spans multiple length scales. In humans, the joint as a whole is a macroscopic structure that may be up to centimeters thick where the cartilage anchors to the underlying SCB via the ZCC: an intermediate, thin layer of mineralized, or calcified, cartilage. The tissues that span this interfacial region are each formed from similar constituent phases, yet are differentially organized at the tissue-level, where the microstructural arrangement contributes to the unique function performed by each tissue. The cell populations in these tissues also vary and are differentially responsive to mechanical loads, disease, and therapeutics for treatment of bone or cartilage disorders.

5.2.1 Anatomy of the Bone–Cartilage Interface

The synovial joint is a well-studied region that contains bone and articular cartilage, has a consistent structure throughout most articular joints, and undergoes significant damage with aging and arthritis. Similarly, the cartilaginous joint brings together two adjacent bones via a continuum of fibrocartilage and hyaline cartilage and often degenerates with age. Despite the prevalent health detriments of disc degeneration, the microstructural and mechanical makeup of the cartilaginous joint's bone–cartilage interface is less well understood as compared to the interface region within the synovial joint.

5.2.1.1 The Synovial Joint

The synovial joint is diarthrotic, or freely moveable, and permits the relative motion via sliding of two adjacent bones that are typically covered with ~1–2 mm thick layer of smooth hyaline articular cartilage (Fig. 5.1). The avascular hyaline cartilage is comprised mainly of Type II collagen and hydrophilic charged proteoglycans that swell with water to provide cushioning. The cartilaginous structures form the primary load-bearing surface of the synovial joint, which varies in microstructure and composition throughout its depth. In superficial layers of cartilage, collagen fibrils are arranged parallel to the surface such that they distribute loads over a greater tissue volume and withstand primarily tensile and shear stresses [38]. As collagen fibrils progress into the deep radial zones of the cartilage, they bend to a direction that lies perpendicular to the calcified cartilage surface. The fibrils maintain this perpendicular orientation as they penetrate into and through the ZCC [39, 40]. Adjoined to the ZCC is a plate of SCB—a cortical-like region of SCB that lacks significant porosity yet is well vascularized. The SCB plate and the adjacent region of the ZCC may undergo remodeling, with ultimate replacement by bone or infilling of bone within the underlying trabecular compartments [41]. The organization of collagen fibrils in synovial joints creates a continuous structure that extends into the ZCC and serves to transmit primarily compressive and shear loads between cartilage, SCB, and the extended bony structure.

5.2.1.2 The Cartilaginous Joint

The cartilaginous joint forms a stabilizing and permanent cartilaginous union between two adjacent bones. These joint structures are slightly moveable, or amphiarthrotic, and occur at locations that include the pubic symphysis and the joints between adjacent vertebral segments. The cartilaginous region is formed by an avascular fibrocartilage disc that attaches to hyaline cartilage-covered bony ends. As an example, the IVD contains a central nucleus pulposus that is encircled by the annulus fibrosis and is sandwiched between two cartilaginous endplates

(Fig. 5.1). Within the IVD, the annulus fibrosis is composed of type I collagen that is organized into lamellae, or highly aligned collagen sheets, of alternating fibril directions in a manner that is similar to a rotating plywood structure [43]. The gelatinous nucleus pulposus consists largely of water and proteoglycans that exist within a network of collagen fibrils [44]. Cartilaginous endplates are formed of hyaline cartilage structures with fibrils that run parallel to the bony endplate, where a mineralized layer forms within the hyaline cartilage and adjacent to the vertebral bone. This layered structure enables a physical, mineralized connection between the bone and the soft tissues [42].

5.2.1.3 Fluids Within the Joint

A fibrous joint capsule, lined with fluid-producing cells within the synovial membrane, encapsulates the joint space between adjacent bones. Within the joint space, viscous fluid bathes the synovial joint's hyaline articular cartilage to lubricate gliding surfaces and deliver nutrients to the cartilaginous cells (i.e., chondrocytes). Loading and unloading of cartilage at low strain rates causes the synovial fluid to exude into the joint space, thus providing additional lubrication, and reabsorb into the cartilage upon unloading. When impacted at high strain rates, the "shock" is absorbed by frictional entrapment of synovial fluid within a charged collagen and proteoglycan matrix [45]; the resulting high apparent stiffness of the cartilage likely reduces the modulus mismatch and consequently facilitates transmission of forces between the bony and cartilaginous tissues.

Within cartilaginous joint tissues, such as within the annulus fibrosus and nucleus pulposis of the IVD, the water-based interstitial fluid contains little mineral content. This fluid facilitates removal of waste products and movement of essential nutrients including oxygen, glucose, and substrates for matrix production [44, 46]. Oxygen concentration and pH vary across the disc, with distance from the nearest blood supply (up to ~7–8 mm), where diffusion drives nutrient and gas exchange [46, 47].

5.2.2 Microscopic Structure of the Bone–Cartilage Interface

Initially, long bones and vertebral bodies lengthen and grow through a process known as endochondral ossification. In this process, the bone lengthens and the leading mineralization front progresses as cartilage at the growth plate becomes calcified to form a secondary center of ossification and the ZCC [48, 49]. Bone remodeling, removal of bone by osteoclasts and replacement with new bone by osteoblasts, occurs in the SCB plate and underlying subchondral trabecular bone (STB) to deposit bone during development and maintain the integrity of bone throughout maturity [41]. Remodeling cells also may invade the underside of the ZCC and create a highly interdigitated interface between the ZCC and SCB.

Thus, hyaline cartilage, calcified cartilage, and SCB form a morphologically continuous transition that is thought to play a major role in preventing large cartilage deformations and facilitating efficient load transfer [50].

5.2.2.1 Hyaline Cartilage

The composition and structure of the hyaline articular cartilage in the synovial joint changes with depth—from the articular surface to its interface with bone [49, 51–57]. Articular cartilage is classified into four zones: the superficial tangential zone (STZ), the middle or radial zone (RZ), the deep zone (DZ), and the ZCC (Fig. 5.1). The STZ, ~10% of the cartilage thickness, contains fine, densely packed and parallel-aligned collagen fibrils that bend to form the outermost articular gliding surface [54, 58, 59]. This zone contains little proteoglycan and may serve to resist shear forces via Type IX collagen bundles that sit perpendicular to and thus reinforce the collagen type II fibers. The middle RZ layer contains a greater proteoglycan component [38]. In this layer, randomly oriented fibers transition shearing forces at the surface into compressive forces within the DZ. In the DZ, proteoglycans are constrained to less than 20% of their free solution volume and trapped within a collagen fibril mesh. The resulting substantial osmotic pressure within the hydrated cartilage creates a high-energy state and loads collagen fibrils in tension [37, 60, 61]. These same DZ fibrils form bundles and assume an orientation that is perpendicular to the mineralized tissue layer as they penetrate the synovial joint's ZCC [62]. Cartilage's microstructural organization thus directs compressive and shear loads from the articulating surface into the ZCC and underlying SCB.

Similarly, collagen fibers within the cartilaginous IVD are primarily loaded in tension [42, 63]. The IVD's cartilaginous endplate forms a barrier between the disc and the subchondral plate and borders the cranial and caudal surfaces of each vertebral body. Unlike the normally penetrating fibrils in the synovial joint, the collagen fibrils in hyaline cartilage lie parallel to the mineralized tissue surface (Fig. 5.1). The orientation of these fibrils as they penetrate into the ZCC, and thus how the soft tissue within the IVD is anchored into the cartilaginous endplate, is not well described in the literature. Further, the cartilage endplate is known to increase in mineral density with aging and disc degeneration, thus exacerbating the property differences between the soft IVD and the mineralized endplate region. This mismatch, in combination with a possible lack of fibrillar anchors into the mineralized tissues, could explain the high failure rate observed at the IVD osteochondral interface.

5.2.2.2 The Zone of Calcified Cartilage

Stresses are thought to be dissipated through the hydrated proteoglycans and collagen fibrils that extend from the hyaline cartilage into the ZCC [64]. The ZCC is formed when mineral-containing fluid exudes from pore spaces in the bone.

In the synovial joint, mineral crystals within the ZCC largely align with the collagen fibrils. Similar structures observed in bone and dental enamel are highly anisotropic with the highest modulus in directions parallel to the long axes of mineral crystals [65, 66]. Unmineralized hyaline cartilage and the ZCC form a continuous, anisotropic, and multilayered structure (Figs. 5.1 and 5.2).

During postnatal development, the ZCC forms via calcification of hyaline cartilage and is a late event in the terminal differentiation of chondrocytes [67, 68]. Mineralization of the hyaline cartilage is initiated within territorial matrix near the cells and spreads throughout the broader extraterritorial matrix [69, 70]. Some chondrocytes survive within the ZCC [71–73]. These cells likely regulate mineralization of the surrounding tissue, as evidenced by highly mineralized regions surrounding necrotic chondrocytes in osteoarthritic human joints [20].

While blood vessels rarely penetrate the interface between ZCC and SCB, pores up to 200 μm in diameter enable some fluid movement across the osteochondral interface [98]. However, due to the poor permeability of the subchondral plate, the deep zones of hyaline cartilage are largely reliant on diffusion of nutrients and gases from the synovial fluid of the joint and interstitial fluid within the neighboring bone. Endplate mineralization increases, while nutrition delivery is diminished, with age in this region, which may contribute to degenerative joint changes in aging and osteoarthritis [49, 99, 100].

Interplay exists between the synovial fluid and the less viscous, mineral-containing interstitial fluid that is contained within the adjacent bones. At the mineralizing front of the ZCC, mechanical strains imparted upon the bony tissues may force mineral-containing, watery interstitial fluid into the adjacent unmineralized cartilage and extend the region occupied by the ZCC. Such mineral apposition into the hyaline cartilage is denoted by a tidemark.

Dense subchondral tissues, including the ZCC and a SCB plate, limit fluid movement between the bone and cartilage [70] (Table 5.2). The dense mineralized endplate structure restricts movement of the bony interstitial fluid—thus preventing mineral deposits within the bulk of healthy soft cartilage and the joint space. However, the ZCC and its tidemarks provide evidence of mineral-filled fluid intrusions into the soft cartilage, and nodules of mineral are commonly found to intrude within osteoarthritic hyaline cartilage and joint spaces [20].

The tidemark, as first described by Fawns and Landells in 1953 [101], forms an undulating surface and represents the most recently calcified border of the ZCC (Fig. 5.2). Tidemark advancement may occur with aging [41, 62, 102, 103], altered loading states [104, 105], and exercise [21, 106]. The waviness of the tidemark may represent differential growth rates of the mineralizing front [62] and reduce stress concentrations as unmineralized collagen fibrils penetrate the ZCC.

Reduplication of the tidemark represents advancement of the ZCC into and thinning of the overlying hyaline cartilage [107]. Multiple basophilic tidemarks are present in healthy tissues, yet excessive tidemark numbers may indicate joint degeneration or osteoarthritis [62]. Thus, the tidemark appears to indicate a mineralization pattern that "starts" and "stops" during normal activities [108] and may be linked with resorption activity within the underlying SCB [109].

Table 5.2 Elastic properties, permeability and porosity of joint tissues (adapted, with permission, from [74])

	Elastic modulus (MPa)	Poisson's ratio	Permeability (m^4/N·s)	Porosity (%)
Hyaline articular cartilage	0.07–1.23 [75] 0.994 ± 0.28 [76] 102 [77]	0.15–0.26 [78]	$2.7 \pm 0.64 \times 10^{-15}$ [79]	65–85% [157, 158]
Articular calcified cartilage	320 [64][a] ≈15,000–22,000 [20, 80, 81][b]			
Subchondral bone	1,150 [82][a] 1,147 [77] 820–1,370 [83] ≈18,000 [20][b]			50–90% [84] 78–92% [85]
Cancellous bone	4,590 [82] 19,800 [6]			4–12.8 [86] <5 [87]
Cortical bone	5,440 [82] 11,800 [88] ≈20,000 [89][b]	0.28 [90]	3.7×10^{-13} [91]	3.8 ± 3.1 (Proximal); 9.3 ± 5.7 (mid-diaphysis); 51.3 ± 7.7 (distal) [92]
Nucleus pulposis	Aggregate compressive: 0.3 [93] Tensile: 0.04 [94]	0.47 [94]	0.2×10^{-15} [93]	0.75 [95]
Annulus fibrosis	Aggregate compressive: 0.56 [93] Tensile: 20 [96]	1 [97]	0.2×10^{-15} [93]	0.70 [95]

[a]Data are collected from bulk beam bending experiments
[b]Data are collected from nanoindentation of plastic-embedded sections

Bone remodeling on the underside of the ZCC securely anchors the hyaline cartilage and ZCC to the underlying SCB via puzzle-like interlocks (Fig. 5.2; arrows) [20, 108]. Remodeling, or resorption of the underside of ZCC by osteoclasts and subsequent infilling of the newly vacant regions with bone by osteoblasts, creates a tortuous, interdigitated interface (Fig. 5.2). While this process may lead to thinning of the hyaline cartilage, healthy joint tissues are observed to maintain a consistent ZCC thickness [110]. This thickness is noted across species to occupy ~6–8% of the total cartilage height [104, 111, 112] and may diminish with aging and disease (e.g., osteoarthritis). However, evidence is lacking to demonstrate that the process of ZCC thinning is normal in healthy, mature cartilage.

5.2.2.3 Subchondral Bone

The layer of relatively uniform, dense SCB plays a critical role in redistributing the diverse stresses from the overlying soft cartilage or IVD and into the subchondral trabecular network [41]. Few, or no, collagen fibers continue across the interface from ZCC to SCB in either synovial or cartilaginous joints [42, 108]. However, the interdigitated interface between the ZCC and SCB serves to anchor the two tissues. A subchondral trabecular network buttresses and transfers loads from the SCB plate into the larger bone structure [41, 113]. The trabeculae in this region are anisotropic and adapt to directions bearing the greatest mechanical loads by remodeling and reorganizing over time. While these two tissues, the SCB plate and the underlying STB, are not well distinguished from each other in the literature, they possess different organization, mechanical properties, and adaptations to mechanical loads [20, 21, 64, 80, 82, 114].

The SCB plate and STB structure are highly sensitive to altered loading states. In exercise or with the disruption of loading patterns observed in osteoarthritis, the marrow spaces within the trabecular bone become infilled with a structurally weak, rapidly deposited woven bone material that possesses low mineral content [115]. Within the spine, regions of SCB that experience high tensile loading due to annular insertion are generally thicker and show more extensive cartilage calcification than other regions of the cartilaginous endplate [43]. The ZCC, SCB, and STB are dynamic structures that change with loading state via normal bone remodeling processes.

5.2.3 Conclusions

While the synovial and cartilaginous joints possess vastly different functions (articulating motion and stability, respectively), the tissues that make up these two joint types possess functional and morphological similarities. For example, the avascular cartilaginous joints that form the IVD between two adjacent spinal vertebral bodies include the cartilaginous endplate, the annulus fibrosis, and the nucleus pulposis. These three structures are generally analogous to the synovial joint's articular cartilage, joint capsule, and synovial fluid, respectively. It is not surprising, then, to find similarities in patterns of interface structure and aging or disease across these two joint types.

The common structural features that define material behavior at the microscopic scale within both hard and soft tissues include the organization, mineralization, and type of collagen fibrils present. The geometry of the calcification front and porosity of the underlying bone also contribute to the structural integrity of the osteochondral interface. The underlying structure and continuity are major factors in predicting and determining behavior of the interface and load transfer.

The response of bone to the stresses from the overlying hyaline cartilage in the synovial joint or in the IVD highlights the interplay between bone and cartilage and mechanisms that regulate remodeling. Further, each tissue within this interface possesses different microstructural and compositional organization and is differentially affected by loading conditions. A complete understanding of the structure, physiology, and function of the individual tissues that make up the osteochondral region can only be accomplished by understanding the differences and interactions between each of the component tissues that make up this complex interface region.

5.3 Materials Within the Bone–Cartilage Interface

The tissues that make up the osteochondral interface are comprised of collagen fibrils, proteoglycans, water, and cells. Additionally, bone and ZCC are dynamic biological composite materials that are strengthened and stiffened with increasing levels of mineralization. This section considers how the composition and microstructural organization within the osteochondral tissues influence the mechanics of the larger joint structure.

Cartilage and bone differ greatly in the organization of their collagenous matrix, type of collagen, and space that is available for infilling by mineral [20, 50]. However, the basic materials that make up these two tissues serve similar biomechanical roles. Tissue organization at the ultra- and micro-scales contributes to a smooth transition between cartilage and bone (Table 5.1). This includes collagen fibril orientation and organization and structural differences between mineralized tissues. It is also at these same length scales that load transfer is predominantly accomplished.

5.3.1 The Organic Phase

Soft tissues within human joints are usually in the form of hyaline cartilage (containing predominately collagen types II and V) or fibrocartilage (collagen types I and II). Both collagen types I and II are fiber forming and possess similar amino acid sequences, yet these proteins possess a different combination of the α-helix strands (type I contains 2 $\alpha1(\text{I})$ and 1 $\alpha2(\text{I})$, type II contains 3 $\alpha1(\text{II})$) [116]. In addition, cartilage tissues contain a high concentration of hydrophilic, charged proteoglycans that provide cushioning and resistance to compression. Other materials include water, inorganic salts, and small amounts of other matrix proteins, glycoproteins, and lipids [45]. The proteoglycans intermingle with collagen fibrils. Proteoglycans form a bottlebrush-like structure via a protein core to which glycosaminoglycans (GAGs) attach. Significant amounts of water inflate this hydrophilic matrix and interact with charged sites on the glycoproteins to contribute to cartilage's osmotic pressure and time-dependent behavior [45]. Cartilage is thus a biocomposite material where, rather than primarily contributing as a matrix component (as occurs in bone), collagen fibers and their cross-links provide fiber reinforcement to the proteoglycan network [37] and align in tension along primary loading directions.

From an engineering perspective, bone can be considered as a particle-reinforced composite composed of a type I collagen fiber matrix, ground substance (consisting mainly of proteoglycans, matrix proteins, and water), and carbonated hydroxyapatite mineral particles [36, 117]. The organic bone matrix imparts toughness (i.e., energy absorption), while the mineral particles provide stiffness and resistance to compressive loads. However, unlike the highly aligned parallel collagen fibrils found within cartilage, bone's organic matrix is less well organized. Material within the ZCC forms a similar biocomposite. In bone and calcified cartilage, anisotropy is typically observed by a preferential orientation of mineralized collagen fibrils and an increased modulus in the principal loading directions [66].

Cells within bone and cartilage both deposit and subsequently regulate the extracellular matrix. In bone, osteocytes trapped within the mineralized matrix regulate mineralization, while osteoblasts and osteoclasts form new bone and remove extant bone, respectively. Chondrocytes produce and maintain the cartilaginous matrix and align with the parallel-aligned collagen fibrils within hyaline articular cartilage [118].

5.3.2 The Mineral Phase

The volume fraction of mineral generally predicts the stiffness of the bone composite. Elastic properties follow particulate composite bounds at macroscopic and microscopic length scales [119, 120]. Other factors that contribute to the properties of bone are mineral platelet size [117, 121, 122], particle orientation with respect to collagen fibrils [50], and hydration of the tissue [123]. However, the mineral composition, organization, and ability to interact with the organic matrix also contribute to the resulting mechanical properties.

The mineral phase of bone consists primarily of an impure form of hydroxyapatite, $Ca_{10}(PO_4)_6(OH)_2$ [124, 125], with substantial substitutions by carbonate (CO_3^{2-}) into the OH^- or PO^{4+} regions of the apatite lattice [124]. Most bone mineral (~98%) exists as small plate-like crystals measuring ~1 × 10 × 15 nm [126–128] with some larger crystals measuring ~40 × 60 × 90 nm [127]. The size and shape of bone mineral may follow the initial crystal formation within the gaps between collagen fibrils in the hole region [129]. However, larger crystals have been observed, via atomic force microscopy (AFM) and transmission electron microscopy (TEM), to exist in the interfibrillar region [127, 130, 131]. The bone mineral surface has been shown, via nuclear magnetic resonance, to interact directly with the collagen fibrils and GAGs within bone's ground substance [121].

The mineral phase of articular calcified cartilage possesses a similar crystal structure to that of bone, with similar dimensional measurements [50]. However, the calcified cartilage can reach higher but more variable mineralization and calcium levels: 1–28 wt% in ZCC vs. 16–26 wt% in SCB [50, 80, 132]. The mineral in the ZCC forms plate-like structures [133] and aligns along the direction of the collagen fibrils [50].

The dimensions and degree of particle alignment in mineralized cartilage also attains values similar to those in SCB [50], yet the mineral volume fraction has been observed in multiple studies to exceed that of the underlying bone [20, 21, 41, 80, 134]. Duer et al. have shown that the connection between the mineral particles and collagen in calcified cartilage is less developed than that in bone, which may be a reflection of increased cartilage hydration and the inherent difference in matrix composition [121]. Unlike bone, a large amount of extrafibrillar space exists in cartilage that is occupied by water [135]. This availability of space, along with the ≈50% decrease in proteoglycan content of the cartilage with mineralization, allows for a high mineral content as compared to bone (~15% greater in ZCC) [136, 137].

The mineral volume fraction throughout the ZCC varies across the tidemarks. Interestingly, the mineral density within the ZCC is often observed to increase with proximity to each tidemark and also with proximity to the hyaline cartilage (Fig. 5.2). The notion that the mineral forms a functional gradient between mineralized and unmineralized tissues at this interface is refuted by such observations, where increased mineralization exacerbates the modulus mismatch between the ZCC and the overlying hyaline cartilage [20, 41, 80].

5.3.3 Conclusions

The analogous structural scales in both bone and cartilage provide a framework for examining the interface between these two tissues. Considering the continuum of material or structures at each hierarchical level demonstrates how the composition and organization at smaller length scales influence material behavior at the macroscopic level [36]. From this perspective, it becomes clear how the unique properties of individual materials form biocomposites, and that these composite materials then combine to form larger, macro-scale hierarchical-based structures that are ideally suited for load transfer across dissimilar material interfaces. Examining the composition of the osteochondral interface from a hierarchical approach that extends from the macro- to the nano-meter length scales provides insight into how these tissues function within the healthy joint. This foundation is critical for understanding how the osteochondral interface is altered by aging or disease and how to ultimately recapitulate key aspects of native tissues with the goal of engineering osteochondral tissues or novel engineered bimaterial systems.

5.4 The Mechanical Properties of Tissues in the Bone–Cartilage Interface

It is generally understood that the tidemark and the ZCC play critical roles in the biomechanical integrity of anchoring cartilage and bone. However, assessing the nature of this role in controlled experiments is complicated by the mismatched material interface. Standard sample processing methods that are typically employed for bone or cartilage samples often fail to address the needs of the entire osteochondral region. Processing methods also cause significant environmental alterations from *in vivo* conditions that introduce bias into native tissue property measurements [1, 20, 21, 62, 80, 138]. Despite these limitations, some work has provided insight into the properties and function of the osteochondral tissues through determination of material properties of the individual tissues and via functional assessment of mechanical interactions between these tissues.

While empirical and observational data on the osteochondral interface tissues reveal information about their collective function, an equal importance lies in quantifying the material properties (e.g., modulus), function, and mechanisms of failure for individual tissues and for the combined osteochondral unit. An accurate representation of material properties of the hyaline cartilage, ZCC, and SCB is needed in order to interpret experimental results from testing whole joint or osteochondral sections, to develop more accurate computational models, to interpret tissue changes that are involved in aging and disease, and to inform processes and strategies for tissue engineering osteochondral replacement materials. However, due to challenges associated with specimen preparation, the heterogeneity and intermingling of tissues, and the small length scales of interface components (e.g., the ZCC), little data exist that accurately characterize the material properties of the tissues in the osteochondral region. Further, the hierarchical construction of these tissues complicates interpretation of results, where data collected at the nano- or micro-scale may only represent the properties of the tissue and compare poorly to the macro-scale. This challenge is consistent with similar challenges in interpreting bone material properties, where properties vary across length scales [82, 139].

Of the osteochondral tissues, the hyaline articular cartilage and the SCB are the most thoroughly characterized. Hyaline cartilage properties vary throughout its depth, but are generally several orders of magnitude below that of the neighboring mineralized tissues (Table 5.2). Determination of SCB properties has been performed by machining and testing a shell, of controlled thickness, from weight-bearing regions of the femoral head [83], machining and testing SCB beams in bending [64, 82], and by performing nanoindentation or AFM on SCB in plastic-embedded sections [20–23, 80, 81]. Similarly, modulus of ZCC has been determined by machining beams of SCB and the ZCC, and then using an analytical approach to determine properties of bulk sections of the ZCC [64], or using nanoindentation and AFM to determine properties at nano- to micro-meter length scales [20, 21, 23, 80, 81].

Modulus values for the bulk SCB and ZCC specimens are lower than the values obtained from nanoindentation or AFM (Table 5.2). Two explanations may exist for this discrepancy. First, modulus values collected at nano- or micro-meter length scales enable high resolution mechanical imaging across very small tissue features due to the small size of most nanoindentation or AFM probes. Testing at such small scales measures the properties of small volumes of material (where regions containing defects are discarded) and may be more sensitive to the nano- or micro-scale construction of the tissue than at the macro-scale, where contributions to the modulus may result from different physical phenomena. Second, probing techniques produce a modulus that represents a multiaxial measurement, unlike what is observed in uniaxial or bending of the bulk specimens. Anisotropy can be observed using multiaxial tests, but its effect is muted and produces modulus values that represent all directions, but with a primary influence from the direction of loading.

Within the literature, most reports cite properties of the ZCC and SCB from a single investigation performed by Mente and Lewis in 1994 [64]. In this study, modulus values were collected from bending tests of beams machined from the ZCC and/or SCB. An analytical approach was then used to determine modulus values for the two individual tissues. This heavily cited study is often used to bolster the argument that the ZCC is less stiff than the SCB, and so must functionally grade properties between bone and cartilage. However, this analysis failed to explicitly consider the anisotropic nature of the material within the ZCC and that the ZCC varies greatly in mineral volume fraction. While directional properties of the ZCC have not been fully characterized, basic composites theory and existing knowledge of other mineralized tissues imply that the modulus would be the greatest in the direction perpendicular to the ZCC surface and the least in the transverse directions (i.e., radially around the joint surface). The modulus that is produced by bending beams machined from transverse sections of the ZCC thus represents the weakest direction of loading where failure would likely occur through detachment of neighboring mineralized collagen fibrils. From this perspective, the modulus that is commonly reported for transverse beams of ZCC does not represent the anisotropic nature of this material. Nor do the low values of modulus, as compared to the adjacent SCB, imply that the ZCC serves to functionally grade loads from the stiff bone to compliant cartilage.

Other studies reporting ZCC properties also fail to capture the anisotropic nature of this mineralized tissue. Nanoindentation measurements provide a glimpse into how the ZCC properties relate to those of the SCB; however, these results are relative and scale-dependent and lack a directional perspective. More advanced testing of the materials in this interface region needs to be performed, perhaps via testing of small, machined specimens to elucidate the material properties at relevant length scales. However, current data in the literature are valuable and provide a starting point to interpret tissue function and identify gaps that can be filled by future studies.

5.4.1 Function of Cartilaginous Tissues

In the deep zone of cartilage, collagen fibrils increase in packing density and perpendicular alignment as they penetrate through the depth of cartilage and into the ZCC [1]. Like fibers that combine to form a rope, the increased packing density

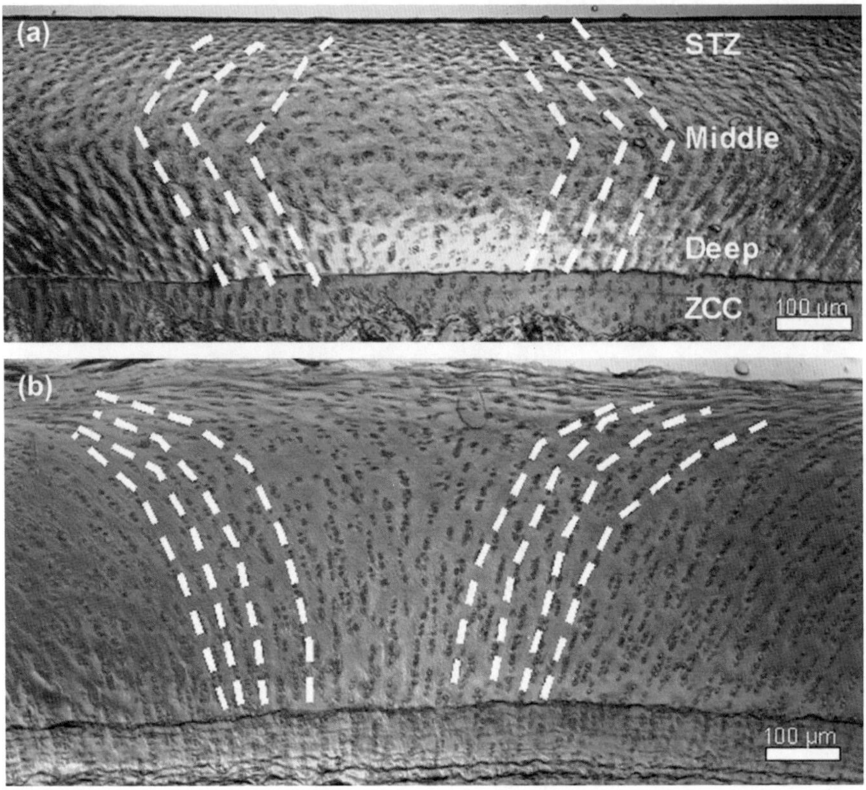

Fig. 5.3 Deformation under compressive loading showing deformation in (**a**) healthy and (**b**) degenerated cartilage. *White dotted lines* illustrate pattern of collagen fibril and chondrocyte deformation. Degenerated and fibrillated cartilage in (**b**) is mechanically weaker and retains less water (adapted, with permission, from [62])

of collagen fibrils forms a mutually supportive fibrous network that can bear more load than many can individually.

Compressive forces applied to the surface of the hyaline cartilage translate into deep shear forces through lateral movement of the radial zone's hyaline cartilage (Fig. 5.3). Under compression, the high osmotic pressure matrix surrounding the fibrils causes matrix stiffening and thus allows only small deformations of the collagen fibrils. The bundled fibrils that continue into the ZCC allow deep zone collagen to better resist lateral shear forces that result from compression of the superficial hyaline articular surface [1, 62, 118]. Large deformations are not observed when simulating physiological loading conditions; significant extension and movement of the collagen fibrils would lead to abrasion and fatigue of the collagen and surrounding matrix [1, 140]. Small deformations of collagen fiber bundles that penetrate into the ZCC likely transmit direct and repeated compressive and shear loads without loss of structural integrity to tissues contained within the interface region [1].

Water is displaced as the matrix consolidates [141]. Fluid that is forced out of the region underneath an applied compressive load first flows in the lateral direction, where the rate of fluid flow depends on the magnitude of the applied stress and the compressive resistance of the cartilage. The intrinsic compressive stiffness of the hyaline cartilage results from the physiochemical linkages between the collagen fibrils and the proteoglycans, which create a matrix that is highly resistant to fluid flow. Water thus serves as an incompressible continuum that communicates compressive strain of the matrix into volumetric dilatation and subsequent poroviscoelastic fluid flow [62]. Excised sections that contain full thickness cartilage and SCB enable visualization of deformation patterns within the collagen matrix with compressive loading of the articular surface [62]. Collagen fibrils are generally aligned with the long axes of chondrocytes, so the cells are used to delineate fibril orientation [142]. Compression of healthy joint tissues shows deformation patterns indicating that strains within the matrix are limited by the radially oriented collagen fibrils in the STZ and the mineralized anchor that is formed by the ZCC. These strain-limiting regions thus control the laterally directed volumetric dilatation within the central regions of the cartilage and resist tissue damage in healthy cartilage. Under compressive loads, collagen fibril orientation at the interface with the ZCC is perpendicular directly under the applied load. In lateral regions, however the collagen fibrils bend to resist shear and maintain the robust anchoring of the hyaline cartilage matrix with the ZCC (Fig. 5.3).

5.4.2 Function of Mineralized Tissues

A notion persists that the ZCC serves to functionally grade properties from the underlying bone to the overlying hyaline cartilage (Table 5.2) [20, 80, 140]; however, the literature lacks substantial evidence to support this claim. As previously mentioned, Mente and Lewis demonstrated that the modulus of calcified cartilage is an order of magnitude less than that of the underlying SCB [64]. Nanoindentation studies of the material property transition in regions spanning bone and calcified cartilage have shown mixed results. Ferguson et al. and Gupta et al. have shown the moduli of calcified cartilage to be lower than adjacent bone in normal and pathologic tissues (i.e., osteoarthritic human or exercised horse tissues) [20, 21, 80]. However, the calcified cartilage modulus is greater than that of bone in other samples in these same studies. The limited number of samples examined in these studies prevents one from making broad statements about the functional role of the ZCC.

The property gradient across the osteochondral interface may depend on many factors, including loading conditions, age of the tissue, activity or exercise level, and disease presence. Indeed, some dispute the role of the ZCC in transitioning, or functionally grading, properties between bone and cartilage [1]. Several functional studies of the osteochondral region, performed by a single research group, show that collagen fiber deformations are constrained by the rigid, high-energy state in the

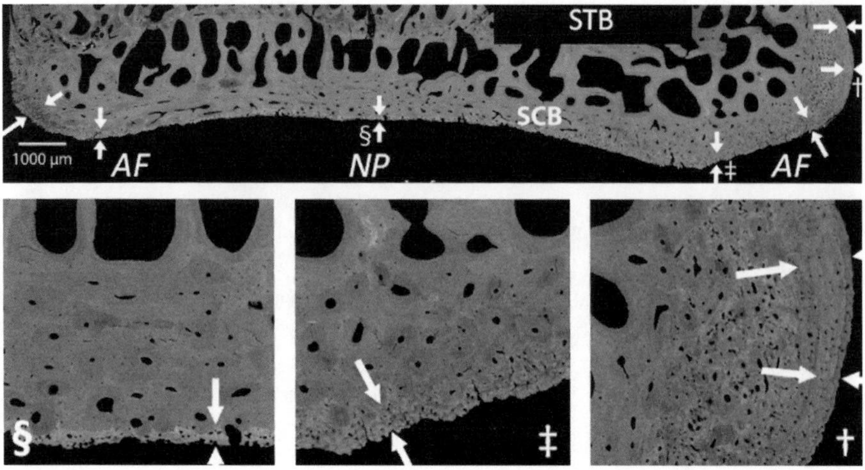

Fig. 5.4 Quantitative backscattered electron (qBSE) image of sagittal hemisection of an ovine lumbar vertebral endplate showing the ZCC (marked with *arrows*) that connects the SCB to the annulus fibrosis and nucleus pulposus tissues (approximate locations shown in *top panel* as "AF" and "NP," respectively). The ZCC is thinnest in the regions that are primarily compressively loaded *in vivo* in regions overlying the NP (§) and the inner AF (‡); also described in [42]. The ZCC is thickest in the outer AF region where joint-stabilizing fibrils insert into the outer AF (†) and apply significant tensile and shear loads; multiple tidemarks exist in this region and indicate that the vertebral ZCC may be dynamic in its response to loading in a manner that is similar to that in articular joints. The thick SCB may transition loads into the underlying struts within the subchondral trabecular bone (STB). Marrow space is shown as *black* (*gray* level = 0) and increasing mineral content shows as shades of *gray* (up to 255)

deepest zone of unmineralized hyaline cartilage [1, 62, 118]. These same studies note that deformations of ZCC were not observed during compressive or shear loading of excised osteochondral sections. The role of the ZCC in transitioning loads from bone to cartilage remains understudied, yet this tissue is undoubtedly critical in the mechanics and mechanobiology of this interfacial region.

The leading tidemark, through which the continuum of collagen fibrils penetrates, forms an abrupt edge between the mineralized material and the adjacent deep zone of the unmineralized hyaline cartilage. BSE and contact resonance-force microscopy images show the interface width, or the distance between high modulus material, ~20 GPa, within the ZCC and the comparably low modulus values, ~10 GPa, in the (PMMA-embedded) hyaline cartilage, is only on the order of 5–10 µm (Figs. 5.2 and 5.4) [22, 23]. The tidemark has sometimes been observed to be of a higher calcium concentration [143] and mineral volume fraction than deeper regions of the ZCC [20, 21, 80]. This abrupt interface and pattern of mineralization can also be visualized at sub-micron resolution in backscattered electron images that are calibrated to exact mineral volume fraction (Figs. 5.2 and 5.4). Such mineralization patterns may exacerbate the modulus mismatch and the abrupt edge at the tissue interface.

Finite element analysis of juxtarticular stresses showed that increased stiffness of the SCB plate (that presumably included the SCB and ZCC) correlated with elevated shear stresses at the bone–cartilage interface [144]. However, similar analyses demonstrated that subchondral stiffening leads only to modest increases in stress within the overlying hyaline cartilage [145, 146]. These results, in combination with the elevated incidence of radial fractures in aged subjects with presumably higher ZCC mineralization, indicates that damage at the osteochondral interface may precede, and ultimately cause, hyaline articular degradation and damage.

How the mineralized cartilage participates in functional grading within the osteochondral region requires further study. An improved understanding of the function of the ZCC and SCB will help to elucidate how alterations in mineralization, porosity, and remodeling of the ZCC and SCB contribute to degeneration with aging and disease in both synovial and cartilaginous joints.

5.4.3 Failure of the Bone–Cartilage Interface

Because the soft, hyaline cartilage forms an abrupt boundary with the underlying ZCC, failure in this region tends to parallel, rather than to penetrate, the interface in synovial joints [147]. However, twisting or dislocation can expose convex joint surfaces to lateral forces and shear-induced lesions or failure within the osteochondral region [148–150]. Osteochondral failure depends mainly on the load intensity and the integrity of the cartilage material—a factor that varies substantially with aging and disease.

Polar forces between water and the negatively charged proteoglycans within the matrix create a significant Donnan pressure effect and thus resist flow—especially at high strain rates such as those most commonly experienced *in vivo* [37, 45]. The total swelling pressure contributes to the high-energy state of the hyaline cartilage and results from a physiochemically derived osmotic pressure and the repulsive charges between closely spaced proteoglycan molecules [37]. Articular cartilage is constrained in its superficial zone by radially oriented (i.e., parallel to the articular surface) collagen fibrils and by the underlying mineral, as evidenced by its immediate expansion upon being cut away from the ZCC and SCB [1, 151, 159].

This complex high-energy state, and the water stored within the cartilage, conveys rigidity and toughness [1]. Yet failure of the tissue enables release of stored potential energy to cause significant tissue damage. For example, adolescent individuals, who lack a substantially calcified cartilage layer, can experience traumatic fractures that transmit deep into the osteochondral junction and penetrate the SCB [152, 153]. In elderly adults, where the ZCC possesses a significant mineral volume fraction, regions of tissue failure tend to locate along, but do not penetrate through, the leading tidemark [154]. In excised human tissues, microcracks often occur in the ZCC from 58- to 75-year-old subjects [155, 156]. Separately, a controlled, *ex vivo* study of shear impact loading of articular cartilage demonstrated age-dependent patterns of osteochondral failure [148]. In immature tissue sections, shear stresses reaching a critical value caused initiation of a large, fast-moving crack of combined modes (mixed-mode I, due to out-of-plane forces and mode II due to in-plane forces) that propagated in the osteochondral region until it arrested. This mixed-mode crack also formed fractures vertically through the articular cartilage. In contrast, mature tissues exhibited smaller cracks that propagated primarily within the tidemark region without vertically oriented damage. The mechanism of failure within the osteochondral region thus changes with development and the consequent increasing mineralization of the developing ZCC.

Less is known about failure in or near the osteochondral interface within the spine. In contrast to the synovial joint, the hyaline cartilage of the cartilaginous endplate consists of collagen fibers that are oriented parallel to the mineralized tissue surface (Fig. 5.1). Anecdotally, orthopaedic surgeons often note that the mature endplate is easy to separate from the underlying bone during surgery. A gap exists in understanding the transfer of mechanical loads and contribution of tissue microstructure to the function of this complex region. Specifically, it is unclear how the parallel orientation of the collagen fibrils sustains function of this interface in the spinal tissues and if this specific construction may be one factor that leads to disc damage and degeneration. Also, how the integration of mineral within this collagen framework causes dissipation of compressive and shear forces within the spinal tissue environment is unknown.

5.5 Concluding Remarks

This chapter both summarizes current knowledge and also highlights gaps in our current understanding of the bone–cartilage interface. Overall, the osteochondral interface forms a complex region that is constructed of multiple tissues and cell types that each respond differently, but not separately, to intrinsic factors including mechanical loading and to extrinsic factors such as drug therapies. In combination with microstructural and compositional differences across the tissues, these factors lead to different mechanical and material properties, mechanosensory responses, and underlying physiology [41]. This complex environment therefore necessitates an improved understanding of the interaction between cell populations, the manner in which mechanical loads are transferred, and how damage and/or altered loading in one tissue may affect the overall unit.

In order to elucidate how alterations in factors such as mineralization, porosity, and remodeling of the ZCC and SCB contribute to degeneration with aging and disease in both synovial and cartilaginous joints, further study on the interface is necessary. Further, an accurate representation of tissue-scale through nano-scale material properties of the hyaline cartilage, ZCC, and SCB is needed in the contexts of hierarchical organization and anisotropy. An improved understanding of this complex, layered, dynamic region will enable interpretation of experimental results from testing whole joint or osteochondral sections, development of more accurate computational models, and understanding of how tissue changes are involved in aging and disease. Further, this knowledge will inform strategies for tissue engineering osteochondral replacement materials and engineering of advanced biomimetic materials that join highly dissimilar materials.

Acknowledgments Support for this work was funded by the National Science Foundation CAREER Award (NSF#1055989), the University of Colorado Innovative Grant Program, and a National Science Foundation graduate fellowship to RCP. Thank you also to Sara E. Campbell at the National Institute of Standards and Technology, Boulder CO USA, for imaging support.

References

1. Broom ND, Poole CA (1982) A functional-morphological study of the tidemark region of articular cartilage maintained in a non-viable physiological condition. J Anat 135(pt 1):65–82
2. Symmons D, Turner G, Webb R, Asten P, Barrett E, Lunt M, Scott D, Silman A (2002) The prevalence of rheumatoid arthritis in the United Kingdom: new estimates for a new century. Rheumatology 41(7):793–800
3. Lawrence RC, Felson DT, Helmick CG, Arnold LM, Choi H, Deyo RA, Gabriel S, Hirsch R, Hochberg MC, Hunder GG, Jordan JM, Katz JN, Kremers HM, Wolfe F (2008) Estimates of the prevalence of arthritis and other rheumatic conditions in the United States. Part II. Arthritis Rheum 58(1):26–35
4. Dang L, Liu Z (2010) A review of current treatment for lumbar disc herniation in children and adolescents. Eur Spine J 19(2):205–214
5. Yang PJ, Temenoff JS (2009) Engineering orthopedic tissue interfaces. Tissue Eng Part B Rev 15(2):127–141
6. Park P, Garton HJ, Gala VC, Hoff JT, McGillicuddy JE (2004) Adjacent segment disease after lumbar or lumbosacral fusion: review of the literature. Spine 29(17):1938–1944
7. Malchau H, Herberts P, Ahnfelt L (1993) Prognosis of total hip replacement in Sweden. Follow-up of 92,675 operations performed 1978–1990. Acta Orthop Scand 64(5):497–506
8. Grayson WL, Chao PH, Marolt D, Kaplan DL, Vunjak-Novakovic G (2008) Engineering custom-designed osteochondral tissue grafts. Trends Biotechnol 26(4):181–189
9. Hung CT, Lima EG, Mauck RL, Takai E, LeRoux MA, Lu HH, Stark RG, Guo XE, Ateshian GA (2003) Anatomically shaped osteochondral constructs for articular cartilage repair. J Biomech 36(12):1853–1864
10. Jiang J, Nicoll SB, Lu HH (2005) Co-culture of osteoblasts and chondrocytes modulates cellular differentiation *in vitro*. Biochem Biophys Res Commun 338(2):762–770
11. Jiang J, Tang A, Ateshian GA, Guo XE, Hung CT, Lu HH (2010) Bioactive stratified polymer ceramic-hydrogel scaffold for integrative osteochondral repair. Ann Biomed Eng 38 (6):2183–2196
12. Murray RC, Blunden TS, Branch MV, Tranquille CA, Dyson SJ, Parkin TD, Goodship AE (2009) Evaluation of age-related changes in the structure of the equine tarsometatarsal osteochondral unit. Am J Vet Res 70(1):30–36
13. Schaefer D, Martin I, Jundt G, Seidel J, Heberer M, Grodzinsky A, Bergin I, Vunjak-Novakovic G, Freed LE (2002) Tissue-engineered composites for the repair of large osteochondral defects. Arthritis Rheum 46(9):2524–2534
14. Shao XX, Hutmacher DW, Ho ST, Goh JC, Lee EH (2006) Evaluation of a hybrid scaffold/cell construct in repair of high-load-bearing osteochondral defects in rabbits. Biomaterials 27(7):1071–1080

15. Kreklau B, Sittinger M, Mensing MB, Voigt C, Berger G, Burmester GR, Rahmanzadeh R, Gross U (1999) Tissue engineering of biphasic joint cartilage transplants. Biomaterials 20 (18):1743–1749
16. Moffat KL, Wang IN, Rodeo SA, Lu HH (2009) Orthopedic interface tissue engineering for the biological fixation of soft tissue grafts. Clin Sports Med 28(1):157–176
17. Spalazzi JP, Dagher E, Doty SB, Guo XE, Rodeo SA, Lu HH (2006) *In vivo* evaluation of a tri-phasic composite scaffold for anterior cruciate ligament-to-bone integration. Conf Proc IEEE Eng Med Biol Soc 1:525–528
18. Harley BA, Lynn AK, Wissner-Gross Z, Bonfield W, Yannas IV, Gibson LJ (2010) Design of a multiphase osteochondral scaffold III: fabrication of layered scaffolds with continuous interfaces. J Biomed Mater Res A 92(3):1078–1093
19. Li X, Xie J, Lipner J, Yuan X, Thomopoulos S, Xia Y (2009) Nanofiber scaffolds with gradations in mineral content for mimicking the tendon-to-bone insertion site. Nano Lett 9(7):2763–2768
20. Ferguson VL, Bushby AJ, Boyde A (2003) Nanomechanical properties and mineral concentration in articular calcified cartilage and subchondral bone. J Anat 203(2):191–202
21. Ferguson VL, Bushby AJ, Firth EC, Howell PG, Boyde A (2008) Exercise does not affect stiffness and mineralisation of third metacarpal condylar subarticular calcified tissues in 2 year old thoroughbred racehorses. Eur Cell Mater 16:40–46; discussion 46
22. Campbell SE, Ferguson VL, Hurley DC (2011) Linking nano- and micromechanical measurements of the bone-cartilage interface. In: Materials Research Society Fall Meeting, Boston, MA, Nov 2011
23. Pak R, Campbell SE, Paietta RC, Ferguson VL (2011) Distribution of nanomechanical properties and mineralization of the osteochondral interface in the femoral head. In: American Society of Mechanical Engineering Summer Bioengineering Conference, Farmington, PA, June 2011
24. Wu ZG, Liu YH (2010) Singular stress field near interface edge in orthotropic/isotropic bi-materials. Int J Solids Struct 47(17):2328–2335
25. Goglio L, Rossetto M (2010) Stress intensity factor in bonded joints: influence of the geometry. Int J Adhes Adhes 30(5):313–321
26. Williams ML (1952) Stress singularities resulting from various boundary conditions in angular corners of plates in extension. J Appl Mech-T Asme 19(4):526–528
27. Shin KC, Kim WS, Lee JJ (2007) Application of stress intensity to design of anisotropic/isotropic bi-materials with a wedge. Int J Solids Struct 44(24):7748–7766
28. Moffat KL, Sun WH, Chahine NO, Pena PE, Doty SB, Hung CT, Ateshian GA, Lu HH (2006) Characterization of the mechanical properties and mineral distribution of the anterior cruciate ligament-to-bone insertion site. Conf Proc IEEE Eng Med Biol Soc 1:2366–2369
29. Thomopoulos S, Marquez JP, Weinberger B, Birman V, Genin GM (2006) Collagen fiber orientation at the tendon to bone insertion and its influence on stress concentrations. J Biomech 39(10):1842–1851
30. Thomopoulos S, Williams GR, Gimbel JA, Favata M, Soslowsky LJ (2003) Variation of biomechanical, structural, and compositional properties along the tendon to bone insertion site. J Orthop Res 21(3):413–419
31. Yao HM, Dao M, Imholt T, Huang JM, Wheeler K, Bonilla A, Suresh S, Ortiz C (2010) Protection mechanisms of the iron-plated armor of a deep-sea hydrothermal vent gastropod. Proc Natl Acad Sci U S A 107(3):987–992
32. Jitcharoen J, Padture NP, Giannakopoulos AE, Suresh S (1998) Hertzian-crack suppression in ceramics with elastic-modulus-graded surfaces. J Am Ceram Soc 81(9):2301–2308
33. Suresh S (2001) Graded materials for resistance to contact deformation and damage. Science 292(5526):2447–2451
34. Chudoba T, Schwarzer N, Linss V, Richter F (2004) Determination of mechanical properties of graded coatings using nanoindentation. Thin Solid Films 469–70:239–247

35. Choi IS, Detor AJ, Schwaiger R, Dao M, Schuh CA, Suresh S (2008) Mechanics of indentation of plastically graded materials—II: experiments on nanocrystalline alloys with grain size gradients. J Mech Phys Solids 56(1):172–183
36. Lakes R (1993) Materials with structural hierarchy. Nature 361(6412):511–515
37. Mow VC, Ratcliffe A, Poole AR (1992) Cartilage and diarthrodial joints as paradigms for hierarchial materials and structures. Biomaterials 13(2):67–97
38. O'Connor P, Orford CR, Gardner DL (1988) Differential response to compressive loads of zones of canine hyaline articular cartilage: micromechanical, light and electron microscopic studies. Ann Rheum Dis 47(5):414–420
39. Weiss C, Rosenberg L, Helfet AJ (1968) An ultrastructural study of normal young adult human articular cartilage. J Bone Joint Surg Am 50(4):663–674
40. Buckwalter JA, Mankin HJ (1998) Articular cartilage: tissue design and chondrocyte-matrix interactions. Instr Course Lect 47:477–486
41. Burr DB (2004) Anatomy and physiology of the mineralized tissues: role in the pathogenesis of osteoarthrosis. Osteoarthr Cartil 12(suppl A):S20–S30
42. Roberts S, Menage J, Urban JPG (1989) Biochemical and structural properties of the cartilage endplate and its relation to the intervertebral disc. Spine 14(2):166–174
43. Roberts S, Evans H, Trivedi J, Menage J (2006) Histology and pathology of the human intervertebral disc. J Bone Joint Surg Am 88A:10–14
44. Eyre DR, Caterson B, Benya P (1991) The intervertebral disc. In: Gordon S, Frymoyer J (eds) New perspectives on low back pain. American Institute of Orthopaedic Surgeons, Philadelphia, PA, pp 147–209
45. Mow VC, Ratcliffe A (1997) Structure and function of articular cartilage and meniscus. In: Mow VC, Hayes WC (eds) Basic orthopaedics biomechanics, 2nd edn. Lippincott-Raven Publishers, Philadelphia, PA, pp 113–177
46. Holm S, Maroudas A, Urban JP, Selstam G, Nachemson A (1981) Nutrition of the intervertebral disc: solute transport and metabolism. Connect Tissue Res 8(2):101–119
47. Urban JP, Holm S, Maroudas A, Nachemson A (1982) Nutrition of the intervertebral disc: effect of fluid flow on solute transport. Clin Orthop Relat Res 170:296–302
48. Glimcher MJ (2006) Bone: nature of the calcium phosphate crystals and cellular, structural, and physical chemical mechanisms in their formation. Med Mineral Geochem 64:223–282
49. Oegema TR, Thompson RC (eds) (1992) The zone of calcified cartilage and its role in osteoarthritis. Articular cartilage and osteoarthritis. Raven, New York
50. Zizak I, Roschger P, Paris O, Misof BM, Berzlanovich A, Bernstorff S, Amenitsch H, Klaushofer K, Fratzl P (2003) Characteristics of mineral particles in the human bone/cartilage interface. J Struct Biol 141(3):208–217
51. Dmitrovsky E, Lane LB, Bullough PG (1978) Characterization of the tidemark in human articular cartilage. Metab Bone Dis Relat Res 1(2):115–118
52. Buckwalter JA, Ehrlich MG, Armstrong AL, Mankin HJ (1987) Electron microscopic analysis of articular cartilage proteoglycan degradation by growth plate enzymes. J Orthop Res 5(1):128–132
53. Campo RD, Romano JE (1986) Changes in cartilage proteoglycans associated with calcification. Calcif Tissue Int 39(3):175–184
54. Lane JM, Weiss C (1975) Review of articular cartilage collagen research. Arthritis Rheum 18(6):553–562
55. Lipshitz H, Etheredge R III, Glimcher MJ (1976) Changes in the hexosamine content and swelling ratio of articular cartilage as functions of depth from the surface. J Bone Joint Surg Am 58(8):1149–1153
56. Muir H, Bullough P, Maroudas A (1970) The distribution of collagen in human articular cartilage with some of its physiological implications. J Bone Joint Surg Br 52(3):554–563
57. Ratcliffe A, Fryer PR, Hardingham TE (1984) The distribution of aggregating proteoglycans in articular cartilage: comparison of quantitative immunoelectron microscopy with radioimmunoassay and biochemical analysis. J Histochem Cytochem 32(2):193–201

58. Clarke IC (1971) Articular cartilage: a review and scanning electron microscope study. 1. The interterritorial fibrillar architecture. J Bone Joint Surg Br 53(4):732–750
59. Redler I, Zimny ML (1970) Scanning electron microscopy of normal and abnormal articular cartilage and synovium. J Bone Joint Surg Am 52(7):1395–1404
60. Hascall VC (1977) Interaction of cartilage proteoglycans with hyaluronic acid. J Supramol Struct 7(1):101–120
61. Muir H (1983) Proteoglycans as organizers of the intercellular matrix. Biochem Soc Trans 11(6):613–622
62. Thambyah A, Broom N (2007) On how degeneration influences load-bearing in the cartilage-bone system: a microstructural and micromechanical study. Osteoarthr Cartil 15(12):1410–1423
63. Urban JP, Roberts S (2003) Degeneration of the intervertebral disc. Arthritis Res Ther 5(3):120–130
64. Mente PL, Lewis JL (1994) Elastic modulus of calcified cartilage is an order of magnitude less than that of subchondral bone. J Orthop Res 12(5):637–647
65. Habelitz S, Marshall SJ, Marshall GW Jr, Balooch M (2001) Mechanical properties of human dental enamel on the nanometre scale. Arch Oral Biol 46(2):173–183
66. Turner CH, Chandran A, Pidaparti RM (1995) The anisotropy of osteonal bone and its ultrastructural implications. Bone 17(1):85–89
67. Mankin HJ (1964) Mitosis in articular cartilage of immature rabbits. A histologic, stathmokinetic (colchicine) and autoradiographic study. Clin Orthop Relat Res 34:170–183
68. Hunziker EB, Quinn TM, Hauselmann HJ (2002) Quantitative structural organization of normal adult human articular cartilage. Osteoarthr Cartil 10(7):564–572
69. Hall BK, Newman S (1991) Cartilage: molecular aspects. CRC Press, Boca Raton, FL
70. Hwang J, Bae WC, Shieu W, Lewis CW, Bugbee WD, Sah RL (2008) Increased hydraulic conductance of human articular cartilage and subchondral bone plate with progression of osteoarthritis. Arthritis Rheum 58(12):3831–3842
71. Hunziker EB (1992) Articular cartilage structure in humans and experimental animals. In: Kuettner KE, Schleyerbach R, Peyron JG, Hascall VC (eds) Articular cartilage and osteoarthritis. Raven, New York, pp 183–189
72. Hunziker EB (1994) Mechanism of longitudinal bone growth and its regulation by growth plate chondrocytes. Microsc Res Tech 28(6):505–519
73. Hunziker EB, Wagner J, Zapf J (1994) Differential effects of insulin-like growth factor I and growth hormone on developmental stages of rat growth plate chondrocytes *in vivo*. J Clin Invest 93(3):1078–1086
74. McMahon LA, O'Brien FJ, Prendergast PJ (2008) Biomechanics and mechanobiology in osteochondral tissues. Regen Med 3(5):743–759
75. Nieminen MT, Toyras J, Laasanen MS, Silvennoinen J, Helminen HJ, Jurvelin JS (2004) Prediction of biomechanical properties of articular cartilage with quantitative magnetic resonance imaging. J Biomech 37(3):321–328
76. Lima EG, Bian L, Ng KW, Mauck RL, Byers BA, Tuan RS, Ateshian GA, Hung CT (2007) The beneficial effect of delayed compressive loading on tissue-engineered cartilage constructs cultured with TGF-beta3. Osteoarthr Cartil 15(9):1025–1033
77. Ding M, Dalstra M, Linde F, Hvid I (1998) Mechanical properties of the normal human tibial cartilage-bone complex in relation to age. Clin Biomech 13(4–5):351–358
78. Korhonen RK, Laasanen MS, Toyras J, Rieppo J, Hirvonen J, Helminen HJ, Jurvelin JS (2002) Comparison of the equilibrium response of articular cartilage in unconfined compression, confined compression and indentation. J Biomech 35(7):903–909
79. Freed LE, Langer R, Martin I, Pellis NR, Vunjak-Novakovic G (1997) Tissue engineering of cartilage in space. Proc Natl Acad Sci U S A 94(25):13885–13890
80. Gupta HS, Schratter S, Tesch W, Roschger P, Berzlanovich A, Schoeberl T, Klaushofer K, Fratzl P (2005) Two different correlations between nanoindentation modulus and mineral content in the bone-cartilage interface. J Struct Biol 149(2):138–148

81. Doube M, Firth EC, Boyde A, Bushby AJ (2010) Combined nanoindentation testing and scanning electron microscopy of bone and articular calcified cartilage in an equine fracture predilection site. Eur Cell Mater 19:242–251
82. Choi K, Kuhn JL, Ciarelli MJ, Goldstein SA (1990) The elastic moduli of human subchondral, trabecular, and cortical bone tissue and the size-dependency of cortical bone modulus. J Biomech 23(11):1103–1113
83. Brown TD, Vrahas MS (1984) The apparent elastic modulus of the juxtarticular subchondral bone of the femoral head. J Orthop Res 2(1):32–38
84. Karageorgiou V, Kaplan D (2005) Porosity of 3D biomaterial scaffolds and osteogenesis. Biomaterials 26(27):5474–5491
85. Grimm MJ, Williams JL (1997) Measurements of permeability in human calcaneal trabecular bone. J Biomech 30(7):743–745
86. Raudenbush D, Sumner DR, Panchal PM, Muehleman C (2003) Subchondral thickness does not vary with cartilage degeneration on the metatarsal. J Am Podiatr Med Assoc 93 (2):104–110
87. Sniekers YH, Intema F, Lafeber FP, van Osch GJ, van Leeuwen JP, Weinans H, Mastbergen SC (2008) A role for subchondral bone changes in the process of osteoarthritis; a micro-CT study of two canine models. BMC Musculoskelet Disord 9:20
88. Duchemin L, Bousson V, Raossanaly C, Bergot C, Laredo JD, Skalli W, Mitton D (2008) Prediction of mechanical properties of cortical bone by quantitative computed tomography. Med Eng Phys 30(3):321–328
89. Ferguson VL, Olesiak SE (2011) Nanoindentation of bone. In: Oyen ML (ed) Handbook of nanoindenation with biological applications. Pan Stanford, Singapore, pp 185–238
90. Pidaparti RM, Vogt A (2002) Experimental investigation of Poisson's ratio as a damage parameter for bone fatigue. J Biomed Mater Res 59(2):282–287
91. Ochoa JA, Hillberry BM (1992) Permeability of bovine cancellous bone. Trans Orthop Res Soc 17:163
92. Basillais A, Bensamoun S, Chappard C, Brunet-Imbault B, Lemineur G, Ilharreborde B, Ho Ba Tho MC, Benhamou CL (2007) Three-dimensional characterization of cortical bone microstructure by microcomputed tomography: validation with ultrasonic and microscopic measurements. J Orthop Sci 12(2):141–148
93. Iatridis JC, Setton LA, Foster RJ, Rawlins BA, Weidenbaum M, Mow VC (1998) Degeneration affects the anisotropic and nonlinear behaviors of human anulus fibrosus in compression. J Biomech 31(6):535–544
94. Panagiotacopulos ND, Pope MH, Krag MH, Bloch R (1987) A mechanical model for the human intervertebral disc. J Biomech 20(9):839–850
95. Antoniou J, Goudsouzian NM, Heathfield TF, Winterbottom N, Steffen T, Poole AR, Aebi M, Alini M (1996) The human lumbar endplate. Evidence of changes in biosynthesis and denaturation of the extracellular matrix with growth, maturation, aging, and degeneration. Spine 21(10):1153–1161
96. Acaroglu ER, Iatridis JC, Setton LA, Foster RJ, Mow VC, Weidenbaum M (1995) Degeneration and aging affect the tensile behavior of human lumbar anulus fibrosus. Spine 20(24):2690–2701
97. Elliott DM, Setton LA (2001) Anisotropic and inhomogeneous tensile behavior of the human annulus fibrosus: experimental measurement and material model predictions. J Biomech Eng 123(3):256–263
98. Boyde A, Firth EC (2004) Articular calcified cartilage canals in the third metacarpal bone of 2-year-old thoroughbred racehorses. J Anat 205(6):491–500
99. Armstrong CG, Mow VC (1982) Variations in the intrinsic mechanical properties of human articular cartilage with age, degeneration, and water content. J Bone Joint Surg Am 64(1):88–94
100. MacLean JJ, Owen JP, Iatridis JC (2007) Role of endplates in contributing to compression behaviors of motion segments and intervertebral discs. J Biomech 40(1):55–63

101. Fawns HT, Landells JW (1953) Histochemical studies of rheumatic conditions. I. Observations on the fine structures of the matrix of normal bone and cartilage. Ann Rheum Dis 12(2):105–113
102. Lane LB, Bullough PG (1980) Age-related changes in the thickness of the calcified zone and the number of tidemarks in adult human articular cartilage. J Bone Joint Surg Br 62 (3):372–375
103. Oegema TR Jr, Johnson SL, Meglitsch T, Carpenter RJ (1996) Prostaglandins and the zone of calcified cartilage in osteoarthritis. Am J Ther 3(2):139–149
104. Muller-Gerbl M, Schulte E, Putz R (1987) The thickness of the calcified layer of articular cartilage: a function of the load supported? J Anat 154:103–111
105. O'Connor KM (1997) Unweighting accelerates tidemark advancement in articular cartilage at the knee joint of rats. J Bone Miner Res 12(4):580–589
106. Doube M, Firth EC, Boyde A (2007) Variations in articular calcified cartilage by site and exercise in the 18-month-old equine distal metacarpal condyle. Osteoarthr Cartil 15(11):1283–1292
107. Karvonen RL, Negendank WG, Teitge RA, Reed AH, Miller PR, Fernandez-Madrid F (1994) Factors affecting articular cartilage thickness in osteoarthritis and aging. J Rheumatol 21(7):1310–1318
108. Oegema TR Jr, Carpenter RJ, Hofmeister F, Thompson RC Jr (1997) The interaction of the zone of calcified cartilage and subchondral bone in osteoarthritis. Microsc Res Tech 37(4):324–332
109. Kiviranta I, Jurvelin J, Tammi M, Saamanen AM, Helminen HJ (1987) Weight bearing controls glycosaminoglycan concentration and articular cartilage thickness in the knee joints of young beagle dogs. Arthritis Rheum 30(7):801–809
110. Green WT Jr, Martin GN, Eanes ED, Sokoloff L (1970) Microradiographic study of the calcified layer of articular cartilage. Arch Pathol 90(2):151–158
111. Kaab MJ, Gwynn IA, Notzli HP (1998) Collagen fibre arrangement in the tibial plateau articular cartilage of man and other mammalian species. J Anat 193(pt 1):23–34
112. Muller-Gerbl M, Schulte E, Putz R (1987) The thickness of the calcified layer in different joints of a single individual. Acta Morphol Neerl Scand 25(1):41–49
113. Laffosse JM, Kinkpe C, Gomez-Brouchet A, Accadbled F, Viguier E, de Gauzy JS, Swider P (2010) Micro-computed tomography study of the subchondral bone of the vertebral endplates in a porcine model: correlations with histomorphometric parameters. Surg Radiol Anat 32(4):335–341
114. Martin RB, Sharkey NA (eds) (2001) Mechanical effects of postmortem changes, preservation, and allograft bone treatments. Bone mechanics handbook, 2nd edn. CRC Press, New York
115. Boyde A (2003) The real response of bone to exercise. J Anat 203(2):173–189
116. Haralson MA, Hassell JR (1995) Extracellular matrix: a practical approach The Practical approach series, vol 151. IRL Press; Oxford University Press, Oxford, New York
117. Fratzl P, Weinkamer R (2007) Nature's hierarchical materials. Prog Mater Sci 52(8):1263–1334
118. Thambyah A, Broom N (2006) Micro-anatomical response of cartilage-on-bone to compression: mechanisms of deformation within and beyond the directly loaded matrix. J Anat 209 (5):611–622
119. Ferguson VL (2009) Deformation partitioning provides insight into elastic, plastic, and viscous contributions to bone material behavior. J Mech Behav Biomed Mater 2(4):364–374
120. Oyen ML, Ko CC (2008) Indentation variability of natural nanocomposite materials. J Mater Res 23(3):760–767
121. Duer MJ, Friscic T, Murray RC, Reid DG, Wise ER (2009) The mineral phase of calcified cartilage: its molecular structure and interface with the organic matrix. Biophys J 96 (8):3372–3378

122. Roschger P, Grabner BM, Rinnerthaler S, Tesch W, Kneissel M, Berzlanovich A, Klaushofer K, Fratzl P (2001) Structural development of the mineralized tissue in the human L4 vertebral body. J Struct Biol 136(2):126–136
123. Bembey AK, Bushby AJ, Boyde A, Ferguson VL, Oyen ML (2006) Hydration effects on the micro-mechanical properties of bone. J Mater Res 21(8):1962–1968
124. Elliott JC (2002) Calcium phosphate biominerals. In: Kohn MJ, Rakovan J, Hughes JM (eds) Phosphates: geochemical, geobiological, and materials importance, vol 48. Reviews in mineralogy & geochemistry. Mineralogical Society of America, Washington, DC, pp 427–453
125. Wilson EE, Awonusi A, Morris MD, Kohn DH, Tecklenburg MMJ, Beck LW (2006) Three structural roles for water in bone observed by solid-state NMR. Biophys J 90(10):3722–3731
126. Ziv V, Weiner S (1994) Bone crystal sizes—a comparison of transmission electron-microscopic and X-ray-diffraction line-width broadening techniques. Connect Tissue Res 30(3):165–175
127. Eppell SJ, Tong WD, Katz JL, Kuhn L, Glimcher MJ (2001) Shape and size of isolated bone mineralites measured using atomic force microscopy. J Orthop Res 19(6):1027–1034
128. Wilson RM, Dowker SEP, Elliott JC (2006) Rietveld refinements and spectroscopic structural studies of a Na-free carbonate apatite made by hydrolysis of monetite. Biomaterials 27 (27):4682–4692
129. Petruska JA, Hodge AJ (1964) Subunit model for tropocollagen macromolecule. Proc Natl Acad Sci U S A 51(5):871–876
130. Landis WJ, Hodgens KJ, Arena J, Song MJ, McEwen BF (1996) Structural relations between collagen and mineral in bone as determined by high voltage electron microscopic tomography. Microsc Res Tech 33(2):192–202
131. Katz EP, Li S (1973) Structure and function of bone collagen fibrils. J Mol Biol 80(1):1–15
132. Zizak I, Paris O, Roschger P, Bernstorff S, Amenitsch H, Klaushofer K, Fratzl P (2000) Investigation of bone and cartilage by synchrotron scanning-SAXS and -WAXD with micrometer spatial resolution. J Appl Crystallogr 33(1):820–823
133. Brown RA, Blunn GW, Salisbury JR, Byers PD (1993) Two patterns of calcification in primary (physeal) and secondary (epiphyseal) growth cartilage. Clin Orthop 294:318–324
134. Reid SA, Boyde A (1987) Changes in the mineral density distribution in human bone with age: image analysis using backscattered electrons in the SEM. J Bone Miner Res 2(1):13–22
135. Ratcliffe A, Mow VC (1996) Articular cartilage. In: Comper WD (ed) Extracellular matrix, vol I. Harwood Academic, Reading, UK, pp 235–302
136. Gong JK, Arnold JS, Cohn SH (1964) Composition of trabecular + cortical bone. Anat Rec 149(3):325–332
137. Lovell TP, Eyre DR (1988) Unique biochemical characteristics of the calcified zone of articular cartilage. Trans Orthop Res Soc 13:511
138. Thambyah A, Broom N (2010) How subtle structural changes associated with maturity and mild degeneration influence the impact-induced failure modes of cartilage-on-bone. Clin Biomech 25(7):737–744
139. Bushby AJ, Ferguson VL, Boyde A (2004) Nanoindentation of bone: comparison of specimens tested in liquid and embedded in polymethylmethacrylate. J Mater Res 19 (1):249–259
140. Redler I, Mow VC, Zimny ML, Mansell J (1975) The ultrastructure and biomechanical significance of the tidemark of articular cartilage. Clin Orthop Relat Res 112:357–362
141. Oloyede A, Broom N (1996) The biomechanics of cartilage load-carriage. Connect Tissue Res 34(2):119–143
142. Kaab MJ, Richards RG, Ito K, ap Gwynn I, Notzli HP (2003) Deformation of chondrocytes in articular cartilage under compressive load: a morphological study. Cells Tissues Organs 175 (3):133–139
143. Hough AJ, Banfield WG, Mottram FC, Sokoloff L (1974) The osteochondral junction of mammalian joints. An ultrastructural and microanalytic study. Lab Invest 31(6):685–695

144. Wei HW, Sun SS, Jao SH, Yeh CR, Cheng CK (2005) The influence of mechanical properties of subchondral plate, femoral head and neck on dynamic stress distribution of the articular cartilage. Med Eng Phys 27(4):295–304
145. Anderson DD, Brown TD, Radin EL (1993) The influence of basal cartilage calcification on dynamic juxtaarticular stress transmission. Clin Orthop Relat Res 286:298–307
146. Brown TD, Radin EL, Martin RB, Burr DB (1984) Finite element studies of some juxtarticular stress changes due to localized subchondral stiffening. J Biomech 17(1):11–24
147. Broom ND (1984) Further insights into the structural principles governing the function of articular cartilage. J Anat 139(pt 2):275–294
148. Flachsmann ER, Broom ND, Oloyede A (1995) A biomechanical investigation of unconstrained shear failure of the osteochondral region under impact loading. Clin Biomech 10 (3):156–165
149. Johnson-Nurse C, Dandy DJ (1985) Fracture-separation of articular cartilage in the adult knee. J Bone Joint Surg Br 67(1):42–43
150. Tomatsu T, Imai N, Takeuchi N, Takahashi K, Kimura N (1992) Experimentally produced fractures of articular cartilage and bone. The effects of shear forces on the pig knee. J Bone Joint Surg Br 74(3):457–462
151. Fry HJ (1974) The interlocked stresses of articular cartilage. Br J Plast Surg 27(4):363–364
152. Matthewson MH, Dandy DJ (1978) Osteochondral fractures of the lateral femoral condyle: a result of indirect violence to the knee. J Bone Joint Surg Br 60-B(2):199–202
153. Rosenberg NJ (1964) Osteochondral fractures of the lateral femoral condyle. J Bone Joint Surg Am 46:1013–1026
154. Meachim G, Bentley G (1978) Horizontal splitting in patellar articular cartilage. Arthritis Rheum 21(6):669–674
155. Mori S, Harruff R, Burr DB (1993) Microcracks in articular calcified cartilage of human femoral heads. Arch Pathol Lab Med 117(2):196–198
156. Sokoloff L (1993) Microcracks in the calcified layer of articular cartilage. Arch Pathol Lab Med 117(2):191–195
157. Freeman MAR (1979) Adult articular cartilage, 2nd edition, p. 560 (Pitman Medical, Kent)
158. Mow VC, Gu WY, Chen FH (2005) Structure and function of articular cartilage and meniscus. Basic orthopaedic biomechanics and mechano-biology (Eds V.C. Mow and R. Huiskes) pp. 181–258 (Lippin- cott Williams & Wilkins, Philadelphia)
159. Setton LA Swelling and curling behaviors of articular cartilage. J Biomech Eng 120(2):355–361

Chapter 6
Muscle–Tendon Interactions in the Absence of Bones: Lessons from the Fruit Fly, *Drosophila*

Talila Volk

6.1 Introduction

Invertebrates provide a unique system in which to study how the musculoskeletal system operates and functions in the absence of bone structures. The fruit fly *Drosophila Melanogaster* has been used as an exciting animal model to study and elucidate various aspects of embryonic development, including the initial steps of muscle and tendon development and patterning [1–3].

Whereas *Drosophila* does not contain cartilage/bone elements, the muscles are connected to specialized muscle attachment cells that are part of the epidermal cell layer, which together with the cuticle, form the exoskeleton [1, 4]. These epidermal cells function as muscle attachment sites and develop into a specialized subset of epidermal cells, referred to as tendons. Despite the fact that these tendon cells appear considerably different from the collagen fiber-rich, multicellular tendons of vertebrates, some of the principles of tendon cell determination, and especially their cross-talk with muscles and the formation of the myotendinous junction (MTJ), appear to be conserved in evolution; therefore, tendon formation in the fly can serve as a paradigm for the corresponding processes in the vertebrate embryo.

Two unique features of the musculoskeletal system in flies that are not present in vertebrates are the absence of bones and the one-to-two relationship between a single muscle cell and its corresponding two tendon cells that connect both ends of the muscle. In such a scenario, the mechanical force produced by muscle contraction is transmitted directly to the two tendon cells at both its ends. Therefore, the structure of these tendons must be robust to resist muscle contractions and to maintain the integrity of the entire ectoderm.

The following chapter describes the origin as well as the differentiation pathway promoting tendon development in *Drosophila* embryonic development,

T. Volk (✉)
Department of Molecular Genetics, Weizmann Institute, Rehovot, Israel
e-mail: talila.volk@weizmann.ac.il

S. Thomopoulos et al. (eds.), *Structural Interfaces and Attachments in Biology*, 119
DOI 10.1007/978-1-4614-3317-0_6, © Springer Science+Business Media New York 2013

the development of the MTJs, and the molecular pathways that determine the structural elements within the fly tendons and provide them with the ability to resist muscle contractions.

6.2 Early Determination of Tendons Is Independent of Muscle Cells

The intricate pattern of tendon cells within the ectoderm emerges in parallel to muscle founder cell determination (Fig. 6.1a). One of the earliest genes that induce tendon progenitor cells within the ectoderm is the EGR-like transcription factor, StripeB, one of the two isoforms produced by the *stripe* gene [5, 6]. The StripeB transcription factor is less active than the alternate StripeA isoform, whose expression is activated at a later developmental stage following the interaction of the tendon with the muscle [7]. StripeB expression is promoted by signaling pathways involved in the patterning of the embryonic ectoderm including Wg- Hh- Notch- and EGFR pathways [8]. Direct Stripe induction is provided by the Wg and Hh signaling pathways, as both TCF and Ci binding sites were shown to be functional in the *stripe* promoter region [9]. StripeB overexpression promotes the beta-gal expression of an enhancer trap inserted in the *stripe* promoter region [10], demonstrating that StripeB positively regulates its own transcription. Once activated, at stage 11–12 of embryonic development, the ectodermal cells are transformed into tendon progenitor cells capable of directing the correct targeting of the muscle cells that migrate towards the Stripe-positive tendon cells (Fig. 6.1b).

Stripe also mediates the induction of adult tendon cells in the fly's thorax [11]. Interestingly, Stripe expression in the thorax antagonizes the expression of AC-S proneural genes, inhibiting sensory organ precursor formation in the areas of future muscle attachment sites. Thus, Stripe expression divides the future adult fly thorax into a Stripe-positive domain, in which tendon cells develop, and a Stripe-negative domain, where sensory bristles form. This mutual exclusion between tendons and neural tissue is conserved in evolution [12].

Several genes involved in muscle targeting to tendon cells are positively regulated by Stripe activity in the embryo, including *slit*, *tsp*, *lrt*, and *slow* [13–17]. Interestingly, although Stripe is sufficient to induce their expression, some of these genes are detected at low expression levels even in *stripe* mutant embryos, raising the possibility that segment polarity genes initially activate a set of tendon-specific genes including StripeB. StripeB then maintains and amplifies the expression of these genes as well as its own transcription, transforming these ectodermal cells into tendon progenitor cells (Fig. 6.2). However, the final differentiation of these progenitor cells depends on their specific interaction with muscles.

Posttranscriptional downregulation of StripeB levels in the tendon progenitor cells is provided by the long isoform of the RNA-binding protein Held Out Wing

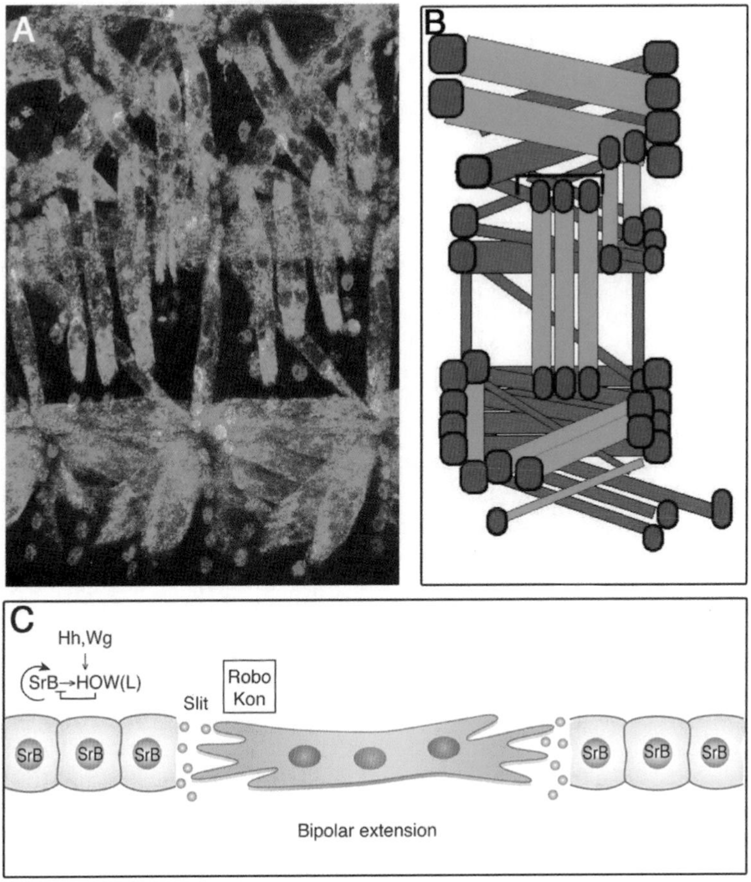

Fig. 6.1 Muscle–tendon interactions in the *Drosophila* embryo. (**a**) Two hemi-abdominal segments of a stage 16 embryo stained for Myosin Heavy Chain (MHC) (*green*) that marks the somatic muscles and for Stripe (*red*) marking the tendon cells. Note that each muscle is associated with two tendon cells at its both ends. (**b**) Schematic representation of a single hemi-abdominal segment showing the 30 types of muscles (*light green* are anterior muscles and *dark green* are more posterior muscles, and their tendon attachment cells are in *red*). (**c**) Scheme of the first stage in tendon assembly; tendon progenitors are defined in the ectoderm by the induction of StripeB (SrB) by segment polarity genes Hh and Wg. StripeB expression is maintained low as a result of posttranscriptional repression of the RNA-binding protein HOW(L). SrB regulates positively its own expression as well as the expression of inhibitor HOW(L). Tendon progenitors secrete Slit and provide initial cues for directing muscle bipolar migration. The muscle responds to Slit through Robo receptors. In addition Kontiki (Kon) contributes to the migration of the muscles

(HOW(L)), which is both necessary and sufficient to reduce *stripe* mRNA levels. HOW(L) itself is a target of StripeB [18, 19]. Thus, HOW(L) creates a negative feedback loop that counteracts StripeB auto-activation, leading to the maintenance of StripeB at low levels in the progenitor tendon cells and inhibiting their subsequent differentiation.

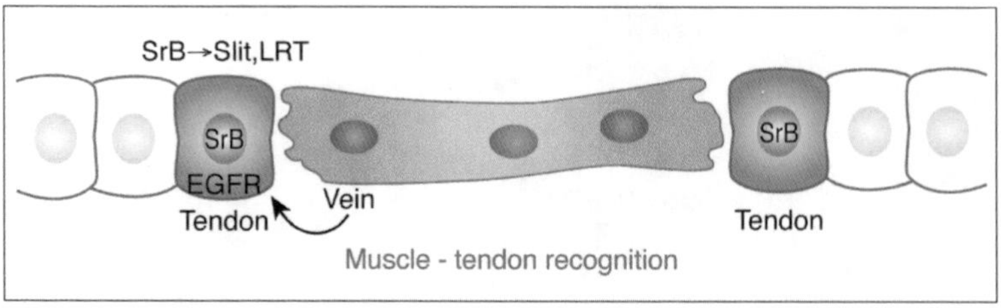

Fig. 6.2 Muscle-tendon recognition. Following the arrival of muscles to their corresponding tendon cells, the muscle signals to the tendon through EGFR activation by means of the neuregulin-like secreted ligand Vein to initiate tendon differentiation and elevate SrB expression. SrB further induces the expression of Slit and LRT, the latter is required to arrest muscle migration. Tendon precursors that do not bind muscles loose SrB expression and become ectoderm cells

The muscle-dependent signal required for differentiation of tendon progenitors into fully mature tendon cells is provided by Vein, a neuregulin-like secreted ligand of the EGF-receptor pathway. Following muscle binding, Vein accumulation at the muscle-tendon junction site specifically activates the EGFR-receptor pathway in the muscle-bound tendon progenitor, driving it to differentiate to a mature tendon cell (Fig. 6.2) [20].

Thus, the initial determination of *Drosophila* tendon progenitor cells in the ectoderm takes place sequentially (Figs. 6.1 and 6.2). The initial weak signal is initiated by segment polarity genes. Then, the signal is strengthened as a result of StripeB activity, which is positively auto-regulated, but also maintained at low levels as a result of the posttranscriptional inhibitory activity of HOW(L). In this manner, the tendon progenitor cells produce the necessary signals for attracting muscle cells towards the attachment sites; however, the cells are not fully committed to a tendon fate, and their final differentiation is still dependent on future interaction with muscles.

6.3 Targeting and Anchoring of Muscles to Tendons and the Formation of the Myotendinous Junction in Drosophila

Whereas the initial determination of muscles and tendons appears to be autonomous in *Drosophila*, targeting of muscles to tendons requires cross-talk between these two tissue types. Muscle migration towards tendons depends on several factors including the initial polarity of the muscle cell, local signals available during muscle migration, target recognition, and signals involved in the migration arrest. Due to the limited amount of information available on these processes in both vertebrates and invertebrates, it is too early to speculate as to the degree of conservation between these processes in the two systems. However, the gradual construction of the MTJ mediated primarily by integrin-dependent adhesion in both

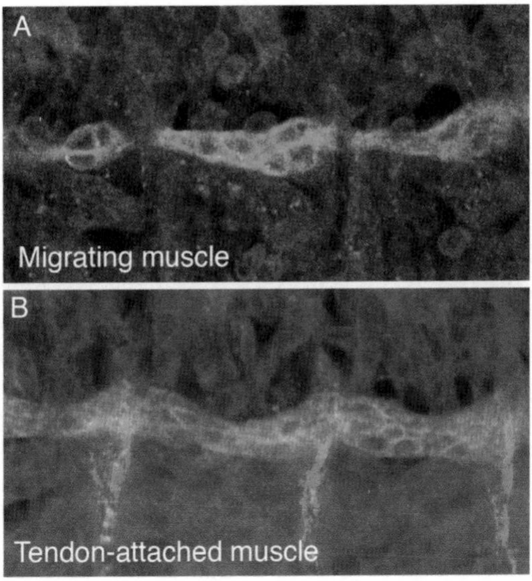

Fig. 6.3 Muscle cell morphology during migration and following attachment to the tendon cell. A single muscle (muscle 12) was labeled with membrane bound GFP (CD8-GFP) and also stained for integrin (*red*). (**a**) At stage 14 the muscle is migrating towards its tendon cell and exhibits a polarized shape. (**b**) At stage 16 the muscle has been attached to tendon cells at its both ends. Its morphology has been changed and integrin (*red line*) is highly detected at the interface between the muscle and the tendon

systems may reflect a high degree of similarity between invertebrates and vertebrates. Below, I discuss what is known regarding muscle targeting and MTJ formation in *Drosophila*.

At stage 12–13 of embryonic development, following fusion of the myoblasts to distinct founder cells, the myotubes acquire characteristic polarity, in which the edges of the cells are directed to either anterior-posterior or dorsal-ventral positions [1]. By detecting individual GFP-labeled myotubes, the migration path of muscle cells towards their targeted tendon cells may be followed (Fig. 6.3). In this manner, it is possible to distinguish between mutations affecting the migration per se, or mutations affecting muscle attachment to tendons. Although both defects result in a phenotype characterized by dissociation between muscles and tendons and the rounding of the muscle cells, defects in muscle migration appear at earlier developmental stages [21].

A unique aspect of muscle migration toward its target tendon cells is its concomitant bipolar extension towards two tendon cells located at its two opposite ends. Imaging of live single muscle cells during their migration suggests a simultaneous bi-directional extension of the muscle cell [1] (Fig. 6.1). How do the muscle ends respond in opposite directions to guiding signals? It is possible that the initial extension of the two muscle ends occurs due to the intrinsic polarity of this cell type independent of any external signals. Only when the two muscle ends are distant enough from each other, might they respond to short-range signals provided by the tendon cells located at the segment border. Such a scenario might take place during vertebrate muscle migration where, in a manner similar to *Drosophila*, the muscles are connected at their two ends to attachment sites.

Several signaling pathways involved in axon guidance were described that mediate muscle guidance toward tendon cells, as well. These include the Slit/

Robo and the Derailed Receptor Tyrosine Kinase pathways [13, 14, 22]. Muscles express the Robo receptors (Robo and Robo2), and Slit is secreted from tendon cells as well as from the ventral cord midline. Interestingly, whereas both Slit/Robo and Derailed pathways repress axon guidance, they appear to mediate attraction of muscles towards their target tendon cells (an exception is the ventral muscles, which are repelled from the ventral midline due to Slit activity secreted at the midline).

Recently, an additional novel protein complex expressed by the ventral longitudinal muscles was demonstrated to mediate muscle migration towards tendon cells. This complex includes the transmembrane protein Kon-Tiki/Perdido, its cytoplasmic partner, the PDZ domain protein, Grip, and the cell surface protein, Echinoid [21, 23–25]. Kon-Tiki and Grip share a similar phenotype, in which mutant muscles do not extend towards the tendon cells during their migration, suggesting that they both mediate a positive attractive cue sensed by the muscle ends. The nature of this signal has not yet been elucidated.

In summary, the unique bipolar extension of the muscle ends might be dependent on short-range signals provided by the tendon cells [26].

6.4 Formation of the Drosophila Myotendinous Junction

In both vertebrates and invertebrates, the correct construction of the MTJ is essential for force transmission and to counteract muscle contraction by the skeletal elements via tendon cells. The MTJ consists of hemi-adherens junctions formed between integrin heterodimers assembled on the muscle and tendon membrane surfaces together with extracellular matrix (ECM) proteins deposited in between these cells [26]. These ECM proteins "glue" both cell types together through integrin receptors associated with the actin cytoskeleton in the cytoplasm of each cell. The glue-like ECM material provides elastic properties to the MTJ, and its unique ultrastructural organization is essential for proper force transmission (Fig. 6.4).

Studies in *Drosophila* revealed the sequence of events associated with MTJ formation. Two types of integrin heterodimers mediate MTJ formation, namely αPS1βPS on the tendon cell and αPS2βPS on the muscle side [27, 28]. They appear to interact with distinct types of ECM proteins; the tendon-specific αPS1bPS interacts with laminin [29, 30], whereas the muscle-specific αPS2βPS interacts with Thrombospondin (Tsp) [15, 31] and with Tiggrin [32] (Fig. 6.4). Laminin as well as Tsp are secreted from the tendon cells, and Tiggrin is secreted from the muscle cell. MTJ dysfunction causes the complete dissociation of muscles from tendons, leading to embryonic lethality. The most severe muscle detachment phenotype is obtained in embryos mutant for either αPS2βPS or its ECM ligand, Tsp. Lack of Laminin, and/or αPS1βPS leads to a less severe muscle detachment phenotype, suggesting that the adhesion of the muscle to the tendon-associated ECM is a critical aspect of the MTJ function.

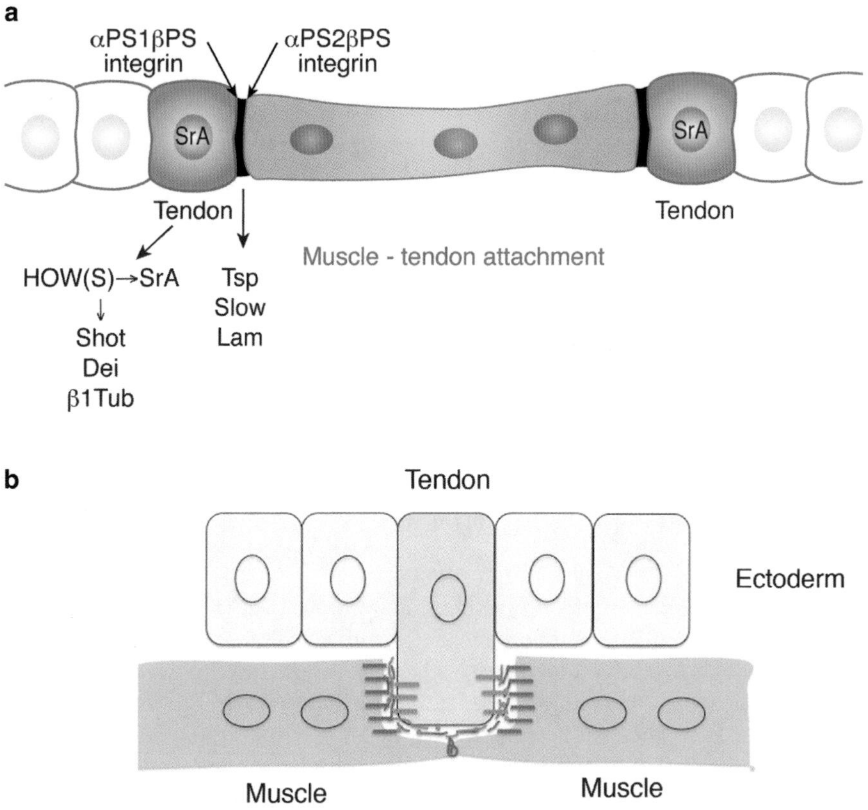

Fig. 6.4 Muscle-tendon interactions following the formation of the MTJ. (**a**) Formation of the MTJ. The MTJ (*black*) is formed through αPS1βPS muscle-specific integrin association with the tendon-secreted ECM component thrombospondin (Tsp), and its regulator Slow. Laminin (Lam) binds the αPS1βPS tendon-specific integrin. At this stage HOW(S) is elevated in the cytoplasm of the tendon cell promoting the formation of StripeA (SrA) essential to induce terminal differentiation by inducing the expression of Shortstop (Shot), Delilah (Dei), and b1tubulin (β1Tub). (**b**) Side view of two muscles from adjacent segments attached to a single tendon cell. *Green* and *orange* are the tendon-specific and muscle-specific integrin receptors. The ECM proteins Tsp and Laminin are deposited between the muscles and tendon cells and the ECM protein Tiggrin is deposited between the two adjacent muscles

The earliest event in the construction of *Drosophila* MTJ is the tendon-specific secretion of Tsp, which precedes muscle attachment and the assembly of PS integrins on the muscle and tendon surfaces. While migrating, the muscle does not respond to Tsp even when ectopically expressed; however, once the muscle ends approach the tendon cell, PS2 integrin gradually accumulates at the muscle ends, presumably as a result of inside-out integrin signaling which, following association of its cytoplasmic tail with Talin, enhances the affinity of its ectodomain to Tsp [27, 33].

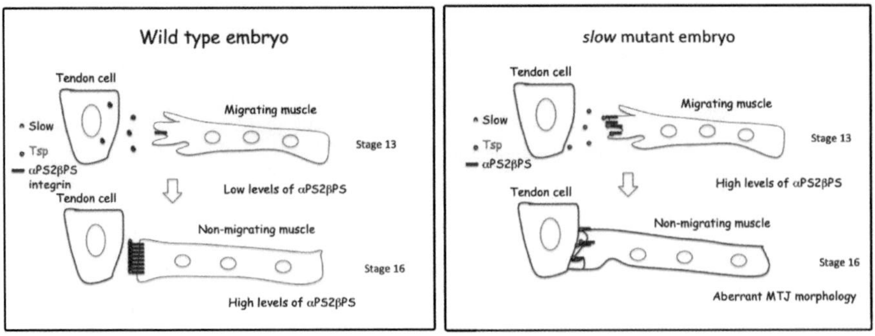

Fig. 6.5 Gradual construction of the MRJ is mediated by Slow activity. *Left panel*—in wild type embryo, Slow and Tsp are secreted from the tendon cell and form a protein complex that inhibits Tsp binding to the muscle integrin receptors prematurely. Only following the arrest of muscle migration, Tsp binds to the integrin receptors, promoting their high accumulation at the muscle ends and a proper formation of MTJ. *Right panel*—in *slow* mutant embryos, integrin receptors accumulate at the leading edge of the muscle prior to the arrest of muscle migration. This leads to aberrant construction of the MTJ that eventually leads to muscle or tendon tearing during larvae movements

Recently, a secreted tendon-specific protein, Slowdown (Slow), was shown to modulate the responsiveness of the muscle integrins to Tsp, presumably through its Tsp association [17]. Lack of *slow* leads to a severe locomotion phenotype in homozygous larvae, and an inability to fly in adult *slow* homozygous mutant escapers. In *slow* mutants, a premature association between Tsp and the muscle αPS2βPS integrin was demonstrated, leading to the accumulation of integrin receptors on the muscle ends prior to the muscle's arrival at the tendon cell. This leads to asymmetric force distribution between muscles and tendons, causing muscle, as well as tendon tearing (Fig. 6.5). Thus, when the interface of the MTJ has not been constructed in a correct manner, both the tendon and the muscle are exposed to aberrant distribution of the mechanical load developed by muscle contraction. This leads to occasional tearing of muscles or tendons, and muscle dysfunction.

Interestingly, a similar phenotype is also obtained when muscle integrin receptors are overexpressed in the muscle cells [33]. Premature "spotty" junctions are detected, and an aberrant MTJ is formed between the muscle and its tendon cell. Therefore, the gradual construction of the MTJ as well as the correct assembly of the ECM is critical for proper musculoskeletal function.

6.5 Arrest of Muscle Migration

The arrival of the muscle cell at the target tendon cell and the formation of the MTJ are temporally and spatially coupled. However, it is not clear how tendon recognition, arrest of muscle migration, and initiation of MTJ formation are coordinated at the molecular level. The transmembrane protein kon-tiki/perdido was shown to interact genetically with the tendon-specific αPS1βPS integrin receptors [23]. Such an interaction might provide the muscle cell with a signal to arrest its migration. The phenotype of *kon-tiki/perdido* is first detected during migration of the muscles; however, an additional role in migration arrest cannot be excluded. LRT, a tendon-specific leucine-rich transmembrane protein, accumulates following muscle arrival and functionally interacts with Robo receptors on the muscle cell. Lack of *lrt* leads to extra membrane extensions, suggesting aberrant muscle targeting and/or defects in the arrest of muscle migration. Moreover, its overexpression stalls muscle extension towards tendon cells, supporting the central role of this molecule in promoting the targeting of muscle to tendon cells [16].

One possible mechanism for the arrest of muscle migration is the initiation of MTJ formation. During muscle migration, the muscle is insensitive to ectopic expression of the ECM protein, Tsp [17]. A possible explanation might be that integrin receptors are not expressed on the membrane of migrating muscle cells. The arrival of the muscle to its target tendon cell leads to the initial accumulation of muscle integrin receptors, responsiveness to Tsp, and the accumulation of integrin at the muscle ends. These initial adhesion events might represent a signal for the muscle to arrest its migratory behavior and to initiate the formation of the MTJ. A finding supporting this possibility is that overexpression of integrin in the muscle during its migration leads to aberrant muscle migratory behavior [17].

In summary, several mechanisms explaining tendon recognition by the muscle and its coupling to the initial formation of the MTJ are based on the function of highly conserved proteins, which may play similar roles during the formation of the MTJ in the vertebrate embryo. Recently, components of the intergin-mediated adhesion machinery, including Talin 1 and Talin 2, as well as the laminin integrin receptors α7β1D and α7Bβ1D were shown to actively mediate vertebrate MTJ, and their absence was shown to lead to myopathies in humans [34, 35].

6.6 The Unique Tendon Cytoskeleton Enables Resistance to Muscle Contractions

Fly tendons utilize the cuticle secreted by the ectoderm as an external skeleton. Specialized proteins connect the tendon plasma membrane to the cuticle, maintaining a tight association between the tendon cell and the exoskeleton [36]. However, the tendon cell itself must resist muscle contraction in a flexible and elastic fashion. In most cases, a single muscle is bound to a single tendon so that the mechanical strength of muscle contraction is transmitted to a single cell and not to multiple tendons, as is the case in vertebrate tendons [4]. Molecular insight into the mechanism enabling the transmission of the contractile forces to the cuticle exoskeleton was deduced from an RNAi-induced knock-down of the *shortstop* (*shot*) gene product in tendon cells. Shortstop is a large evolutionarily conserved protein containing a microtubule binding sequence at its C' terminal domain, a large spectrin repeat domain, and plakin and

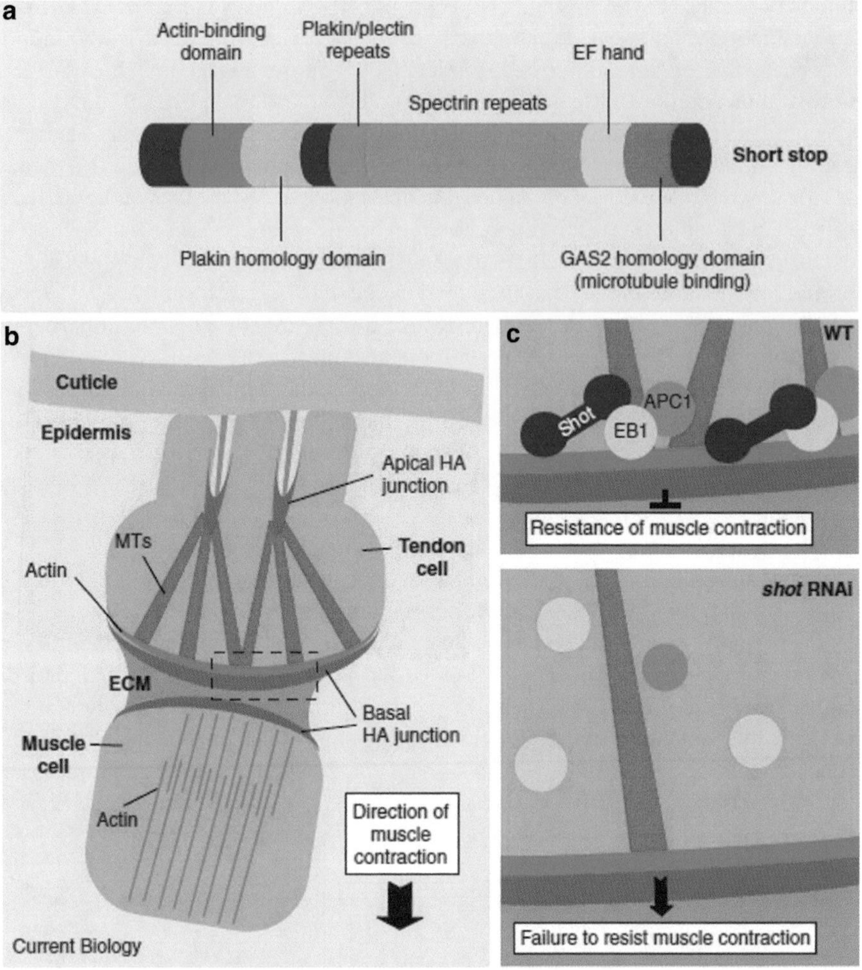

Fig. 6.6 *Drosophila* Shot links the actin and microtubule cytoskeletons. (**a**) Diagram of the various domains of the Shot protein. (**b**) Schematic depicting the tendon cell linking muscle cells to the exoskeleton. Region outlined with a dotted box represents the region that is enlarged in (**c**). *MTs* microtubules; *ECM* extracellular matrix; *HA* hemi-adherens junction. (**c**) Model of Shot function. In the wild type (WT), Shot binds EB1, recruiting it and APC1 to microtubule plus ends, resulting in resistance to muscle contraction. In the absence of Shot (*shot* RNAi), EB1 and APC1 are lost from microtubule plus ends, and tendon cells fail to resist muscle contraction (note that some microtubules detach in *shot* RNAi mutants)

claponin-actin binding motifs at its N-terminal domain [37, 38]. Shortstop is highly expressed in tendon cells, neurons, and ectodermal cells. A tendon-specific knock-down of Shot using the *stripe-gal4* driver leads to larvae that hatch but are incapable of developing to the third instar larval stage, eventually leading to larval lethality [39]. The tendon cells of these larvae are highly elongated, and often tear apart while maintaining the MTJ (Fig. 6.6). Molecular analysis has shown that Shot accumulates at the cytoplasmic faces of the tendon-cell MTJ, where it promotes the polarized organization of the plus ends of microtubules that are stretched between the MTJ and the cuticle. Reduction at the levels of Shot leads to dissociation of the MT plus ends from the MTJ and extensive elongation of the tendon cell. These results suggest that the polarized array of MT within the tendon cells is critical for the tendon cell to resist muscle contraction.

6.7 Conclusions

Analysis of the fly musculoskeletal system reveals unique solutions to overcome issues shared with musculoskeletal assembly and function in vertebrates. For example, instead of multiple tendon cells in vertebrates that share the muscle-generated forces between many cell units, in *Drosophila*, the force is divided between multiple MT-fibers within a single cell. Analysis of the fly musculoskeleton enables us to define the critical phases essential for the correct functionality of this system. These include: (a) the precise encounter between muscles and their corresponding tendon cells; (b) the critical role of the integrin receptors in the formation of the MTJ, and the gradual construction of the MTJ to accommodate the final morphology of the muscle and tendon ends; (c) the elasticity of the tendon cells that is maintained by the MT system; and (d) the essential role of the ECM and its precise assembly and deposition during MTJ formation.

Acknowledgment The studies described in this review were supported by a grant from the Israel Science Foundation to T. Volk and a previous grant from the Minerva Foundation with funding from the Federal German Ministry of Education and Research to T. Volk. I also thank S. Schwarzbaum for her English corrections of this chapter.

References

1. Schnorrer F, Dickson BJ (2004) Muscle building; mechanisms of myotube guidance and attachment site selection. Dev Cell 7(1):9–20
2. Beckett K, Baylies MK (2006) The development of the Drosophila larval body wall muscles. Int Rev Neurobiol 75:55–70
3. Schweitzer R, Zelzer E, Volk T (2010) Connecting muscles to tendons: tendons and musculoskeletal development in flies and vertebrates. Development 137(17):2807–2817
4. Volk T (1999) Singling out Drosophila tendon cells: a dialogue between two distinct cell types. Trends Genet 15(11):448–453
5. Frommer G, Vorbruggen G, Pasca G, Jackle H, Volk T (1996) Epidermal egr-like zinc finger protein of Drosophila participates in myotube guidance. EMBO J 15(7):1642–1649
6. Volk T, VijayRaghavan K (1994) A central role for epidermal segment border cells in the induction of muscle patterning in the Drosophila embryo. Development 120(1):59–70
7. Volohonsky G, Edenfeld G, Klambt C, Volk T (2007) Muscle-dependent maturation of tendon cells is induced by post-transcriptional regulation of stripeA. Development 134(2):347–356

8. Hatini V, DiNardo S (2001) Divide and conquer: pattern formation in Drosophila embryonic epidermis. Trends Genet 17(10):574–579
9. Piepenburg O, Vorbruggen G, Jackle H (2000) Drosophila segment borders result from unilateral repression of hedgehog activity by wingless signaling. Mol Cell 6(1):203–209
10. Becker S, Pasca G, Strumpf D, Min L, Volk T (1997) Reciprocal signaling between Drosophila epidermal muscle attachment cells and their corresponding muscles. Development 124(13): 2615–2622
11. Fernandes JJ, Celniker SE, VijayRaghavan K (1996) Development of the indirect flight muscle attachment sites in Drosophila: role of the PS integrins and the stripe gene. Dev Biol 176(2): 166–184
12. Usui K, Pistillo D, Simpson P (2004) Mutual exclusion of sensory bristles and tendons on the notum of dipteran flies. Curr Biol 14(12):1047–1055
13. Chanana B, Steigemann P, Jackle H, Vorbruggen G (2009) Reception of Slit requires only the chondroitin-sulphate-modified extracellular domain of Syndecan at the target cell surface. Proc Natl Acad Sci U S A 106(29):11984–11988
14. Kramer SG, Kidd T, Simpson JH, Goodman CS (2001) Switching repulsion to attraction: changing responses to slit during transition in mesoderm migration. Science 292(5517): 737–740
15. Subramanian A, Wayburn B, Bunch T, Volk T (2007) Thrombospondin-mediated adhesion is essential for the formation of the myotendinous junction in Drosophila. Development 134(7): 1269–1278
16. Wayburn B, Volk T (2009) LRT, a tendon-specific leucine-rich repeat protein, promotes muscle-tendon targeting through its interaction with Robo. Development 136(21):3607–3615
17. Gilsohn E, Volk T (2010) Slowdown promotes muscle integrity by modulating integrin-mediated adhesion at the myotendinous junction. Development 137(5):785–794
18. Nabel-Rosen H, Dorevitch N, Reuveny A, Volk T (1999) The balance between two isoforms of the Drosophila RNA-binding protein how controls tendon cell differentiation. Mol Cell 4(4):573–584
19. Nabel-Rosen H, Volohonsky G, Reuveny A, Zaidel-Bar R, Volk T (2002) Two isoforms of the Drosophila RNA binding protein, how, act in opposing directions to regulate tendon cell differentiation. Dev Cell 2(2):183–193
20. Yarnitzky T, Min L, Volk T (1997) The Drosophila neuregulin homolog Vein mediates inductive interactions between myotubes and their epidermal attachment cells. Genes Dev 11(20):2691–2700
21. Schnorrer F, Kalchhauser I, Dickson BJ (2007) The transmembrane protein Kon-tiki couples to Dgrip to mediate myotube targeting in Drosophila. Dev Cell 12(5):751–766
22. Callahan CA, Bonkovsky JL, Scully AL, Thomas JB (1996) Derailed is required for muscle attachment site selection in Drosophila. Development 122(9):2761–2767
23. Estrada B, Gisselbrecht SS, Michelson AM (2007) The transmembrane protein Perdido interacts with Grip and integrins to mediate myotube projection and attachment in the Drosophila embryo. Development 134(24):4469–4478
24. Swan LE, Wichmann C, Prange U, Schmid A, Schmidt M, Schwarz T, Ponimaskin E, Madeo F, Vorbruggen G, Sigrist SJ (2004) A glutamate receptor-interacting protein homolog organizes muscle guidance in Drosophila. Genes Dev 18(2):223–237
25. Swan LE, Schmidt M, Schwarz T, Ponimaskin E, Prange U, Boeckers T, Thomas U, Sigrist SJ (2006) Complex interaction of Drosophila GRIP PDZ domains and Echinoid during muscle morphogenesis. EMBO J 25(15):3640–3651
26. Brown NH (2000) Cell-cell adhesion via the ECM: integrin genetics in fly and worm. Matrix Biol 19(3):191–201
27. Bokel C, Brown NH (2002) Integrins in development: moving on, responding to, and sticking to the extracellular matrix. Dev Cell 3(3):311–321
28. Brown NH (2000) An integrin chicken and egg problem: which comes first, the extracellular matrix or the cytoskeleton? Curr Opin Cell Biol 12(5):629–633

29. Martin-Bermudo MD, Brown NH (1999) Uncoupling integrin adhesion and signaling: the betaPS cytoplasmic domain is sufficient to regulate gene expression in the Drosophila embryo. Genes Dev 13(6):729–739
30. Gotwals PJ, Fessler LI, Wehrli M, Hynes RO (1994) Drosophila PS1 integrin is a laminin receptor and differs in ligand specificity from PS2. Proc Natl Acad Sci USA 91(24): 11447–11451
31. Chanana B, Graf R, Koledachkina T, Pflanz R, Vorbruggen G (2007) AlphaPS2 integrin-mediated muscle attachment in Drosophila requires the ECM protein Thrombospondin. Mech Dev 124(6):463–475
32. Fogerty FJ, Fessler LI, Bunch TA, Yaron Y, Parker CG, Nelson RE, Brower DL, Gullberg D, Fessler JH (1994) Tiggrin, a novel Drosophila extracellular matrix protein that functions as a ligand for Drosophila alpha PS2 beta PS integrins. Development 120(7):1747–1758
33. Tanentzapf G, Brown NH (2006) An interaction between integrin and the talin FERM domain mediates integrin activation but not linkage to the cytoskeleton. Nat Cell Biol 8(6):601–606
34. Conti FJ, Monkley SJ, Wood MR, Critchley DR, Muller U (2009) Talin 1 and 2 are required for myoblast fusion, sarcomere assembly and the maintenance of myotendinous junctions. Development 136(21):3597–3606
35. Conti FJ, Felder A, Monkley S, Schwander M, Wood MR, Lieber R, Critchley D, Muller U (2008) Progressive myopathy and defects in the maintenance of myotendinous junctions in mice that lack talin 1 in skeletal muscle. Development 135(11):2043–2053
36. Bokel C, Prokop A, Brown NH (2005) Papillote and Piopio: Drosophila ZP-domain proteins required for cell adhesion to the apical extracellular matrix and microtubule organization. J Cell Sci 118(Pt 3):633–642
37. Brown NH (2008) Spectraplakins: the cytoskeleton's Swiss army knife. Cell 135(1):16–18
38. Sonnenberg A, Liem RK (2007) Plakins in development and disease. Exp Cell Res 313(10): 2189–2203
39. Subramanian A, Prokop A, Yamamoto M, Sugimura K, Uemura T, Betschinger J, Knoblich JA, Volk T (2003) Shortstop recruits EB1/APC1 and promotes microtubule assembly at the muscle-tendon junction. Curr Biol 13(13):1086–1095

Chapter 7
Dentin/Adhesive Interface in Teeth

Paulette Spencer, Qiang Ye, Jonggu Park, Ranganathan Parthasarathy, Orestes Marangos, Anil Misra, Brenda S. Bohaty, Viraj Singh, and Jennifer S. Laurence

7.1 Posterior Composite Restorations

In 2005, 166 million dental restorations were placed in the United States [1] and clinical studies suggest that more than half were replacements for failed restorations [2]. Replacement of failed restorations consumes 60% of the average dentist's practice time (NIDCR 13-DE-102) and this emphasis on replacement therapy is expected to increase as concerns about mercury release from dental amalgam force dentists to select alternative materials. Resin composite is the most commonly used alternative [3], but moderate-to-large composite restorations have higher failure rates, more recurrent caries, and increased frequency of replacement as compared to amalgam [2–8].

Results from clinical studies suggest that, after 8 years, the failure rate for posterior composite restorations was at least 50% greater than that for high copper

P. Spencer (✉)
Department of Mechanical Engineering, Bioengineering Research Center, University of Kansas, Lawrence, KS, USA
e-mail: pspencer@ku.edu

Q. Ye • J. Park • R. Parthasarathy • O. Marangos
Bioengineering Research Center, University of Kansas, Lawrence, KS, USA

A. Misra
Department of Civil, Environmental, and Architectural Engineering, Bioengineering Research Center, University of Kansas, Lawrence, KS, USA

B.S. Bohaty
Department of Pediatric Dentistry, University of Missouri-Kansas City, Kansas City, MO, USA

V. Singh
Department of Mechanical Engineering, University of Kansas, Lawrence, KS, USA

J.S. Laurence
Department of Pharmaceutical Chemistry, University of Kansas, Lawrence, KS, USA

S. Thomopoulos et al. (eds.), *Structural Interfaces and Attachments in Biology*,
DOI 10.1007/978-1-4614-3317-0_7,

amalgam restorations [9]. At 5 years, the need for additional treatment was 50% greater in children receiving composite restorations as compared to children treated with dental amalgam [5]. Based on a review of dental records from 3,071 subjects, Simecek and colleagues reported in 2009 a significantly higher risk of replacement for posterior composite restorations as compared to amalgam [4]. In a study of amalgam and composite restorations placed by 243 Norwegian dentists, the mean age of failed amalgam was ~11 years, while the mean age for failed composite was significantly lower at 6 years [7]. Indeed, after nearly five decades of research, the clinical lifetime of large-to-moderate posterior composite restorations continues to be approximately one-half of that of dental amalgam [10].

The reduced clinical lifetime of moderate-to-large class II composite restorations can be particularly detrimental for patients because removal of these restorations can lead to extensive loss of sound tooth structure. For example, the removal of composite restorations produced significantly greater increases in cavity volume in comparison to the removal of amalgam [11]. The increase in cavity volume and increased frequency of replacement means that significantly greater amounts of tooth structure will be lost with treatment and re-treatment of class II composite restorations [11]. Over the lifetime of the patient, the additional loss of tooth structure will translate to more complex restorations and eventually total tooth loss. The reduced longevity, increased frequency of replacement, and the need for a more complex restoration mean increased costs to the patient in terms of both time and money [12].

The premature failure of moderate-to-large composite restorations can be traced to a breakdown of the bond at the tooth surface/composite material interface [9, 10, 13–17] and increased levels of the cariogenic bacteria, Streptococcus mutans, at the perimeter of these materials [18–22]. The composite is too viscous to bond directly to the tooth and thus, a low viscosity adhesive must be used to form a bond between the tooth and composite. The breakdown of the composite/tooth bond has been linked to the failure of current adhesives to consistently seal and adhere to the dentin [2, 17–26]. Acid etching provides effective mechanical bonding between enamel and adhesive, but bonding to dentin has been fraught with problems.

7.2 Dental Substrate

Dentin is the hydrated composite structure that constitutes the body of each tooth, providing both a protective covering for the pulp and serving as a support for the overlying enamel. Enamel, with its exceptionally high mineral content, is a very brittle tissue. Without the support of the more resilient dentin structure, enamel would fracture when exposed to the forces of mastication. Dentin supports, as well as compensates, for the brittle nature of the enamel.

Dentin is composed of approximately 50% inorganic material, 30% organic material, and 20% water by volume [27]. Dentin mineral is a carbonate rich, calcium deficient apatite [28, 29]. The organic component is predominantly type I collagen, with minor contributions from phosphoproteins, glycoproteins, proteoglycans, and some plasma proteins [30]. The composition of dentinal fluid is reportedly similar to plasma [29].

Features of the dentin structure include the tubules that traverse the structure from the pulp cavity to the region just below the dentin-enamel junction (DEJ) or the dentin-cementum junction. The tubules, which could be modeled as narrow tunnels a few microns or less in diameter, represent the tracks taken by the odontoblastic cells from the pulp chamber to the respective junctions. Dentinal tubule diameter measures approximately 2.5 μm near the pulp and 0.9 μm near the DEJ [31]. Tubule density and orientation vary from location to location; density is lowest at the DEJ and highest at the predentin surface at the junction to the pulp chamber.

The number of tubules in young premolar and molar teeth ranges from 50,000 to 75,000 per square millimeter at the pulpal surface to approximately half as many per square millimeter in the proximity of the DEJ [27]. The content of the tubules include fluid and odontoblast processes for all or part of their course. In contrast to root dentin, the tubules in coronal dentin are surrounded by a collar of highly mineralized peritubular dentin [32].

The composition of the peritubular dentin is carbonate apatite with very small amounts of organic matrix, whereas intertubular dentin, i.e., the dentin separating the tubules, is type I collagen matrix reinforced with apatite. Thus, the composition of intertubular dentin is primarily mineralized collagen fibrils; the fibrils are described as a composite of a collagen framework and thin plate-shaped carbonated apatite crystals whose c-axes are aligned with the collagen fibril axis [33]. In healthy dentin, the majority of the mineralized collagen fibrils are perpendicular to the tubules [34]. It is important to recognize that the composition of dentin is not static. It is influenced by the relative position of the dentin within the tooth, the age of the dentin, and the presence and/or absence of disease [29].

7.2.1 Altered Forms of Dentin

In contrast to enamel, dentin is a vital tissue containing the cell processes of odontoblasts and neurons. Since the odontoblasts can be stimulated to deposit more dentin, this tissue is capable of limited repair. The structure–property relationships of dentin vary with location, physiological, aging, and disease processes.

The composition, mineralization, and structure are different between normal and altered forms of dentin [27, 29, 31, 33]. A wide variety of terms have been used to describe the types of dentin associated with physiological aging and disease processes. Descriptors such as secondary, tertiary, sclerotic, and transparent dentin have all been used. In general, secondary dentin forms as a result of normal physiologic stimuli, whereas tertiary or reparative dentin forms as a result of a pathologic process such as caries. The rate of secondary dentin deposition is generally slower than the rate associated with primary or initial dentin deposition.

It is suggested that the rate of secondary dentin deposition depends upon the individual's diet and occlusal forces [4]. Secondary dentin deposition results in gradual narrowing of the pulp chamber.

Tertiary dentin, also referred to as reparative, irregular secondary, irritation, response, or reactionary dentin, is formed in response to an insult such as caries or abrasion [29]. This tissue, which appears to represent a protective response, has a less regular structure with fewer and less well-aligned tubules as compared to primary dentin [35]. Reparative dentin is formed by new odontoblast-like cells, while reactionary dentin is formed by surviving odontoblasts subjacent to damaged or diseased dentin [22]. For example, pulpal injury leads to the proliferation, migration, and differentiation of odontoblast-like cells from the pulp, giving rise to the secretion of reparative dentin [36]. In comparison, mild injuries stimulate the surviving postmitotic odontoblasts at the site of the injury to secrete reactionary dentin [37]. It has been suggested that fibroblasts or undifferentiated cells in the pulpal tissue are the likely progenitor cells of the new odontoblast-like cells [38].

The terms sclerotic and transparent dentin are often used interchangeably to describe dentin that has altered mineralization. As an example, sclerotic dentin describes tissue that exhibits obliteration of the dentin tubule as a result of progressive deposition of peritubular dentin [29]. This type of dentin is generally found in the roots, especially near the apex and the amount of sclerosed dentin increases with age [4, 35].

Carious dentin is characteristically described as consisting of infected and affected layers. The infected layer is removed prior to reparative procedures with synthetic materials. The affected layer is generally not removed during treatment and, based on structural features, this layer is subdivided into the following: turbid or discolored layer, transparent zone, and subtransparent zone [11, 39]. The transparent zone occupies the largest proportion of the carious dentin [40]. Transparent dentin has been characterized as hypermineralized, but results from a recent study suggest that only a limited number of carious lesions with transparent dentin develop hypermineralized intertubular regions [31]. However, investigators agree that, in contrast to normal, healthy dentin, the tubules within the caries-affected dentin are frequently occluded by acid-resistant mineral deposits [11, 31, 39].

7.3 Failure of Posterior Composite Restorations and Dentin/Adhesive Bonding

The primary factor in the premature failure of moderate-to-large composite restorations is secondary decay at the margins of the restorations [7]. For example, in a study of radiographs from 459 adults, age 18–19 years, the investigators reported that among 650 interproximal restorations the failure rate as a result of secondary or recurrent decay was 43% for composite compared to 8% for amalgam [6]. In a separate study of amalgam and composite restorations

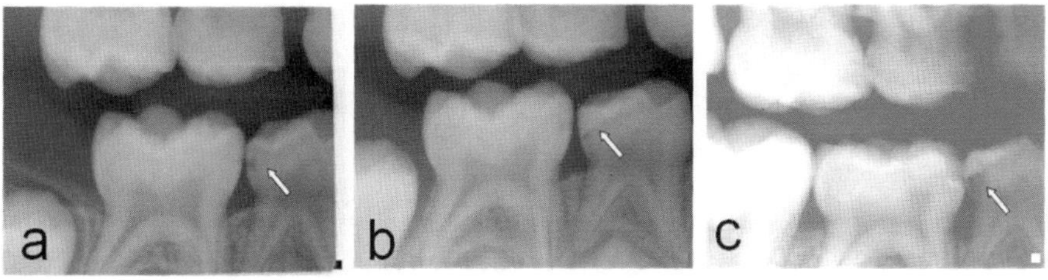

Fig. 7.1 Radiographic image of primary teeth on *right side*. (**a**) The *arrow* denotes carious lesion on the proximal surface of mandibular right first primary molar. (**b**) The *arrow* denotes the composite restoration on first primary molar. (**c**) Radiographic image of primary teeth on right side, 2 years after figure (**b**). The *arrow* denotes the failed class II composite restoration because of extensive decay

placed in 8–12-year-old children, the primary reason for failure of both materials was secondary decay; secondary decay was 3.5 times higher in composite restorations [4].

In moderate-to-large class II composite restorations, secondary decay is most often localized gingivally (Fig. 7.1). Secondary decay at the gingival margin is linked to failure of the bond between the tooth and composite and increased levels of the cariogenic bacteria, Streptococcus mutans, at the perimeter of these materials [20, 21, 41]. For clarification, class I restorations involve the biting surface only while class II restorations involve the biting surface and one or more proximal surfaces.

As described earlier, the composite is too viscous to bond directly to the tooth surface. A low viscosity adhesive is used to form a bond between the tooth and composite. Acid etching leads to effective mechanical bonding at the interface between enamel and adhesive, but bonding to dentin has been fraught with challenges and problems.

Clinicians frequently find very little enamel available for bonding at the gingival margin of class II composite restorations and thus, the bond at the gingival margin depends on the integrity of the seal formed with dentin. Under clinical conditions, one can frequently detect a separation between the composite material and the tooth surface at the gingival margin [38]. These marginal gaps have been related to technique-sensitive and unreliable bonding between the adhesive and dentin [38, 42].

At the vulnerable gingival margin, the adhesive may be the primary barrier between the prepared tooth and the surrounding environment. A failed adhesive means that there are gaps between the tooth and composite. Bacterial enzymes, oral fluids, and bacteria can infiltrate these gaps, and this activity will lead to recurrent decay, hypersensitivity, pulpal inflammation, and restoration failure [2, 17, 23, 40, 43]. The lack of durable dentin adhesives is considered one of the major problems with the use of composites in direct restorative dentistry [44].

7.4 Dentin/Adhesive Bond and the Hybrid Layer

The two fundamental processes involved in bonding an etch-and-rinse adhesive to dentin are: removal of the mineral phase from the dentin substrate without altering the collagen matrix and filling the voids left by the mineral with adhesive that undergoes complete in situ polymerization, i.e., the formation of a resin-reinforced or hybrid layer. The ideal hybrid layer would be characterized as a 3-dimensional polymer/collagen network that provides both a continuous and stable link between the bulk adhesive and dentin substrate. Numerous studies indicate that this ideal objective has not been achieved [25, 45–55].

The hybrid layer is formed when an adhesive resin penetrates a demineralized or acid-etched dentin surface and infiltrates the exposed collagen fibrils. During acid etching, the mineral phase is extracted from a zone that measures between 1 and ~10 μm of the dentin surface [35, 56, 57]. The composition of the exposed substrate differs radically from mineralized dentin. For example, mineralized dentin is 50% mineral, 30% collagen, and 20% water by volume [39], whereas demineralized dentin is 30% collagen and 70% water [58, 59]. With removal of the mineral phase, the collagen fibers are suspended in water. If there is a substantial zone of demineralization and the water supporting the collagen network is removed either by air drying or the action of an air syringe, the collagen will collapse [59, 60]. A collapsed collagen network reduces the porosity and inhibits resin penetration through the demineralized layer [59]. It forms a barrier between the demineralized layer and the underlying intact or unreacted dentin surface [61, 62]. A collapsed collagen network severely compromises the dentin/adhesive (d/a) bond [58, 60, 61].

7.4.1 Wet Bonding

In the early 1990s, wet bonding was introduced to counteract the problems of collagen collapse [46, 63–66]. Wet bonding means that the dentin is kept fully hydrated throughout the bonding procedure; the surface morphology of the demineralized layer does not change because the water supporting the collagen matrix is not removed [67]. Bond strength results [46, 63–66] with "wet" bonding support these findings, that is, the higher bond strengths with this technique reflect the minimal collapse of "wet" vs. air-dried dentin collagen [59]. It is speculated that moist dentin provides a more porous collagen network and that increased porosity means more space for adhesive infiltration [59, 61, 63–65, 68].

With wet bonding techniques, the channels between the demineralized dentin collagen fibrils are filled with water, solvent, conditioner, and/or oral fluids [59]. The only mechanism available for adhesive resin infiltration is diffusion of the resin into whatever fluid is in the spaces of the substrate and along the collagen fibrils. Ideally, the solvent in combination with hydrophilic monomers (e.g., hydroxyethyl methacrylate (HEMA)) conditions the collagen to remain expanded during adhesive infiltration. However, HEMA, a primary component in many single bottle commercial dentin adhesives, can dramatically reduce the evaporation of water [69]. Hydrophobic monomers, such as 2,2-bis[4(2-hydroxy-3-methacryloyloxy-propyloxy)-phenyl] propane (BisGMA), would resist diffusing into these sites where there is residual water [25, 50, 70–72]. Under *in vivo* conditions, there is little control over the amount of water left on the tooth. As a result, it is possible to leave the dentin surface so wet that the adhesive undergoes physical separation into hydrophobic and hydrophilic-rich phases [71].

Results from our laboratory indicated that excess moisture prohibited the formation of an impervious, structurally integrated d/a bond at the gingival margin of Class II composite restorations [25, 26]. Clinicians must routinely attempt to bond to naturally wet substrates such as caries-affected dentin [73] or deep dentin [36, 37, 74, 75]. The water content of caries-affected dentin has been reported to be 2.7 times greater than that of normal dentin [73]. In deep dentin, 22% of the surface area is exposed tubules while exposed tubules account for 1% of the surface area of dentin close to the DEJ [76]. The large increase in surface area attributable to tubules means that in deep dentin, pulpal fluid will contribute additional moisture to that already present within the demineralized dentin matrix. Since our current adhesives are very sensitive to excess moisture, bonding to these clinically relevant substrates is a formidable challenge [26, 77–79].

7.4.2 Extrinsic and Intrinsic Water Absorption

Absorption of extrinsic water leads to plasticization of the adhesive and loss of interfacial d/a bond strength as a result of water attack. One example of the effect of water absorption on chemically cured poly-HEMA specimens is the dramatic decrease in physical properties after 24 h aqueous storage; the tensile properties were reduced to an almost gum-like quality [80]. The mean values for tensile strength of dry and wet poly-HEMA specimens were ~18 and 1 MPa, respectively. This reduction was attributed to water sorption after polymerization and/or extraction of water-soluble unreacted monomers or oligomers. As a result of water uptake into the poly-HEMA specimens, the percent elongation increased from ~20 to 220%. The authors suggested that since there is no cross-linking in the poly-HEMA, the water allowed the linear chains to slide over one another, thus resulting in a tenfold increase in percent elongation. In this investigation, intrinsic water at concentrations >5 vol% inhibited the light polymerization of HEMA, even with a tenfold increase in the initiators camphorquinone (CQ)/dimethylaminoethyl methacrylate (DMAEMA).

A study from our laboratory showed that at water concentrations ≥25 vol%, BisGMA-based adhesive/water solutions mimicked oil and water mixtures in that they separated into distinct phases immediately following sonication [71]. At 25 vol % water the adhesive separates into particles whose composition is primarily BisGMA; the composition of the surrounding matrix material is primarily HEMA that exhibited limited monomer/polymer conversion. The limited conversion of the HEMA-rich phase suggests that either the photoinitiator is localized to the hydrophobic phase or it is incompatible with the hydrophilic HEMA [81–83].

In the absence of water, HEMA is a good solvent for BisGMA, so a relatively homogeneous solution can be formed. Water is also a good solvent for HEMA but a nonsolvent for BisGMA. With increasing water concentration, the adhesive may experience phase separation. Based on our previous work [84], a water concentration of at least 10% is required for visible macro-phase separation in HEMA/BisGMA formulations with a mass ratio of 45/55. A related study from our laboratory has provided direct evidence that with phase separation, there is minimal distribution of BisGMA and the hydrophobic photoinitiators camphorquinone (CQ) and ethyl 4-(dimethylamino)benzoate (EDMAB) in the aqueous phase [85].

Studies from our laboratory have shown spectral evidence of phase separation in a commercial total-etch BisGMA/HEMA adhesive bonded to wet, demineralized dentin matrices [35, 52, 72]. Ethanol is the solvent in this commercial adhesive. The primary function of the solvent is to displace the water from the wet, demineralized dentin matrix, but the spectroscopic results indicate that there is enough water present to promote detrimental adhesive phase separation. In this study, the majority of the intertubular d/a interface was characterized by collagen fibrils from the demineralized dentin matrix with limited spectral contribution from the critical dimethacrylate component (BisGMA). Thus, the demineralized dentin matrix is primarily infiltrated by HEMA. HEMA has a low cross-link density and thus, it will tend to absorb extraneous water, leading to plasticization and breakdown of the adhesive. In this study, the HEMA exhibited limited monomer/polymer conversion and it is expected that the unreacted components would be released in the mouth [86].

The sensitivity of our current adhesives to excess moisture is also reflected in the water-blisters that form in adhesives placed on over-wet surfaces [87–89]. The optimum amount of wetness varies as a function of the adhesive system [90]. Additionally, it is impossible to simultaneously achieve uniform wetness on all of the walls of the cavity preparation [91]. Wet bonding is, in short, a very technique-sensitive procedure and optimum bonding with our current commercial adhesives occurs over a very narrow range of conditions, e.g., water content [74].

One suggested approach to solve these problems is "ethanol-wet bonding" [92, 93]. A concern with this method is that, in the clinical setting, this solvent may be diluted because of repeated exposure of the material to the atmosphere or concentrated because of separation of the bonding liquids into layers within the bottle. Results from our laboratory have shown an inverse relationship between mechanical and thermal properties and the concentration of ethanol that is present during photopolymerization of model BisGMA-based adhesives [82]. In addition, the hybridization process is very sensitive to the ethanol content in the adhesive system [79]. Although the effect of "ethanol-wet bonding" on durability is not known, results from our laboratory suggest that this approach will not overcome the clinical challenges associated with forming a durable bond at the dentin/adhesive interface [94, 95].

Current strategies to promote bonding of the resinous materials to intrinsically wet substrates also include the incorporation of ionic and hydrophilic monomers into the adhesive [96]. These adhesives etch and prime simultaneously, thus addressing the problems of collagen collapse and simplifying the bonding protocol. Unfortunately, the hydrophilic nature of these components enhances water sorption and hydrolytic breakdown in the mouth [91, 96–99]. With these systems, the bonded interface lacks a nonsolvated hydrophobic resin coating and thus, the resultant hybrid layers behave as semipermeable membranes permitting water movement throughout the bonded interface even after adhesive polymerization [93]. The higher concentration of hydrophilic monomers in these systems is associated with decreased structural integrity at the d/a interface [93, 100]. *In vivo* aging studies have reported degradation of the d/a bond at 1-year even when the bonded dentin was protected by enamel from direct exposure to the oral environment [101]. These results suggest that hydrophilicity and hydrolytic stability of resin monomers are generally antagonistic [91].

7.5 Hybrid Layer Degradation

It has been hypothesized that the *in vivo* degradation of the hybrid layer follows a cascade of events that begins when the dentin is acid-etched [102]. Disruption of the tooth structure by drilling stimulates proteolytic enzymes such as matrix metall-oproteinases (MMPs), which can degrade the exposed collagen component of the hybrid layer [103]. Degradation by MMPs is expected to be most important acutely in the period following adhesive application. Chronic deterioration of the hybrid layer involves hydrolysis and leaching of the adhesive that has infiltrated the demineralized dentin matrix [25, 72]. Leaching is facilitated by water ingress into the loosely cross-linked or hydrophilic domains of the adhesive. The hydrophilic domain exhibits limited monomer/polymer conversion because of adhesive phase separation [71] and lack of compatibility between the photoinitiator and hydrophilic phase [83]. The poorly polymerized hydrophilic phase degrades rapidly in the aqueous environment. The previously resin-infiltrated collagen matrix is exposed and vulnerable to attack by proteolytic enzymes [103, 104].

The structure of methacrylate adhesives suggests a general mechanism for their chemical and enzymatic degradation in oral fluids. Water initially enters the adhesive matrix by diffusion into loosely cross-linked or hydrophilic domains or may be trapped within the matrix during photopolymerization in the moist oral environment [105, 106]. Portions of the matrix may be directly exposed to oral fluids, e.g., the gingival margin of Class II and V composite restorations. The presence of water promotes the chemical hydrolysis of ester bonds in methacrylate materials. This reaction is expected to be relatively slow at the neutral pH typical of saliva, but excursions in pH caused by food or cariogenic bacteria may lead to transient acid or base catalysis. The carboxylate and alcohol degradation products of ester hydrolysis are more hydrophilic than the parent ester, further enhancing the local ingress of water. With time, local domains of the methacrylate network may become sufficiently degraded and/or hydrophilic to permit access by esterases, which greatly accelerate ester bond hydrolysis. The esterase-catalyzed degradation of monomethacrylates, dimethacrylates, and commercial dental resins has been documented in solution [107–110], in saliva [109, 111, 112], and *in vivo* [101]. The breaking of covalent bonds by addition of water to ester bonds is considered to be one of the main reasons for resin degradation within the hybrid layer [90, 91]. Degradation of methacrylate ester groups produces carboxylic acids—the same functional group that is the culprit in lactic acid-induced decay.

7.6 Water-Compatible Esterase-Resistant Adhesives

Water is ubiquitous in the mouths of healthy patients and thus it is imperative that we develop restorative materials that can function adequately in the presence of water. Forty years ago, researchers were discussing the detrimental effect of water on bonding dental materials to the tooth; to date, this problem has not been resolved [113]. One approach to the problem of bonding to wet dentin has been to increase the relative hydrophilicity of dentin adhesives with a goal of promoting increased wetting of the collagen. However, hydrophilic polymers absorb more water than more hydrophobic resins [91]; the consequence of this increased water sorption is lowered mechanical properties [105] and increased degradation under wet conditions [98, 101, 114].

There are several strategies for reducing hydrolytic degradation of methacrylate adhesives. One strategy involves selectively modifying methacrylate side chains so that they are both water-compatible and esterase-resistant [115–117]. This can be accomplished by the use of bulky and/or branched functional groups that are poor esterase substrates but are sufficiently hydrophilic to be water-compatible (e.g., by incorporating polar functional groups such as –OH). Published reports on the reduced esterase susceptibility of urethane-modified BisGMA [108] and of acrylates with branched or aromatic side chains [110] support this approach. Another strategy involves increasing matrix hydrophobicity following initial monomer penetration into the dentin layer. Secondary cross-linking of polar functional groups on methacrylate side chains could be employed to achieve this goal. Increasing the extent of conversion of methacrylate resins will reduce susceptibility to esterase hydrolysis by reducing the number of unreacted pendant groups [81, 118].

Adhesive phase separation causes incomplete and differential infiltration of the demineralized dentin matrix [71, 119]. The collagen fibrils are not completely protected by the hydrophobic resin polymers and they will be susceptible to degradation [25, 44, 49, 120, 121]. Water-compatible components in adhesive formulations have to be considered, especially the partition of these components in the aqueous environment when phase separation occurs. In our laboratory, several approaches, such as new monomers with branch structure [115, 117, 122], solubility enhancer [70, 123], and water-soluble photoinitiators [81, 83], have been utilized to improve adhesive performance. Therefore, future adhesive systems need to be designed carefully to achieve a more homogeneous monomer distribution and conversion within the hybrid layer to overcome the defects associated with phase separation.

Any change in the chemical structure intended to increase esterase resistance and water compatibility will likely alter other chemical and physical properties of the adhesive. Under clinical function, the methacrylate-based dentin adhesives are subjected to both chemical and mechanical stresses. The interplay between the two forms of stress is expected to result in an alteration of the adhesive mechanical properties with time [124, 125].

The mechanical property change results from a variety of mechanisms, including: (1) change in the chemical nature of the polymer in the form of either plasticization, strain hardening, embrittlement, or crystallization, and (2) proliferation of surface and subsurface flaws due to combined effect of mechanical loads and chemical stress, e.g., biologic fouling, exposure to lactic acid (produced by S. mutans). The change in adhesive properties has a significant effect on the mechanical performance and durability of the d/a interface, which is a complex construct of different material phases at the micro-scale. Based on micro-scale structure–property measurements, our group has developed an idealized microstructural representation of the d/a interface [126] that can be utilized to perform micromechanical stress analyses using 3D micro-scale finite element (μFE) models [127]. Figure 7.2 shows a 3D micro-scale finite element model based on the idealized representation. We can see from Fig. 7.2 that the different material phases at the d/a interface will experience different stress amplitudes under functional load [126, 128]. Therefore, they reach their failure strength at different overall stress levels. As a consequence, the overall failure behavior of the d/a interface is not necessarily determined by the weakest component. Instead, the component whose stress concentration is closest to its failure strength determines the failure.

We have used micromechanical stress-analysis to show the effect of such stress concentrations on the mechanisms that govern the overall fatigue failure behavior of the d/a interface [44]. Fatigue-life (durability) curves were obtained for a number of d/a interface conditions as shown in Fig. 7.3. It was found that d/a interfaces with graded adhesive infiltration and thick hybrid layer exhibit lower durability. Predictions were compared to experimental data [129] to illustrate the predictive power of our methodology [44].

7.7 Dentin/Adhesive Interface: The Weak Link in Composite Restorations

In summary, the d/a bond can be the first defense against substances that may penetrate and ultimately undermine the composite restoration *in vivo*. However, as indicated in a recent review of dental composite, the properties of the materials are

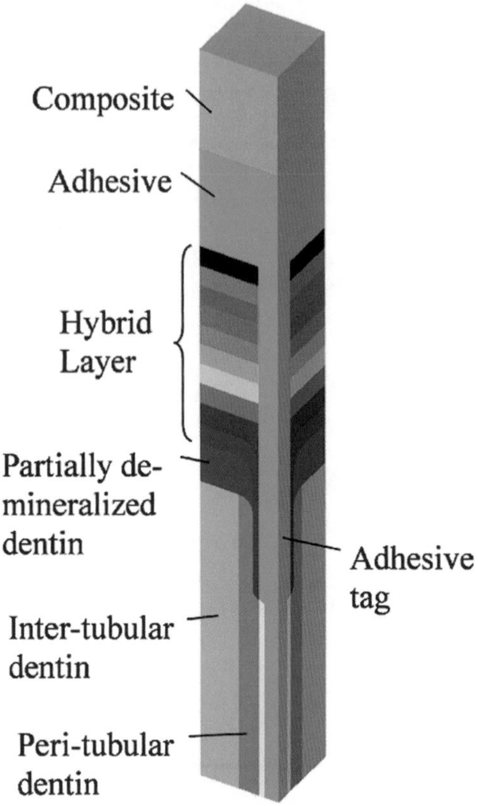

Fig. 7.2 3-d μFE model of d/a interface computational cell

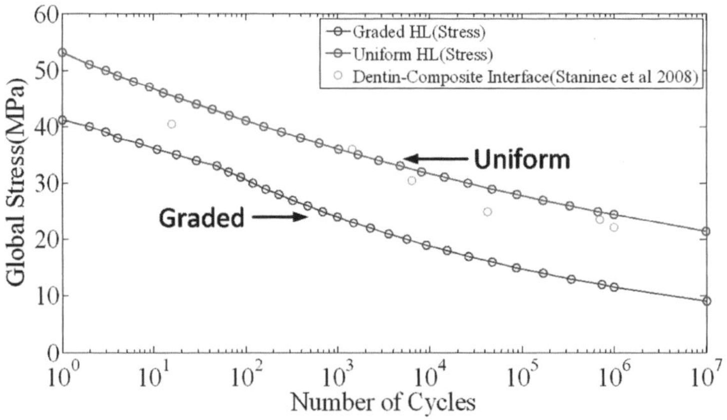

Fig. 7.3 Master SN curves for d/a interface under stress boundary conditions along with measured data (HL: Hybrid Layer; reproduced, with permission, from [44])

one part of a complex problem [130]. The success of clinical restorations depends on a variety of factors, including proper technique, appropriate materials, and proper patient selection [130].

In vitro and *in vivo* studies have suggested that several factors inhibit the formation of a durable d/a bond. These factors include: (1) water sorption and hydrolysis of the adhesive resin; (2) inadequate monomer/polymer conversion of the infiltrating adhesive; (3) incomplete resin infiltration; and (4) incomplete solvent evaporation [79, 82, 86, 93]. One strategy for reducing hydrolytic degradation involves selectively modifying methacrylate side chains so that they are both water-compatible and esterase-resistant [115–117, 122, 131, 132].

Inadequate monomer/polymer conversion may be addressed by including photoinitiators that are compatible with the hydrophilic components [81]. It is clear that full realization of our efforts to develop durable dentin adhesives demands quantitative information about solubility, water miscibility, distribution ratio, and phase partitioning behavior [85, 133].

The failure of the d/a bond, in concert with reports of increased levels of cariogenic bacteria at the perimeter of composite materials, points to an interesting interplay between microbiology and adhesive degradation as key elements in the premature failure of moderate-to-large composite restorations. Adhesion of S. mutans to surfaces in the mouth creates an environment that supports the subsequent attachment and growth of other bacterial species, ultimately forming a micro-ecosystem known as a biofilm. Dental plaque biofilm cannot be eliminated [134]. It may, however, be possible to reduce the pathogenic impact of the biofilm at the margin of the composite restoration by engineering novel, durable dentin adhesives [135].

Acknowledgements The authors gratefully acknowledge research support from NIH/NIDCR grants DE014392 (PS), DE022054 (PS, JSL), and K23DE/HD00468 (BSB). The authors gratefully acknowledge the numerous oral surgeons and their staff who assisted us with these projects.

References

1. Beazoglou T, Eklund S, Heffley D, Meiers J, Brown LJ, Bailit H (2007) Economic impact of regulating the use of amalgam restorations. Public Health Rep 122(5):657–663
2. Murray PE, Windsor LJ, Smyth TW, Hafez AA, Cox CF (2002) Analysis of pulpal reactions to restorative procedures, materials, pulp capping, and future therapies. Crit Rev Oral Biol Med 13(6):509–520
3. Simecek JW, Diefenderfer KE, Cohen ME (2009) An evaluation of replacement rates for posterior resin-based composite and amalgam restorations in US Navy and Marine Corps recruits. J Am Dent Assoc 140(2):200–209
4. Bernardo M, Luis H, Martin MD, Leroux BG, Rue T, Leitao J, DeRouen TA (2007) Survival and reasons for failure of amalgam versus composite posterior restorations placed in a randomized clinical trial. J Am Dent Assoc 138(6):775–783
5. DeRouen TA, Martin MD, Leroux BG, Townes BD, Woods JS, Leitao J, Castro-Caldas A, Luis H, Bernardo M, Rosenbaum G, Martins IP (2006) Neurobehavioral effects of dental amalgam in children: a randomized clinical trial. JAMA 295(15):1784–1792

6. Levin L, Coval M, Geiger SB (2007) Cross-sectional radiographic survey of amalgam and resin-based composite posterior restorations. Quintessence Int 38(6):511–514
7. Mjor IA, Dahl JE, Moorhead JE (2000) Age of restorations at replacement in permanent teeth in general dental practice. Acta Odontol Scand 58(3):97–101
8. Soncini JA, Maserejian NN, Trachtenberg F, Tavares M, Hayes C (2007) The longevity of amalgam versus compomer/composite restorations in posterior primary and permanent teeth: findings From the New England Children's Amalgam Trial. J Am Dent Assoc 138 (6):763–772
9. Collins CJ, Bryant RW, Hodge KL (1998) A clinical evaluation of posterior composite resin restorations: 8-year findings. J Dent 26(4):311–317
10. Van Nieuwenhuysen JP, D'Hoore W, Carvalho J, Qvist V (2003) Long-term evaluation of extensive restorations in permanent teeth. J Dent 31(6):395–405
11. Hunter AR, Treasue ET, Hunter AJ (1995) Increases in cavity volume associated with the removal of class 2 amalgam and composite restorations. Oper Dent 20:2–6
12. Tobi H, Kreulen CM, Vondeling H, van Amerongen WE (1999) Cost-effectiveness of composite resins and amalgam in the replacement of amalgam class II restorations. Community Dent Oral Epidemiol 27:137–143
13. Mair LH (1998) Ten-year clinical assessment of three posterior resin composites and two amalgams. Quintessence Int 29:483–490
14. Mjor IA, Dahl JE, Moorhead JE (2002) Placement and replacement of restorations in primary teeth. Acta Odontol Scand 60(1):25–28
15. Nordbo H, Leirskar J, von der Fehr FR (1998) Saucer-shaped cavity preparations for posterior approximal resin composite restorations: observations up to 10 years. Quintessence Int 29:5–11
16. Owens BM, Johnson WW (2005) Effect of insertion technique and adhesive system on microleakage of Class V resin composite restorations. J Adhes Dent 7:303–308
17. Van Meerbeek B, Van Landuyt K, De Munck J, Hashimoto M, Peumans M, Lambrechts P, Yoshida Y, Inoue S, Suzuki K (2005) Technique-sensitivity of contemporary adhesives. Dent Mater J 24(1):1–13
18. Anusavice KJ (1998) Management of dental caries as a chronic infectious disease. J Dent Educ 62:791–802
19. Dunne SM, Gainsford ID, Wilson NHF (1997) Current materials and techniques for direct restorations in posterior teeth. Part 1: silver amalgam. Int Dent J 47:123–136
20. Hansel C, Leyhausen G, Mai UE, Geurtsen W (1998) Effects of various resin composite (co) monomers and extracts on two caries-associated micro-organisms *in vitro*. J Dent Res 77:60–67
21. Santerre JP, Shajii L, Leung BW (2001) Relation of dental composite formulations to their degradation and the release of hydrolyzed polymeric-resin-derived products. Crit Rev Oral Biol Med 12:136–151
22. Svanberg M, Mjor IA, Orstavik D (1990) Mutans streptococci in plaque from margins of amalgam composite, and glass-ionomer restorations. J Dent Res 69(3):861–864
23. Hashimoto M, Ohno H, Kaga M, Endo K, Sano H, Oguchi H (2001) Resin-tooth adhesive interfaces after long-term function. Am J Dent 14(4):211–215
24. Meiers JC, Kresin J (1996) Cavity disinfectants and dentin bonding. Oper Dent 21:153–159
25. Spencer P, Wang Y, Bohaty B (2006) Interfacial chemistry of moisture-aged class II composite restorations. J Biomed Mater Res B Appl Biomater 77(2):234–240
26. Wang Y, Spencer P (2005) Interfacial chemistry of class II composite restoration: structure analysis. J Biomed Mater Res A 75(3):580–587
27. Ten Cate AR (1994) Repair and regeneration of dental tissue. In: Ten Cate AR (ed) Oral histology. Development, structure, and function, 4th edn. Mosby, St. Louis, pp 456–468
28. LeGeros RZ (1991) Calcium phosphates in oral biology and medicine. In: Meyers HM (ed) Monographs in oral science, vol 15. Karger, Basel, p 121

29. Marshall GW, Marshall SJ, Kinney JH, Balooch M (1997) The dentin substrate: structure and properties related to bonding. J Dent 25:441–458
30. Butler WT (1992) Dentin extracellular matrix and dentinogenesis. Oper Dent suppl 5:18–23
31. Ten Cate AR (1994) Oral histology. Development, structure, and function. In: 4th edn. Mosby, St. Louis, pp 174
32. Wang R, Weiner S (1998) Human root dentin: structure anistropy and vickers microhardness isotropy. Connect Tissue Res 39:269–279
33. Weiner S, Veis A, Beniash E, Arad T, Dillon JW, Sabsay B, Siddiqui F (1999) Peritubular dentin formation: crystal organization and the macromolecular constituents in human teeth. J Struct Biol 126(1):27–41
34. Kinney JH, Pople JA, Marshall GW, Marshall SJ (2001) Collagen orientation and crystallite size in human dentin: a small angle X-ray scattering study. Calcif Tissue Int 69:31–37
35. Wang Y, Spencer P (2002) Quantifying adhesive penetration in adhesive/dentin interface using confocal raman microspectroscopy. J Biomed Mater Res 59:46–55
36. Marshall GW, Inai N, Magidi ICW, Balooch M, Kinney JH, Tagami J, Marshall SJ (1997) Dentin demineralization: effects of dentin depth, PH and different acids. Dent Mater 13:338–343
37. Pereira PNR, Okuda M, Sano H, Yoshikawa T, Burrow MF, Tagami J (1999) Effect of intrinsic wetness and regional difference on dentin bond strength. Dent Mater 15:46–53
38. Roulet JF (1997) Benefits and disadvantages of tooth-coloured alternatives to amalgam. J Dent 25:459–473
39. Marshall J, GW (1993) Dentin: microstructure and characterization. Quint Int 24:606–617
40. Brannstrom M (1984) Communication between the oral cavity and the dental pulp associated with restorative treatment. Oper Dent 9(57–68)
41. Leinfelder KF (2000) Do restorations made of amalgam outlast those made of resin-based composite? J Am Dent Assoc 131(8):1186–1187
42. Kleverlaan CJ, Feilzer AJ (2005) Polymerization shrinkage and contraction stress of dental resin composites. Dent Mater 21:1150–1157
43. Andersson-Wenckert IE, van Dijken JW, Kieri C (2004) Durability of extensive Class II open-sandwich restorations with a resin-modified glass ionomer cement after 6 years. Am J Dent 17:43–50
44. Spencer P, Ye Q, Park J, Topp EM, Misra A, Marangos O, Wang Y, Bohaty BS, Singh V, Sene F, Eslick J, Camarda K, Katz JL (2010) Adhesive/Dentin interface: the weak link in the composite restoration. Ann Biomed Eng 38(6):1989–2003
45. Burrow MF, Satoh M, Tagami J (1996) Dentin durability after three years using a dentin bonding agent with and without priming. Dent Mater 12:302–307
46. Hashimoto M, Ohno H, Kaga M, Endo K, Sano H, Oguchi H (2000) *In vivo* degradation of resin-dentin bonds in humans over 1 to 3 years. J Dent Res 79:1385–1391
47. Hashimoto M, Ohno H, Sano H, Tay FR, Kaga M, Kudou Y, Oguchi H, Araki Y, Kubota M (2002) Micromorphological changes in resin-dentin bonds after 1 year of water storage. J Biomed Mater Res Appl Biomater 63:306–311
48. Sano H, Yoshikawa T, Pereira PNR, Kanemura N, Morigami M, Tagami J, Pashley DH (1999) Long-term durability of dentin bonds made with a self-etching primer, *in vivo*. J Dent Res 78(4):906–911
49. Spencer P, Swafford JR (1999) Unprotected protein at the dentin-adhesive interface. Quintessence Int 30(7):501–507
50. Spencer P, Wang Y, Walker MP, Wieliczka DM, Swafford JR (2000) Interfacial chemistry of the dentin/adhesive bond. J Dent Res 79(7):1458–1463
51. Wang Y, Spencer P (2005) Continuing etching of an all-in-one adhesive in wet dentin tubules. J Dent Res 84:350–354
52. Spencer P, Katz JL, Tabib-Azar M, Wang Y, Wagh A, Nomura T (2003) Hyperspectral analysis of collagen infused with BisGMA-based polymeric adhesive. In: Lewandrowski KU,

Trantolo DJ, Hasirci V, Yaszemski M, Altobelli DE (eds) Tissue engineering and novel delivery systems. Marcel Decker, New York, pp 599–632
53. Wang Y, Spencer P (2004) Overestimating hybrid layer quality in polished adhesive/dentin interfaces. J Biomed Mater Res 68A:735–746
54. Wang Y, Spencer P (2004) Physicochemical interactions at the interfaces between self-etch adhesive systems and dentin. J Dent 32:567–579
55. Wang Y, Spencer P, Yao X (2006) Micro-raman imaging analysis of monomer/mineral distribution in intertubular region of adhesive/dentin interfaces. J Biomed Optics 11:024005–024001 to 024005–024007
56. Eick JD, Gwinnet AJ, Pashley DH, Robinson SJ (1997) Current concepts on adhesion to dentin. Crit Rev Oral Biol Med 8:306–335
57. Wang Y, Spencer P (2004) Effect of acid etching time and techniques on interfacial characteristics of the adhesive-dentin bond using differential staining. Eur J Oral Sci 112:293–299
58. Eick JD, Cobb CM, Chappell RP, Spencer P, Robinson SJ (1993) The dentinal surface: its influence on dentinal adhesion. Part III. Quintessence Int 24:571–582
59. Pashley DH, Ciucchi B, Sano H, Horner JA (1993) Permeability of dentin to adhesive agents. Quintessence Int 24:618–631
60. Gwinnett AJ (1993) Quantitative contribution of resin infiltration/hybridization to dentin bonding. Am J Dent 6:7–9
61. Tam LE, Pilliar RM (1994) Fracture surface characterization of dentin-bonded interfacial fracture toughness specimens. J Dent Res 73(3):607–619
62. Wieliczka DM, Kruger MB, Spencer P (1997) Raman imaging of dental adhesive diffusion. Appl Spectrosc 51:1593–1596
63. Gwinnett AJ (1994) Dentin bond strength after air drying and rewetting. Am J Dent 7:144–148
64. Gwinnett AJ (1994) Altered tissue contribution to interfacial bond strength with acid conditioned dentin. Am J Dent 7:243–246
65. Gwinnett AJ, Yu S (1995) Effect of long-term water storage on dentin bonding. Am J Dent 8 (2):109–111
66. Kanca J (1992) Improved bond strength through acid etching of dentin and bonding to wet dentin surfaces. J Am Dent Assoc 123:235–243
67. Kinney JH, Balooch M, Marshall SJ, Marshall GW (1993) Atomic force microscope study of dimensional changes in dentine during drying. Arch Oral Biol 38:1003–1007
68. Gwinnett AJ (1994) Chemically conditioned dentin: a comparison of conventional and environmental scanning electron microscopy findings. Dent Mater 10:150–155
69. Pashley EL, Zhang Y, Lockwood PE, Rueggeberg FA, Pashley DH (1998) Effects of HEMA on water evaporation from water-HEMA mixtures. Dent Mater 14(1):6–10
70. Guo X, Spencer P, Wang Y, Ye Q, Yao X, Williams K (2007) Effects of a solubility enhancer on penetration of hydrophobic component in model adhesives into wet demineralized dentin. Dent Mater 23(12):1473–1481
71. Spencer P, Wang Y (2002) Adhesive phase separation at the dentin interface under wet bonding conditions. J Biomed Mater Res 62(3):447–456
72. Wang Y, Spencer P (2003) Hybridization efficiency of the adhesive dentin interface with wet bonding. J Dent Res 82:141–145
73. Ito S, Saito T, Tay FR, Carvalho RM, Yoshiyama M, Pashley DH (2005) Water content and apparent stiffness of non-caries versus caries-affected human dentin. J Biomed Mater Res B Appl Biomater 72(1):109–116
74. Roulet JF, Degrange M (eds) (1999) Adhesion: the silent revolution in dentistry, 1st edn. Quintessence Publishing Co, Inc, Berlin
75. Wang Y, Spencer P (2005) Evaluation of the Interface between one-bottle adhesive systems and dentin by Goldner's Trichrome Stain. Am J Dent 18:66–72
76. Pashley DH (1989) Dentin: a dynamic substrate in dentistry. Scanning Microsc 3:161–176

77. Spencer P, Wang Y, Katz JL, Misra A (2005) Physicochemical interactions at the dentin/adhesive interface using FTIR chemical imaging. J Biomed Opt 10(3):031104
78. Wang Y, Spencer P, Hager C, Bohaty B (2006) Comparison of interfacial characteristics of adhesive bonding to superficial versus deep dentin using SEM and staining techniques. J Dent 34:26–34
79. Wang Y, Spencer P, Yao X, Brenda B (2007) Effect of solvent content on resin hybridization in wet dentin bonding. J Biomed Mater Res A 82(4):975–983
80. Paul SJ, Leach M, Rueggeberg FA, Pashley DH (1999) Effect of water content on the physical properties of model dentine primer and bonding resins. J Dent 27:209–214
81. Ye Q, Park J, Topp E, Spencer P (2009) Effect of photoinitiators on the *in vitro* performance of a dentin adhesive exposed to simulated oral environment. Dent Mater 25(4):452–458
82. Ye Q, Spencer P, Wang Y, Misra A (2007) Relationship of solvent to the photopolymerization process, properties, and structure in model dentin adhesives. J Biomed Mater Res A 80(2):342–350
83. Wang Y, Spencer P, Yao X, Ye Q (2006) Effect of coinitiator and water on the photoreactivity and photopolymerization of HEMA/camphoquinone-based reactant mixtures. J Biomed Mater Res A 78(4):721–728
84. Ye Q, Wang Y, Spencer P (2009) Nanophase separation of polymers exposed to simulated bonding conditions. J Biomed Mater Res B Appl Biomater 88(2):339–348
85. Ye Q, Park J, Pamatmat F, Misra A, Laurence JS, Parthasarathy R, Marangos O, Spencer P (2012) Quantitative analysis of aqueous phase composition of model dentin adhesives experiencing phase separation. J Biomed Mater Res B Appl Biomater 100B:1086–1992
86. Ferracane JL (2006) Hygroscopic and hydrolytic effects in dental polymer networks. Dent Mater 22(3):211–222
87. Tay FR, Gwinnett AJ, Pang KM, Wei SHY (1996) An optical, micromorphological study of surface moisture in the total etched resin-dentin interface. Am J Dent 9:43–48
88. Tay FR, Gwinnett AJ, Wei SHY (1996) The overwet phenomenon: a transmission electron microscopic study of surface moisture in the acid-conditioned, resin-dentin interface. Am J Dent 9:161–166
89. Tay FR, Gwinnett AJ, Wei SHY (1996) Micromophological spectrum from overdrying to overwetting acid-conditioned dentin in water-free, acetone-based, single-bottle primer/adhesives. Dent Mater 12:236–244
90. Tay FR, Pashley DH (2003) Water treeing—a potential mechanism for degradation of dentin adhesives. Am J Dent 16(1):6–12
91. Tay FR, Pashley DH (2003) Have dentin adhesives become too hydrophilic? J Can Dent Assoc 69(11):726–731
92. Nishitani Y, Yoshiyama M, Donnelly AM, Agee KA, Sword J, Tay FR, Pashley DH (2006) Effects of resin hydrophilicity on dentin bond strength. J Dent Res 85(11):1016–1021
93. Breschi L, Mazzoni A, Ruggeri A, Cadenaro M, Di Lenarda R, De Stefano DE (2008) Dental adhesion review: aging and stability of the bonded interface. Dent Mater 24(1):90–101
94. Marangos O, Misra A, Spencer P, Bohaty B, Katz JL (2009) Physico-mechanical properties determination using microscale homotopic measurements: application to sound and caries-affected primary tooth dentin. Acta Biomater 5(4):1338–1348
95. Marangos O, Misra A, Spencer P, Katz JL (2011) Scanning acoustic microscopy investigation of frequency-dependent reflectance of acid- etched human dentin using homotopic measurements. IEEE Trans Ultrason Ferroelectr Freq Control 58(3):585–595
96. Hebling J, Pashley DH, Tjaderhane L, Tay FR (2005) Chlorhexidine arrests subclinical degradation of dentin hydbrid layers *in vivo*. J Dent Res 84(8):741–746
97. Frankenberger R, Pashley DH, Reich SM, Lohbauer U, Petschelt A, Tay FR (2005) Characterisation of resin-dentine interfaces by compressive cyclic loading. Biomaterials 26 (14):2043–2052
98. Okuda M, Pereira PN, Nakajima M, Tagami J, Pashley DH (2002) Long-term durability of resin dentin interface: nanoleakage vs. microtensile bond strength. Oper Dent 27:289–296

99. Yiu CK, King NM, Pashley DH, Suh BI, Carvalho RM, Carrilho MR, Tay FR (2004) Effect of resin hydrophilicity and water storage on resin strength. Biomaterials 25(26):5789–5796
100. Peumans M, Kanumilli P, De Munck J, Van Landuyt K, Lambrechts P, Van Meerbeek B (2005) Clinical effectiveness of contemporary adhesives: a systematic review of current clinical trials. Dent Mater 21(9):864–881
101. Donmez N, Belli S, Pashley DH, Tay FR (2005) Ultrastructural correlates of *in vivo*/*in vitro* bond degradation in self-etch adhesives. J Dent Res 84(4):355–359
102. Sano H (2006) Microtensile testing, nanoleakage, and biodegradation of resin-dentin bonds. J Dent Res 85:11–14
103. Pashley DH, Tay FR, Yiu C, Hashimoto M, Breschi L, Carvalho RM, Ito S (2004) Collagen degradation by host-derived enzymes during aging. J Dent Res 83(3):216–221
104. De Munck J, Van Landuyt K, Peumans M, Poitevin A, Lambrechts P, Braem M, Van Meerbeek B (2005) A critical review of the durability of adhesion to tooth tissue: methods and results. J Dent Res 84(2):118–132
105. Ito S, Hashimoto M, Wadgaonkar B, Svizero N, Carvalho RM, Yiu C et al (2005) Effect of resin hydrophilicity on water sorption and changes in modulus of elasticity. Biomaterials 26:6449–6459
106. Yoshida E, Uno S, Nodasaka Y, Kaga M, Hirano S (2007) Relationship between water status in dentin and interfacial morphology in all-in-one adhesives. Dent Mater 23(5):556–560
107. Finer Y, Jaffer F, Santerre JP (2004) Mutual influence of cholesterol esterase and pseudocholinesterase on the biodegradation of dental composites. Biomaterials 25:1787–1793
108. Finer Y, Santerre JP (2004) The influence of resin chemistry on a dental composite's biodegradation. J Biomed Mater Res 69A:233–246
109. Finer Y, Santerre JP (2004) Salivary esterase activity and its association with the biodegradation of dental composites. J Dent Res 83:22–26
110. Yourtee DM, Smith RE, Russo KA, Burmaster S, Cannon JM, Eick JD, Kostoryz EL (2001) The stability of methacrylate biomaterials when enzyme challenged: kinetic and systematic evaluations. J Biomed Mater Res 57(4):523–531
111. Hagio M, Kawaguchi M, Motokawa W, Mizayaki K (2006) Degradation of methacrylate monomers in human saliva. Dent Mater J 25(2):241–246
112. Munksgaard EC, Freund M (1990) Enzymatic hydrolysis of (di)methacrylates and their polymers. Scand J Dent Res 98:261–267
113. Kugel G, Ferrari M (2000) The science of bonding: from first to sixth generation. JADA 131:20s–25s
114. Wadgaonkar B, Ito S, Svizero N, Elrod D, Foulger S, Rodgers R, Oshida Y, Kirkland K, Sword J, Rueggeberg F, Tay F, Pashley D (2006) Evaluation of the effect of water-uptake on the impedance of dental resins. Biomaterials 27:3287–3294
115. Park JG, Ye Q, Topp EM, Kostoryz EL, Wang Y, Kieweg SL, Spencer P (2008) Preparation and properties of novel dentin adhesives with esterase resistance. J Appl Polymer Sci 107 (6):3588–3597
116. Park JG, Ye Q, Topp EM, Lee CH, Kostoryz EL, Misra A, Spencer P (2009) Dynamic mechanical analysis and esterase degradation of dentin adhesives containing a branched methacrylate. J Biomed Mater Res B Appl Biomater 91(1):61–70
117. Park JG, Ye Q, Topp EM, Spencer P (2009) Enzyme-catalyzed hydrolysis of dentin adhesives containing a new urethane-based trimethacrylate monomer. J Biomed Mater Res B Appl Biomater 91(2):562–571
118. Kostoryz EL, Dharmala K, Ye Q, Wang Y, Huber J, Park JG, Snider G, Katz JL, Spencer P (2009) Enzymatic biodegradation of HEMA/bisGMA adhesives formulated with different water content. J Biomed Mater Res B Appl Biomater 88(2):394–401
119. Finger WJ, Shao B, Hoffmann M, Kanehira M, Endo T, Komatsu M (2007) Does application of phase-separated self-etching adhesives affect bond strength? J Adhes Dent 9(2):169–173
120. Carvalho RM, Chersoni S, Frankenberger R, Pashley DH, Prati C, Tay FR (2005) A challenge to the conventional wisdom that simultaneous etching and resin infiltration always occurs in self-etch adhesives. Biomaterials 26(9):1035–1042

121. Garcia-Godoy F, Tay FR, Pashley DH, Feilzer A, Tjaderhane L, Pashley EL (2007) Degradation of resin-bonded human dentin after 3 years of storage. Am J Dent 20(2):109–113
122. Park JG, Ye Q, Topp EM, Misra A, Spencer P (2009) Water sorption and dynamic mechanical properties of dentin adhesives with a urethane-based multifunctional methacrylate monomer. Dent Mater 25(12):1569–1575
123. Guo X, Wang Y, Spencer P, Ye Q, Yao X (2008) Effects of water content and initiator composition on photopolymerization of a model BisGMA/HEMA resin. Dent Mater 24 (6):824–831
124. Singh V, Misra A, Marangos O, Park J, Ye Q, Kieweg SL, Spencer P (2010) Viscoelastic and fatigue properties of model methacrylate-based dentin adhesives. J Biomed Mater Res B Appl Biomater 95(2):283–290
125. Singh V, Misra A, Marangos O, Park J, Ye Q, Kieweg SL, Spencer P (2011) Fatigue life prediction of dentin-adhesive interface using micromechanical stress analysis. Dent Mater 27 (9):e187–e195
126. Misra A, Spencer P, Marangos O, Wang Y, Katz JL (2005) Parametric study of the effect of phase anisotropy on the micromechanical behavior of dentin/adhesive interfaces. J R Soc Interface 2:145–157
127. Singh V (2009) Viscoelastic and fatigue properties of dental adhesives and their impact on dentin-adhesive interface durability. Master of Science, University of Kansas, Lawrence
128. Misra A, Spencer P, Marangos O, Wang Y, Katz JL (2004) Micromechanical analysis of dentin/adhesive interface using finite element method. J Biomed Mater Res 70B:56–65
129. Staninec M, Kim P, Marshall GW, Ritchie RO, Marshall SJ (2008) Fatigue of dentin-composite interfaces with four-point bend. Dent Mater 24(6):799–803
130. Drummond JL (2008) Degradation, fatigue, and failure of resin dental composite materials. J Dent Res 87(8):710–719
131. Park J, Ye Q, Topp EM, Misra A, Kieweg SL, Spencer P (2010) Effect of photoinitiator system and water content on dynamic mechanical properties of a light-cured bisGMA/HEMA dental resin. J Biomed Mater Res A 93(4):1245–1251
132. Park J, Eslick J, Ye Q, Misra A, Spencer P (2011) The influence of chemical structure on the properties in methacrylate-based dentin adhesives. Dent Mater 27:1086–1093
133. Ye Q, Park J, Laurence JS, Parthasarathy R, Misra A, Spencer P (2011) Ternary phase diagram of model dentin adhesive exposed to over-wet environments. J Dent Res 90(12): 1434–1438
134. Thomas JG, Nakaishi LA (2006) Managing the complexity of a dynamic biofilm. J Am Dent Assoc 137:10S–15S
135. Park J, Ye Q, Spencer P, Laurence JS (2012) Determination of neutralization capacity and stability of a basic methacrylate monomer using NMR. Int J Polymer Mater 61:144–153

Chapter 8
Specific Adhesion of Soft Elastic Materials

Jizeng Wang

8.1 Introduction

Cell adhesion plays a central role in many biological functions, such as cell migration, spreading, differentiation, and growth. The capability to control cell-substrate and cell-cell interactions, for which a quantitative description of cell adhesion is a critical step, is essential for tissue and cellular engineering. A continuum treatment of cell adhesion at the focal adhesion level might be inappropriate, as the typical focal adhesion size is only about ten times larger than molecular bond spacing. Rupture of even one molecular bond may lead to apparent changes in adhesion stress. As a result, the stochastic association/dissociation processes of discrete molecular bonds will significantly influence the strength of a focal adhesion. This adds a new phenomenon of direct relevance to the traditional continuum treatment of elastic adhesion. A key objective of this chapter is to link stochastic theories of ligand-receptor bonds and continuum mechanics descriptions of dissimilar soft elastic materials contacted via specific interactions of molecular bonds. Although overly simplified in a number of aspects, we show in this chapter that such a model seems to give predictions that are consistent with relevant experimental observations on focal adhesion dynamics.

8.2 Facts on Cellular Adhesions

Biological cells actively adhere to their extracellular matrix (ECM) and to other cells through a large variety of ligand-receptor bonds that engage various energy-consuming motor, signaling, and internalization pathways. This adhesion plays a

J. Wang (✉)
Key Laboratory of Mechanics on Disaster and Environment in Western China
Lanzhou University, Lanzhou, Gansu, China
e-mail: jzwang@lzu.edu.cn

S. Thomopoulos et al. (eds.), *Structural Interfaces and Attachments in Biology*,
DOI 10.1007/978-1-4614-3317-0_8,

critical role in cell migration, spreading, differentiation, growth, motility, apoptosis, and tissue formation [1]. Cells adhere to substrates through the formation of focal complexes (FXs), focal adhesions (FAs), and related ECM adhesions. The FXs are small, dot-like, clusters of ligand-receptor bonds that can further develop into FAs, which are micron-sized, complex multi-molecular assemblies linked on one side to the ECM via membrane-bound receptors and on the other side to actin stress fibers in the cytoskeleton. FAs can be dissociated when strong mechanical forces are applied. Importantly, recent experiments also show that cells use mechanical force as a signal to strengthen initial integrin-ECM adhesions into FXs [2]. The FXs are usually continuously formed and turned over under the protruding lamellipodia [3], which may or may not further develop into mature FAs. The size, assembly, and stability of FAs depend on the mechanical forces applied to them [4–6], as well as to the mechanical properties of the ECM [7, 8] and actin cytoskeleton [9]. A typical cell will attach and apply traction forces to the ECM [10] via myosin II motor proteins on the actin filament system that link directly to adhesion sites. Inhibition of myosin II leads to accumulation of immature FXs and to the disappearance of mature FAs [6, 11–14], while activation of myosin II induces FA assembly [15–17]. On the other hand, application of external forces to FAs is found to stimulate their growth in the direction of the force even when myosin II activity is suppressed [18]. Therefore, irrespective of their origin, mechanical forces seem to play a key role in the growth and stability of FAs.

The size of mature FAs on hard substrates can reversibly increase or decrease in response to the applied force, with stress maintained near a constant value of ~5.5 kPa independent of cell type [19] but dependent upon matrix stiffness. Force affects FA dynamics most strongly when the substrate is sufficiently stiff; large FAs cannot be formed on very soft substrates [7, 20, 21]. Traction forces transmitted through focal adhesions generate significant substrate displacements when the substrate is compliant, and various gel systems have emerged that allow not only quantitative study of the tractions but also reveal wide-ranging and surprising biological effects of matrix elasticity, not only on motility and proliferation, but even on stem cell differentiation [22].

Details about these mechanical, chemical, and biological interactions in single cells and biomolecules remain elusive [23]. Despite many fascinating studies on cell adhesion, there is still no theoretical framework to understand the different experimental observations and complex interplay between the physical properties of the cell's environment, including the role of matrix properties, in directing the cell's behavior. Consequently, our understanding of the mechanics of cell adhesion is still quite fragmented in terms of theoretical models. It will be challenging to develop theoretical models that explain experimental observations about the effects of cellular contractile or applied forces, substrate stiffness, and adhesion size on the stability and growth/shrinkage of FAs as well as other adhesion assemblies.

8.3 Modeling Strategy

Like most engineering materials, cells deform when subjected to external forces, and focal adhesions (FAs) can be dissociated when strong mechanical forces are applied. However, does cell adhesion behave like a continuous or discrete multi-scale-system? Or, should cell adhesion be modeled mechanically as a continuum or a discrete multi-scale system? It may seem contradictive, but the answer largely depends on the relevant biological tissues and scales involved. The underlying assumption for treating a material as a continuum is that the smallest dimension to be considered is much larger than the space over which structures and properties may vary significantly. In biological cells, adhesion is mediated by the formation and rupture of specific molecular bonds between ligands and receptors. As the typical FA size is only about ten times larger than the bond spacing, the random association/dissociation processes of these discrete binder molecules may significantly change the distribution of adhesion stress and adhesion strength. This effect reflects the coupling between the elastic deformation of the cell-ECM system and the variance of bond number, adding a new phenomenon of direct relevance to either the continuum or pure stochastic treatment of adhesion.

We recall the continuum modeling of adhesion between elastic media, which has been an active research topic in contact mechanics for a few decades. For the adhesive contacts of elastic spheres, the JKR [24] and DMT [25] models are very useful in modeling the adhesive contact at two opposite extremes, whether surface forces are short-ranged compared to resulting elastic deformations [26]. The Maugis–Dugdale model [27], which is based on a cohesive description of the surface forces, describes the transition between the JKR and DMT theories.

To maintain a stable adhesion state, one usually needs to know the strength of a particular adhesion between two elastic media. In the case of a pulling load applied to the adhered elastic bodies (Fig. 8.1), a stress concentration is expected to occur at the edge of the contacting region. An increase of the load then enlarges the intensity of stress concentration and eventually drives the edge cracks to propagate and break the joint. In this case, the carrying capacity of the joint is not used most efficiently because only a small fraction of material is highly stressed at any instant of loading, and failure occurs by incremental crack propagation. The maximum strength should correspond to an optimal adhesion state that at pull-off, the interfacial stress is uniformly distributed over the contact region with a magnitude equal to the theoretical adhesion strength. Gao and Yao [28] suggest that a robust, shape-insensitive optimal adhesion becomes possible only when the adhesion size is small enough. Below a critical structural size, the material fails no longer by propagation of a pre-existing crack, but by uniform rupture at the limiting strength of the binding molecules.

At the other extreme, from a statistical mechanics point of view, a single molecular bond has only a finite lifetime. The time scale associated with individual association/dissociation events takes minutes under small stretching forces, e.g., below 5 pN for biotin-streptavidin bonds [29, 30]. Recent single molecule

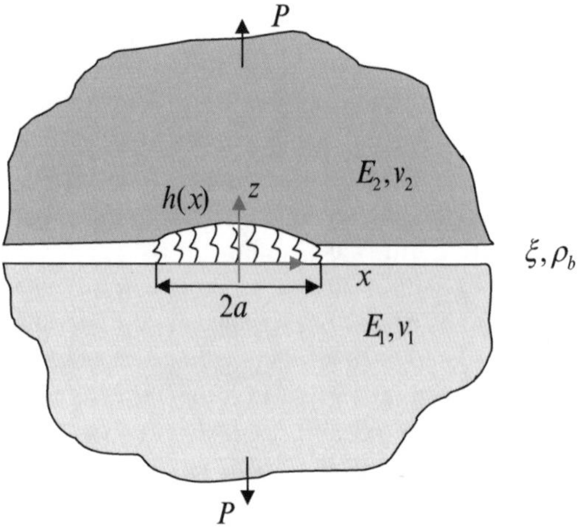

Fig. 8.1 Model of an adhesive patch of molecular bonds between two elastic bodies subject to an applied tensile load

experiments for activated $\alpha_5\beta_1$-integrin binding to fibronectin under low loading rates have indicated that the characteristic time scale for ligand-receptor binding/dissociation is on the order of 100 s (e.g., Li et al. [31]). Although a single bond has only a limited lifetime, a cluster of bonds can survive for much longer due to collective effects in a stochastic ensemble. A common assumption of the existing models on molecular cluster adhesion is equally sharing of applied load among all closed bonds. Based on this assumption, Erdmann and Schwarz [32] predict that the cluster lifetime monotonically increases as the cluster size grows: the larger the cluster, the more stable it is. When the cluster becomes large enough, constant adhesion strength will be reached. This finding is similar to FXs that are subject to frequent turnover, and large clusters tend to have a much longer lifetime similar to FAs.

It seems that the theories of classical contact mechanics and molecular clusters suggest two opposite tendencies for the adhesion strength as a function of adhesion size. In cell adhesion, both the cell and ECM can be regarded as elastic media in a relative limited time scale, while the molecular bonds are subject to frequent rupture and rebinding. Such a system couples the elastic deformation of contacting media and stochastic processes of binder molecules. It is expected that the optimal strength will be achieved at a finite size. As an implication, experimental observations have shown in general that focal adhesion size is limited to around a few microns [33].

In order to provide unification of the elasticity description of adhesive contact at large scales and the statistical description of single-bond behavior at small scales, we developed an idealized model [34–41] of an adhesive patch of molecular bonds between two elastic bodies subject to an applied tensile load to realize the coupling between elasticity of the adhesion system and statistical behaviors of molecular bonds. In this model, one side of the adhesion is an elastic medium and can be viewed as the body of a cell (actin cytoskeleton), and the other side is an elastic substrate with a surface profile $h(x)$ representing ECM. The Young's modulus and Poisson's ratio are E_1, ν_1 for the cell body and E_2, ν_2 for the substrate. Following the convention in contact mechanics, we define a reduced modulus E^* such that $1/E^* = (1-\nu_1^2)/E_1 + (1-\nu_2^2)/E_2$. The distribution of interfacial stress is governed by classical elasticity equations in contact mechanics while the rupture and rebinding of molecular bonds obey stochastic equations in molecular mechanics. The effects of elastic moduli, adhesion size, and bond rebinding rate on the cluster lifetime and strength can be studied in the presence of strongly non-uniform distribution of interfacial stress.

8.4 Adhesion of Rigid Media

For a limiting case, adhesion of rigid media via ligand-receptor bonds has been well studied [32], in which case molecular bonds are uniformly loaded. Note that the bond breaking/reforming are discrete Markov events; we have the one-step master equation for the number of closed bonds n as [42, 43]

$$\mathrm{d}p_n/\mathrm{d}t = g_{n-1}p_{n-1} + r_{n+1}p_{n+1} - (r_n + g_n)p_n \tag{8.1}$$

where $p_n(t)$ represents the probability that n bonds are closed at time t, and r_n and g_n are the dissociation and association rates, respectively. A quantity of large interest is the average property of closed bonds. Define the kth moment as

$$<n^k> = \sum_{n=0}^{N_t} n^k p_n(t) \tag{8.2}$$

For the average number of the bonds $<n>$, if we multiply the master equation by n and sum both sides over n, we can obtain [44, 45],

$$\frac{\mathrm{d}}{\mathrm{d}t}<n> = <g_n> - <r_n> \tag{8.3}$$

As r_n is usually a nonlinear function of n, the deterministic equation of $<n>$ is usually achieved by approximately expanding $<r_n>$ around $n = <n>$. For example, a first order approximation can lead to the Bell equation [32]

$$d<n>/\mathrm{d}t = k_0\gamma(N_t - <n>) - k_0<n>\exp(P/<n>F_\mathrm{b}) \tag{8.4}$$

where $r_n = k_0 n \exp(P/nF_\mathrm{b})$, $g_n = k_0\gamma(N_t - n)$, N_t is the total bond number, P/n is the force applied to each bond, and k_0 and F_b are the rate and force constants, respectively.

In the stochastic description of cluster adhesion, cluster lifetime can be identified by the time at which the last bond ruptures. This is exactly the concept of mean first passage time from an initial state with number of closed bonds $n = N_t$ to the state without closed bonds, $n = 0$. Analytical solutions of mean first passage time for different boundaries are available in Honerkamp's book [42]. On the other hand, numerical results can be obtained by Monte Carlo stochastic simulations as demonstrated by Erdmann and Schwarz [32] for the bond clusters with equally shared loading. In detail, for each set of parameter values of N_t, r_n, and g_n, they compute many different trajectories. Thus, averaging for given time t over the different simulation trajectories yields the desired results. Following this analysis, Erdmann and Schwarz [32] have demonstrated that, under a given value of the applied force, there exists a critical cluster size beyond which the system behaves like a macroscopic adhesion patch with a much-prolonged lifetime; below this critical size, the cluster behaves as a single molecular bond with a finite lifetime for a given force.

8.5 Adhesion of Elastic Media

8.5.1 Interfacial Bond Distribution

The uniform distribution of adhesion molecules along the adhesion interface is intrinsically unstable. In order to answer why molecular bonds need to be clustered to stabilize the cellular adhesion, we consider an elasticity-diffusion description of the adhesion system, which consists of two elastic half-spaces, each covered with a lipid membrane, joined together by mobile molecular bonds that diffuse, along with unbonded binder molecules, in the interface under the combined action of a layer of glycocalyx repellers and an applied stress. We assume that ρ_{t} is the total number of available molecular sites per unit area, which is distributed among ρ_{b} of closed bonds, ρ_{L} of free ligands, ρ_{R} of free receptors, and $\rho_{\mathrm{t}} - \rho_{\mathrm{b}} - \rho_{\mathrm{L}} - \rho_{\mathrm{R}}$ of empty sites. The glycocalyx repellers are assumed to be immobile with a constant area density equal to ρ_{g}.

As the characteristic time scale for certain ligand-receptor binding/dissociation can be on the order of 100 s [31], which is two orders of magnitude larger than that of protein molecules in a lipid membrane to diffuse a distance on the order of 1 μm by Brownian motion [44–46], we assume that the total number of ligand-receptor bonds remains constant in the analysis of bond clustering due to diffusion.

We induce small perturbations to the densities of molecular bonds and free binders [41], which cause non-uniform elastic deformation in the two elastic solids. The perturbation-induced energy change of the system per unit area of interface consists of three terms: the strain energy in the two solids and two membranes, the binding energy in the stressed molecular bonds and repeller molecules, and the change in configurational entropy due to the molecular density perturbations. We have derived this change of total free energy per unit area of interface energy as [41]

$$G = \rho_{b\varepsilon}^2 \frac{\xi_b^2 (h_0 - l_b)^2}{4(\rho_0 \xi_b + \rho_g \xi_g)} \left(\beta - \frac{\lambda^7 \lambda_1 + 2\lambda^4 \lambda_2^4}{\lambda^7 \lambda_1 + \lambda^6 \lambda_0 \lambda_1 + 2\lambda^4 \lambda_2^4 + \lambda^3 \lambda_1 \lambda_2^4 + \lambda_2^8} \right) \tag{8.5}$$

where $\lambda_0 = \pi E^*/(\rho_0 \xi_b + \rho_g \xi_g)$, $\lambda_1 = \lambda_0 [E_1/(1 - v_1^2) + E_2/(1 - v_2^2)]/E^*$, $\lambda_2 = 2\pi (\lambda_0 \kappa / \pi E^*)^{1/4}$, $\beta = \pi k_B T \rho_t E^* / [\lambda_0 \xi_b^2 \rho_0 (h_0 - l_b)^2 (\rho_t - \rho_0)]$, ξ_b and ξ_g the spring constants of molecular bonds and glycocalyx repellers, κ the membrane-bending stiffness, $h_0 - l_b$ the bond deformation, and $\rho_{b\varepsilon}$ the perturbation amplitude of bond density. Equation (8.5) can be used to investigate the stability of the reference state of homogeneous bond distribution. For a given perturbation wavelength, a negative free energy change, i.e., $G < 0$, will imply that the reference state is unstable with respect to this wavelength of perturbation.

In the case that deformation energy of the membrane is neglected, in which case $\kappa = 0$ and $\lambda_2 = 0$, then $G > 0$ gives

$$\frac{\lambda_0}{\lambda_0 + \lambda} - 1 + \beta > 0 \tag{8.6}$$

Since λ is positive, this condition is satisfied for all perturbation wavelengths if $\beta \geq 1$, implying that the homogeneous bond distribution is stable. If $1 > \beta > 0$, the reference state is stable against perturbations with small wavelengths but unstable against those with wavelengths exceeding a critical value given by $\lambda_c = \lambda_0 \beta / (1 - \beta)$. In the absence of an applied stress, the condition $1 > \beta > 0$ is valid for bond density values in the range determined through

$$\frac{(\rho_0 \xi_b + \rho_g \xi_g)^3}{\rho_0 (\rho_t - \rho_0)} < \frac{\rho_g^2 \xi_b^2 \xi_g^2 (l_b - l_g)^2}{k_B T \rho_t} \tag{8.7}$$

The elastic deformation energies in the bulk and membrane always tend to destabilize while the configurational entropy always favors a uniform bond distribution. For $1 > \beta > 0$, the perturbation-induced change in elastic energies is large enough to overcome the entropic change, in which case bond clustering results in a net decrease in free energy.

In living cells, the density of glycocalyx molecules with a typical equilibrium length between 10 and 30 nm [47], a persistence length p about 0.6 nm and a contour length from 0.4 to 1.6 μm [48], is on the order of ~$10^4/\mu m^2$ [49]. The spring constant of a flexible polymer can be estimated as $3k_B T/2$ pL [50], which predicts $\xi_g = 0.01$ pN/nm for glycocalyx, if the contour length L of the glycocalyx molecules is taken to be 1 μm. A typical ligand-receptor bond, the integrin-fibronectin pair, has a spring constant of $\xi_b = 0.25$ pN/nm and an equilibrium

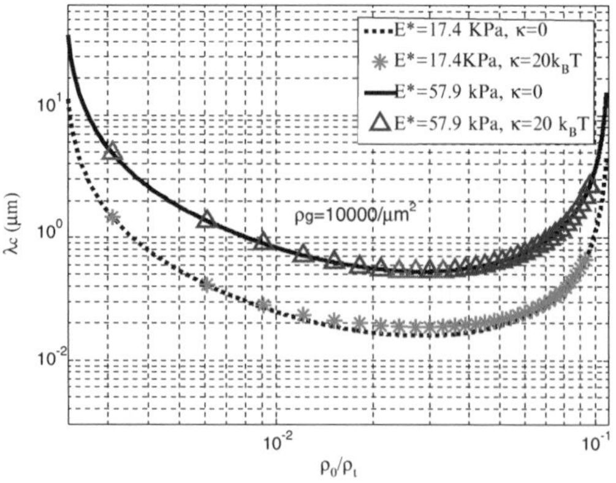

Fig. 8.2 The critical perturbation wavelength, λ_c, as a function of ρ_0/ρ_t. Other parameter choices: $E_1 = E_2$, $\xi_g = 0.01$ pN/nm, $\xi_b = 0.25$ pN/nm, $v_1 = v_2 = 0.37$, $\rho_t = 10000/\ \mu m^2$, $l_b = 11$ nm, $l_g = 30$ nm, $T = 300$ K

length about 11 nm [51]. The Young's modulus of cells has been reported between 4 and 230 kPa [52] and Poisson's ratio around 0.36–0.38 [53].

We have demonstrated in [41] that the condition $0<\beta<1$ is satisfied if the number of receptors in cell membrane as observed in experiments is 50–500/μm^2 [54–56], corresponding to the range of relative bond density of 0.01–0.1 in which clustering instability occurs. For this range of ρ_0/ρ_t values, Fig. 8.2 plots the critical wavelength λ_c as a function of the relative bond density ρ_0/ρ_t for different values of Young's modulus with or without including the membrane deformation, i.e., $\kappa = 0$ or $\kappa = 20\,k_B T$. Figure 8.2 shows that, for bond density values in the instability range, the critical wavelength is generally on the order of 1 μm for realistic values of cell modulus. This length scale is in broad agreement with experimentally observed adhesion plaques in cell adhesion [57].

8.5.2 Stochastic-Elasticity Coupling

Consider the adhesion of molecular bonds grouped in an adhesion cluster of size $2a$ between two dissimilar elastic media subjected to a tensile force P, as shown in Fig. 8.1. We focus on the situation that interfacial adhesion arises solely from the ligand-receptor bonds which are assumed to have a finite stiffness ξ and can statistically transit between open and closed states, as described by Bell [58]. For simplicity, we consider a slice of the system with out-of-plane thickness b, corresponding to the so-called plane-strain problem in elasticity. Within each cluster, individual molecular bonds are periodically distributed at a spacing of b, corresponding to a bond density of $\rho_0 = 1/b^2$ and a total number of $N_t = 2a/b$. The normal interfacial traction, $\sigma(x)$, is related to the surface separation u as $\sigma(x) = \rho_b\, \xi u$. Using the elastic Green's functions for semi-infinite media [59], it can be shown that u obeys the following integral equations [35]

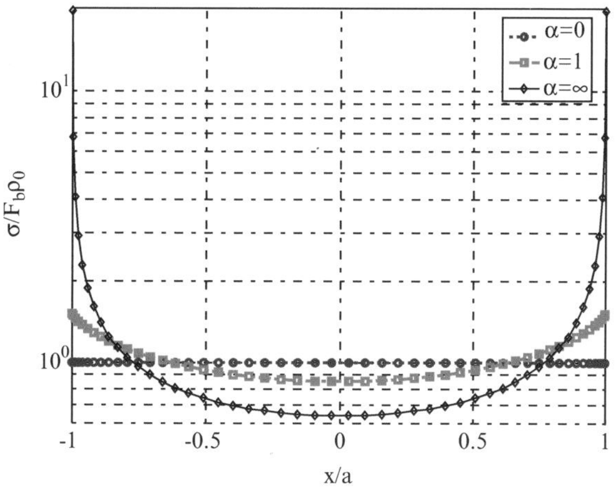

Fig. 8.3 Normalized interfacial traction distribution for different values of the stress concentration index (SCI) for an adhesion patch with all bonds closed. The normalized pulling force $P/aF_b\rho_0 = 2$

$$\frac{\partial \hat{u}}{\partial r} = -\frac{2\alpha}{\pi}\int_{-1}^{1}\frac{\hat{\rho}\hat{u}}{r-s}\mathrm{d}s \tag{8.8}$$

where $\hat{u} = u\xi/F_b$, $r = x/a$, $\hat{\rho} = \rho_b/\rho_0$, $\hat{\sigma} = \sigma/\xi F_b\rho_0 = \hat{\rho}\hat{u}$, and

$$\alpha = \frac{a\rho_0\xi}{E^*} \tag{8.9}$$

The effect of α can be immediately understood from the solutions to (8.8) in extreme cases. In the limit $\alpha \to 0$, the solution is $\sigma(x) = \text{constant}$ for a constant bond distribution within the adhesion domain $-a \le x \le a$, indicating a uniform distribution of interfacial traction independent of the bond location x. In this limit, the interfacial traction is equally shared among all bonds. In the opposite limit when $\alpha \to \infty$, the solution to (8.8) becomes

$$\sigma(x) = \frac{P}{\pi a}\frac{1}{\sqrt{1 - x^2/a^2}} \tag{8.10}$$

This is the classical singular solution for a 2D external crack [60]. For the intermediate range $0<\alpha<\infty$, the maximum traction generally occurs at the edge of adhesion and the minimum at the center. In the case that $\rho_b = \rho_0$, Fig. 8.3 shows that the interfacial traction is nearly uniform for small α values, while crack-like stress concentration emerges near the adhesion edge for large α. Therefore, we refer to α as the stress concentration index (SCI) [40]. Equation (8.9) shows that α is linearly proportional to the adhesion size, the bond density, and stiffness and inversely proportional to the reduced elastic modulus of cell and substrate. All these factors play a role in controlling the distribution of interfacial traction within the adhesion domain. In particular, we note that the stiffness of both cell and substrate needs to be sufficiently large in order to keep α small.

For any instantaneous bond configuration during the stochastic process of bond breaking/reforming, one can determine the interfacial traction using the appropriate elastic Green's functions [59]. The force acting on each closed bond and surface separation at each open bond are critical factors to determine the bond reaction rates at any instant. We consider a cluster with all bonds closed initially. The bonds undergo stochastic breaking or rebinding described by the master equation (8.1). If all of the n closed bonds equally share the total applied load P, then $r_n = ne^{P/n}$ and $g_n = \gamma(N_t - n)$. However, elastic deformation of the system makes the load P to be shared non-uniformly among closed bonds, the total dissociation rate becomes

$$r_n = \sum_{i=1}^{n} \mathrm{e}^{P_i}, \quad \sum_{i=1}^{n} P_i = P \tag{8.11}$$

Thus, the behavior of stochastic-elasticity coupling of the adhesion system can be governed by (8.1), (8.8), and (8.11). Monte Carlo simulations have been conducted by Qian et al. [36, 40] to solve these equations, where each bond location x_i is considered as an independent reaction site where the next event will be bond rupture at rate $k_{\mathrm{off}}(x_i) = r_n/k_0$ if the bond is currently closed, and bond rebinding at rate $k_{\mathrm{on}}(x_i) = g_n/k_0$ if the bond is currently open. The reaction rates, $k_{\mathrm{on}}(x_i)$ and $k_{\mathrm{off}}(x_i)$, are computed from the elastic solution of forces at closed bonds and surface separations at open bonds. The so-called first reaction method of Gillespie's algorithm is used in the simulations [36, 40]. When the binding state of any bond (open vs. closed) has undergone a change, an update of the force and surface separation at all bonds is re-calculated using the associated elastic Green's function, and the results are used to determine the next reaction events. This coupling between elasticity and stochastic events starts at an initial state when all bonds are assumed to be closed and the process proceeds until all bonds within the adhesion domain become open. The total elapsed time t is recorded as the lifetime of the cluster.

Figure 8.4 shows the normalized lifetime of the cluster as a function of the cluster size for different values of the reduced elastic modulus E^* and rebinding rate γ. The simulation results indicate that a size-window exists for stable adhesion. In all cases, the traction distribution along the adhesion interface is non-uniform and the failure becomes increasingly crack-like at increasing cluster size. Very small clusters resemble single molecule behavior with limited lifetime and large clusters fail by severe stress concentration near the adhesion edge. Increasing the reduced elastic modulus tends to stabilize and strengthen the adhesion by alleviating stress concentration within the FAs domain. We observe that the size-window of stable adhesion shifts and broadens as the cell and substrate stiffen, which can be understood from the point of view that large values of E^* decrease the SCI toward the regime of uniform interfacial traction. The concept of a size-window for stable adhesion should be a general feature of molecular adhesion

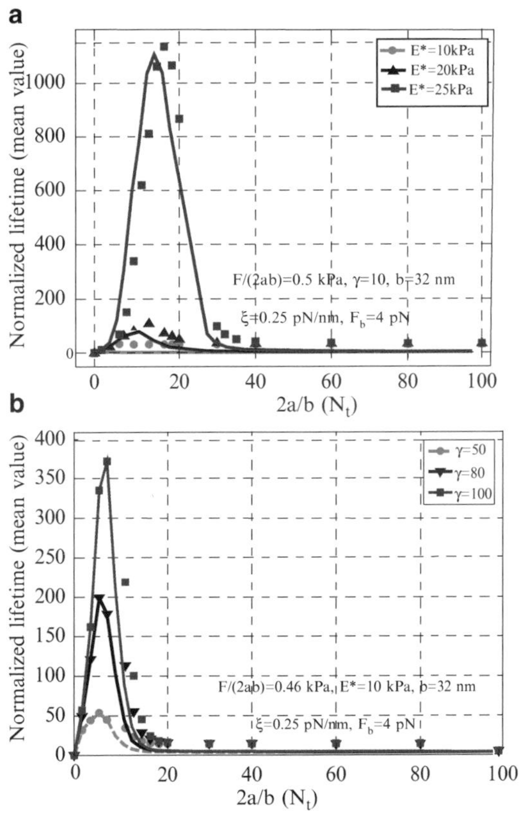

Fig. 8.4 The normalized lifetime of the adhesion cluster as a function of the cluster size N_t for different values of: (**a**) the reduced elastic modulus E^*, and (**b**) the rebinding rate γ

clusters between elastic media because stochastic effects are expected to dominate at small scales and crack-like failure dominates at large scales. Increasing adhesion size or decreasing material modulus tends to increase α toward the regime of crack-like stress concentration, hence reducing the lifetime and stability of adhesion.

8.5.3 Critical Bond Spacing for Stable Adhesion

An interesting phenomenon on receptor-independent adhesion has been reported by Spatz and co-workers [61, 62]. They showed that stable FAs on substrates prepared with precisely controlled ligand distribution can be formed only if the ligand spacing is below 58 nm and no adhesion is possible for ligand spacing above 73 nm, and that these critical spacings seem to be insensitive to cell types [61]. A feasible explanation of this phenomenon has been provided by Lin et al. [63] by considering the competition between thermal fluctuations of cell membranes and ligand-receptor binding. However, as it has been experimentally confirmed that cell adhesion can be significantly influenced by glycocalyx [64–66], we hypothesize that cell surface repellers such as glycocalyx may also play a role in the phenomenon of critical bond spacing. To address this issue, we considered an alternative model of cell adhesion via opposing forces induced by polymer repellers and ligand-receptor bonds, where we treat repellers and binders as worm-like chains confined in a nanoslit in which ligand-receptor bonds transition stochastically between open and closed states.

When a free polymer chain of contour length L, persistence length p, and mean-squared radius of gyration R_g^2 [67] to be confined inside a nanoslit of separation h, a force f will be imposed on the opposing parallel walls. This force can be derived based on the free energy expression given by Chen and Sullivan [68], which appears as a repulsive force when $h \ll L$.

In the case that the two ends of the polymer chain are tethered to the opposing walls of the slit, the effect of end tethering is expected to be small for $h \rightarrow 0$. In the opposite limit of $h \rightarrow L$, the chain becomes strongly stretched, and its force-separation relationship can be given by the classical Marko and Siggia formula [69]. For the intermediate range $0 < h < L$, we propose an interpolating formula on the force-separation relation [39]:

$$f(h,p,L) = \frac{k_B T}{p}\left[\frac{1}{4(1-h/L)^2} - \frac{1}{4} - \frac{h}{2L}\right] - \pi^2 R_g^2 k_B T \times \frac{2 + c_1(p/h) + c_2(p/h)^2}{6h^3[1 + c_3(p/h) + c_4(p/h)^2]^{5/3}} \tag{8.12}$$

It can be easily verified that (8.12) matches the above-mentioned two limiting cases of $h \rightarrow 0$ and $h \rightarrow L$.

Similar to the model as shown in Fig. 8.1, we consider the molecular adhesion mediated by polymer repellers of density ρ_g and binders of density ρ_0, among which ρ_b of them are actually closed. We adopt a rebinding rate per unit area of $g = k_0\gamma(\rho_0 - \rho_b)$. Thus, (8.4) at steady state can be changed into

$$\gamma(\rho_0 - \rho_b) = e^{f(h_{eq},L,p)/F_b}\rho_b \tag{8.13}$$

On the other hand, the stability of adhesion is considered as a competition between attractive interactions of ligand-receptor binding and repulsive forces due to the size mismatch between repellers and binders. According to (8.12), the repulsive stress of polymer repellers and the attractive stress of the molecular bonds can be expressed as $\sigma_g = \rho_g f(h_{eq}, p_g, L_g)$ and $\sigma_b = \rho_b f(h_{eq}, p_b, L_b)$, which must balance, i.e.,

$$\sigma_b = \sigma_g \tag{8.14}$$

From this relation, we can calculate the equilibrium density of closed ligand-receptor bonds.

In cell adhesion, a common type of polymer repellers is glycocalyx, one kind of which has the contour length around 1 μm, and the number density $\rho_g = 3000/\ \mu m^2$. For typical values, we take $p_g/L_b = 1/100$, $L_g/L_b = 5$, $\gamma = 1$, and $F_b = 4$ pN in numerically solving (8.13) and (8.14). For a typical ligand-receptor pair, we consider binding between activated $\alpha_5\beta_1$ integrin to fibronectin, for which recent single molecule experiments have shown parameter values of $k_0 = 0.012$ Hz and $F_b \approx 9$ pN, corresponding to a binding energy about $24k_BT$. The rebinding rate thus can be estimated to be ~$\gamma = 0.2$. Using these parameters, Wang et al. [39] have shown that there exists a critical initial bond density of 288/μm^2, corresponding to a critical ligand spacing about 59 nm, which is very close to the experimentally observed critical spacing [61, 62]. These results indicate that polymer repellers can play a significant role in the stability of cell adhesion and their effect can potentially explain the phenomenon of critical ligand spacing in cell adhesion. In contrast to the membrane fluctuation model of Lin et al. [63], the present model focused on the critical conditions under which molecular adhesion can be stabilized against the nonspecific repulsive forces of glycocalyx. It seems that both the membrane fluctuation model of Lin et al. [63] and the present model can quantitatively explain the observed critical ligand spacing, indicating considerable uncertainties in model building as well as parameter selections in this area of research.

8.5.4 Effects of Surface Topography

Cell adhesion involves coordinated actions of many biological molecules [70, 71], and topographic features of these molecules may influence the attachment and adhesion of mammalian cells [72]. On the other hand, adhesion strength and alignment of cells can also be affected by nano-patterning and surface roughness of substrates as experimentally demonstrated in [73–75].

For nonspecific adhesion of materials, to maintain stable adhesion, one usually needs to determine the strength of a particular configuration of adhesive contact. In the case of a pulling force applied on two adhered elastic bodies, a stress concentration is expected to occur near the edge of the contact region. Usually, increasing the load enlarges the intensity of the stress concentration, eventually driving crack propagation at the edge to break the joint. In this case, the carrying capacity of the joint is not used most efficiently because only a small fraction of material is highly stressed at any instant of loading, and failure occurs by incremental crack propagation. The maximum strength should correspond to an optimal adhesion state in which the interfacial stress is uniformly distributed over the contact region, with magnitude equal to the theoretical adhesion strength at pull-off. Gao and Yao [28] suggest that such optimal adhesion can be achieved by either size reduction, or by optimization of the shape of the contact surfaces. For macroscopic adhesion, the state of optimal adhesion achieved by change in contact shape is not robust against small deviations from the optimal shape. A robust, shape-insensitive optimal adhesion becomes possible only when the adhesion size is small enough. In this case, the material fails no longer by propagation of a pre-existing crack, but by uniform rupture at the limiting strength of the binding molecules.

Different from the adhesion of materials through nonspecific interactions such as van der Waals forces, cells adhere on substrates through the formation of noncovalent bonds between ligand and receptor molecules on opposing surfaces. In cell adhesion, both cells and the ECM can be regarded as soft elastic materials (within a certain time scale) joined by binding molecules subject to frequent rupture and rebinding. Here, we use the analytical model of stochastic-elastic coupling, as shown in Fig. 8.1, to investigate how the adhesion strength between two soft elastic materials depends on the size of bond clusters and the shape of the contact surfaces, where only specific adhesion via ligand-receptor linkages is considered, and secondary nonspecific interactions such as van der Waals forces are neglected.

Taking into account the surface shape, $h(x)$, similar to (8.8), we have

$$\frac{\partial \hat{u}}{\partial r} = -\frac{2\alpha}{\pi}\int_{-1}^{1}\frac{\hat{\rho}\hat{u}}{r-s}\mathrm{d}s + \beta\alpha\frac{\mathrm{d}\hat{h}}{\mathrm{d}r} \tag{8.15}$$

where, in addition to (8.8), we denote $\hat{h} = h/a, \beta = E^*/\rho_0 F_\mathrm{b}$.

By adopting a rebinding rate of exponential type,

$$g(\tau) = k_0\gamma[\rho_0 - \rho_\mathrm{b}(x,\tau)]\exp\left(-\eta\frac{\xi u^2}{2k_\mathrm{B}T}\right) \tag{8.16}$$

where η is a dimensionless parameter characterizing how strong the rebinding rate depends on the separation between a pair of open bonds, based on (8.3), we can derive

$$\frac{\mathrm{d}\hat{\rho}}{\mathrm{d}\tau} = -\hat{\rho}\exp(\hat{u}) + \gamma(1-\hat{\rho})\exp(-\lambda\hat{u}^2) \tag{8.17}$$

where $\lambda = \eta F_\mathrm{b}^2/2k_\mathrm{B}T\xi$.

At steady state, in the case of $\hat{h} = 0$ and $\alpha \to \infty$, it follows from (8.10) that the stress field near the edge of the contact area, $x \to \pm a$, has a square-root singularity with stress intensity factor $K_\mathrm{I} = P/\sqrt{\pi a}$. The critical condition for crack initiation at the adhesion edge is governed by the Griffith condition $G = 2\gamma_\mathrm{ad}$, where γ_ad is the fracture surface energy and G is the energy release rate, $G = 2K_\mathrm{I}^2/E^* = 2P^2/\pi a E^*$. At the critical point of onset of crack motion, the energy released per unit area of crack growth must be equal to the energy associated with interfacial debonding. For adhesive contact problems, the Griffith condition is often written as $G \geq W_\mathrm{ad}$, where W_ad is the work of adhesion, and the critical pull-off stress can be determined as

$$\sigma_\mathrm{Griffith} = \frac{P_\mathrm{Pull-off}}{2a} = \sqrt{\frac{\pi E^* W_\mathrm{ad}}{8a}} \tag{8.18}$$

For adhesion via molecular bonds, the work of adhesion can be estimated as

$$W_{\mathrm{ad}} \sim \rho_0\left(\frac{1}{2}\xi u_{\max}^2\right) \sim \rho_0\left[\frac{1}{2}\xi\left(\frac{F_{\mathrm{b}}}{\xi}\right)^2\right] = \frac{\rho_0 F_{\mathrm{b}}^2}{2\xi} \tag{8.19}$$

where $u_{\max}$ is the maximum deformation allowed for each bond, and F_{b}/ξ is the typical length scale of bond deformation. From (8.18) and (8.19), we can estimate the dimensionless pull-off stress as

$$\frac{\sigma_{\mathrm{Griffith}}}{\rho_0 F_{\mathrm{b}}} = C_{\mathrm{G}}\frac{\sqrt{\pi}}{4}\sqrt{\frac{E^*}{\rho_0\xi a}} \tag{8.20}$$

It follows from (8.20) that the pull-off stress is proportional to $1/\sqrt{a}$. As the adhesion size a is reduced, (8.20) predicts an increasing pull-off stress, approaching infinity as a goes to zero. However, this trend cannot continue forever, since stress cannot exceed the strength of molecular adhesion. This suggests a critical adhesion size below which adhesion strength can no longer be described by the Griffith theory. Similar arguments of transition between Griffith fracture and failure at theoretical strength have been made for mineral pieces in bone [76] and fibrillar adhesion in gecko [28].

On the other hand, the strength of molecular adhesion can be estimated as

$$\frac{\sigma_{\mathrm{Bell}}}{\rho_0 F_{\mathrm{b}}} = C_{\mathrm{B}}\frac{\gamma}{1+\gamma} \tag{8.21}$$

where C_{B} is a prefactor. Thus a critical adhesion size can be identified by equating the adhesion strengths in both Griffith and Bell regimes as $a_{\mathrm{cr}} \sim E^*/\rho_0\xi$ or $\alpha_{\mathrm{cr}} \sim 1$.

Here, we use the coupled elastic-stochastic model to investigate whether the continuum theory based on the Griffith concept is applicable in the case of molecular adhesion. The normalized pull-off stress is plotted as a function of the normalized cluster size or SCI in Fig. 8.5 for a rebinding rate of $\gamma = 2$. In the plot, we include the predictions of Griffith's theory and Bell's theory by using (8.20) and (8.21) with pre-factors $C_{\mathrm{G}} = 3.3$, $C_{\mathrm{B}} = 0.7$. It can be seen from Fig. 8.5 that the normalized pull-off stress is well predicted by Griffith's theory for large adhesion size, corresponding to a large SCI α, and that reduction of adhesion size or α results in deviation from Griffith's theory and eventually adhesion failure at the adhesion strength determined from Bell's theory.

Gao and Yao [28] have previously shown that, for adhesive contact between a cylindrical punch and a substrate via van der Waals interaction, optimal adhesion could be achieved by a combination of size reduction and shape optimization. At small contact sizes, the shape of the contact surfaces does not play an important role. At large contact sizes, optimal adhesion becomes sensitive to small variations in contact surface shape, with the theoretical adhesion strength attained only if the

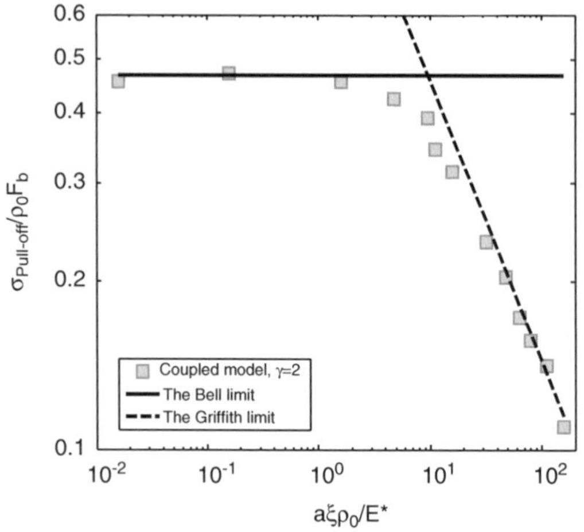

Fig. 8.5 The normalized pull-off stress as a function of the normalized adhesion size, also referred to as the SCI

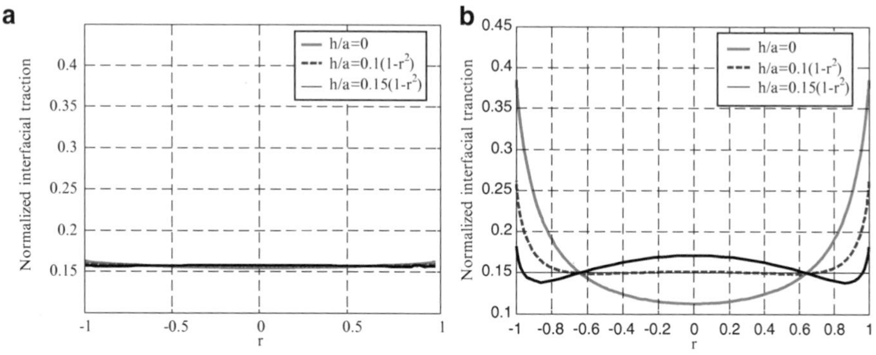

Fig. 8.6 The normalized interfacial traction distributions under different values of the contact shape when the SCI is taken as (**a**) $\alpha = 0.1$, (**b**) $\alpha = 10$ and the rebinding rate and the normalized remote load as $\gamma = 2$ and $P/a\rho_0 F_b = 0.1$

shape can be manufactured exactly. The present analysis confirms that these conclusions are also valid for adhesion via molecular bonds. For example, Fig. 8.6 shows interfacial stress distribution for different contact surface shapes. The stress concentration near the adhesion edge decreases as the shape depth increases, indicating that variations in contact surface shape can significantly reduce α and increase the adhesion strength when the contact size or SCI is large. On the other hand, when the contact size or α is small, the interfacial stress distribution becomes insensitive to variations in contact surface shape, as shown in Fig. 8.6b, where interfacial stress distributions are seen to remain nearly

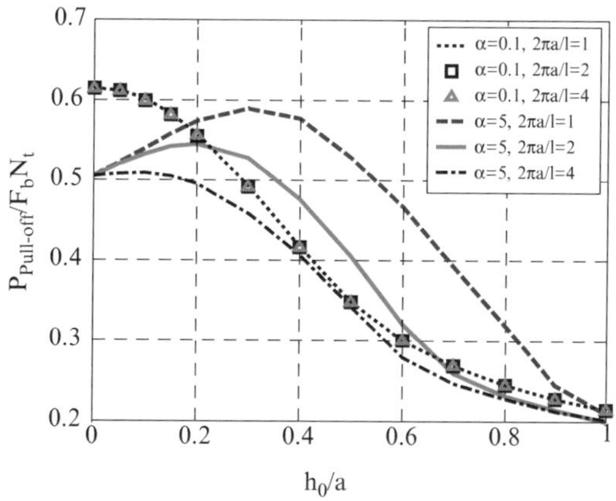

Fig. 8.7 The normalized pull-off force as a function of the normalized surface undulation amplitude under different values of the SCI and wave numbers. Other selected parameters are $\gamma = 2$, $\lambda = 2.576$, and $\beta = 1$

uniform at $\alpha = 0.1$ for different shapes. This analysis of specific adhesion via receptor-ligand bond clusters demonstrates that optimal adhesion can be achieved at any length scale by designing the shape of the contact surfaces. However, the robustness of optimal adhesion against random shape variations can only be achieved at sufficiently small contact size or for a small SCI, α.

In order to investigate the specific adhesion of a soft elastic body on a wavy surface via a patch of molecular bonds, we consider a wavy surface profile, $h(x) = h_0[1 + \cos(2\pi x/l)]$. By solving (8.15) and (8.17) at steady state, Fig. 8.7 shows the normalized pull-off force as a function of the amplitude of surface undulation for different magnitudes of surface wavelength and SCI, α. It can be seen from Fig. 8.7 that for relatively small adhesion size or SCI, the adhesion strength tends to decrease monotonically as the surface amplitude increases. This can be understood from the point of view that increasing surface amplitude leads to more non-uniform stress distribution within the contact patch. For relatively large adhesion size or SCI, there exists an optimal surface topography with a finite undulating amplitude and an optimal wavelength on the same scale as the adhesion patch size for the maximum adhesion strength.

8.5.5 Active Control of Focal Adhesions

Analysis of the SCI has shown that, depending on system parameters, there is a transition between uniform stress (equal load sharing) and crack-like singular stress distribution along the contact interface. It seems that an important parameter under control by the cell is the stiffness of the cell body, as contractile forces can stiffen or soften the actin network of the cytoskeleton, allowing the cell to modulate stress distribution along the cell-substrate interface and, in so doing, control the stability and growth/shrinkage of FAs.

Cells can modulate dynamic interactions between semiflexible polymers such as actin filaments or protein microtubules by using various binding proteins. Depending on the binding proteins, F-actin strands at medium concentration can form both chemical (cross-linked) and physical (entangled) networks with different elastic properties [77–80]. One type of cross-linked chemical polymer network is the parallel actin bundle, which can serve as stress fibers to mediate cell adhesions [77]. In [34], we have investigated the hyperelastic behavior of an F-actin bundle based on the behavior of a confined worm-like chain [81, 82]. By treating each chain in the bundle as a harmonically confined worm-like chain, we obtained closed-form expressions for the axial stress–strain relation. This revealed a strongly nonlinear, hyperelastic behavior for these bundles under stretch. According to this result, a contractile stress of 5.5 kPa [19], which has been reported for stress fibers near a focal adhesion, would lead to local stiffness orders of magnitude larger than that of the cell as a whole. Based on the concept of the SCI discussed above, we expect that the hyperelastic property of stress fibers may play a very important role in stability control of focal adhesions.

Acknowledgments This work was supported by grants from the National Natural Science Foundation of China (11032006, 11072094, and 11121202), a grant from the Ph.D. Program Foundation of Ministry of Education of China (20100211110022), the program for New Century Excellent Talents in University (NCET-10-0445), and the Fundamental Research Funds for the Central Universities (lzujbky-2012-k06).

References

1. Crawford JM (2003) Cell adhesion molecules in inflammation and immunity: relevance to periodontal diseases. Crit Rev Oral Biol Med 5:91–123
2. Galbraith CG (2002) The relationship between force and focal complex development. J Cell Biol 159:695–705
3. Nobes CD, Hall A (1995) Rho, Rac, and Cdc42 GTPases regulate the assembly of multimolecular focal complexes associated with actin stress fibers, lamellipodia, and filopodia. Cell 81:53–62
4. Balaban NQ, Schwarz US, Riveline D, Goichberg P et al (2001) Force and focal adhesion assembly: a close relationship studied using elastic micropatterned substrates. Nat Cell Biol 3:466–472
5. Burridge K, Chrzanowska-Wodnicka M (1996) Focal adhesions, contractility, and signalling. Annu Rev Cell Dev Biol 12:463–518
6. Helfman DM, Levy ET, Berthier C, Shtutman M et al (1999) Caldesmon inhibits nonmuscle cell contractility and interferes with the formation of focal adhesions. Mol Biol Cell 10:3097–3112
7. Pelham RJ, Wang Y-L (1997) Cell locomotion and focal adhesions are regulated by substrate flexibility. Proc Natl Acad Sci 94:13661–13665
8. Discher DE, Janmey P, Wang Y (2005) Tissue cells fell and response to the stiffness of their substrate. Science 310:1139–1143
9. Bar-Ziv R, Tlusty T, Moses E, Safran SA, Bershadsky AD (1999) Pearling in cells: a clue to understanding cell shape. Proc Natl Acad Sci 96:10140–10145

10. Harris AK, Wild P, Stopak D (1980) Silicone rubber substrata: a new wrinkle in the study of cell locomotion. Science 208:177–179
11. Grosheva I, Vittitow JL, Goichberg P, Gabelt BT, Kaufman PL, Borras T, Geiger B, Bershadsky AD (2006) Caldesmon effects on the actin cytoskeleton and cell adhesion in cultured HTM cells. Exp Eye Res 82:945–958
12. Totsukawa G, Wu Y, Sasaki Y, Hartshorne DJ, Yamakita Y, Yamashiro S, Matsumura F (2004) Distinct roles of MLCK and ROCK in the regulation of membrane protrusions and focal adhesion dynamics during cell migration of fibroblasts. J Cell Biol 164:427–439
13. Chrzanowska-Wodnicka M, Burridge K (1996) Rho-stimulated contractility drives the formation of stress fibers and focal adhesions. J Cell Biol 133:1403–1415
14. Volberg T, Geiger B, Citi B, Bershadsky AD (1994) Effect of protein kinase inhibitor H-7 on the contractility, integrity, and membrane anchorage of the microfilament system. Cell Motil Cytoskeleton 29:321–338
15. Leopoldt D, Yee HF, Rozengurt E (2001) Calyculin-A induces focal adhesion assembly and tyrosine phosphorylation of p125(Fak), p130(Cas), and paxillin in Swiss 3T3 cells. J Cell Physiol 188:106–119
16. Xia D, Stull JT, Kamm KE (2005) Myosin phosphatase targeting subunit 1 affects cell migration by regulating myosin phosphorylation and actin assembly. Exp Cell Res 304:506–517
17. Bershadsky AD, Kozlov M, Geiger B (2006) Adhesion-mediated mechanosensitivity: a time to experiment, and a time to theorize. Curr Opin Cell Biol 18:472–481
18. Riveline D, Zamir E, Balaban NQ, Schwarz US, Ishizaki T, Narumiya S, Kam Z, Geiger B, Bershadsky AD (2001) Focal contacts as mechanosensors: externally applied local mechanical force induces growth of focal contacts by an mDia1-dependent and ROCK-independent mechanism. J Cell Biol 153:1175–1186
19. Tan JL, Tien J, Pirone DM, Gray DS, Bhadriraju K, Chen CS (2003) Cells lying on a bed of microneedles: an approach to isolate mechanical force. Proc Natl Acad Sci USA 100:1484–1489
20. Saez A, Buguin A, Silberzan P, Ladoux B (2005) Is the mechanical activity of epithelial cells controlled by deformations or forces? Biophys J 89:L52–L54
21. Engler AJ, Bacakova L, Newman C, Hategan A, Griffin M, Discher DE (2004) Substrate compliance versus ligand density in cell on gel responses. Biophys J 86:617–628
22. Engler AJ, Sen S, Sweeney HL, Discher DE (2006) Matrix elasticity directs stem cell lineage specification. Cell 126:677–689
23. Bao G, Suresh S (2003) Cell and molecular mechanics of biological materials. Nat Mater 2:715–725
24. Johnson KL, Kendall K, Roberts AD (1971) Surface energy and contact of elastic solids. Proc R Soc Lond A 324:301–313
25. Derjaguin BV, Muller VM, Toporov YP (1975) Effect of contact deformations on the adhesion of particle. J Colloid Interf Sci 53:314–326
26. Greenwood JA (1997) Adhesion of elastic spheres. Proc R Soc Lond A 453:1277–1297
27. Maugis D (1992) Adhesion of spheres: the JKR-DMT transition using dugdale model. J Colloid Interf Sci 150:243–269
28. Gao H, Yao H (2004) Shape insensitive optimal adhesion of nanoscale fibrillar structures. Proc Natl Acad Sci 101:7851–7856
29. Evans E (2001) Probing the relation between force-lifetime-and chemistry in single molecular bonds. Annu Rev Biophys Biomol Struct 30:105–128
30. Merkel R, Nassoy P, Leung A, Ritchie K, Evans E (1999) Energy landscapes of receptor-ligand bonds explored with dynamic force spectroscopy. Nature 397:50–53
31. Li F, Redick SD, Erickson HP, Moy VT (2003) Force measurements of the integrin-fibronectin interaction. Biophys J 84:1252–1262
32. Erdmann T, Schwarz US (2004) Stochastic dynamics of adhesion clusters under shared constant force and with rebinding. J Chem Phys 121:8997–9017

33. Zaidel-Bar R, Cohen M, Addadi L, Geiger B (2004) Hierarchical assembly of cell-matrix adhesion complexes. Biochem Soc Trans 32:416–420
34. Wang J, Gao H (2011) On hyperelastic stress–strain law of F-actin bundles. Theor Appl Mech Lett 1:014003
35. Wang J, Gao H (2010) Size and shape dependent steady-state pull-off force in molecular adhesion between soft elastic materials. Int J Fract 166:13–19
36. Qian J, Wang J, Lin Y, Gao H (2009) Lifetime and strength of periodic bond clusters between elastic media under inclined loading. Biophys J 97:2438–2445
37. Wang J, Qian J, Gao H (2009) Effects of capillary condensation in adhesion between rough surfaces. Langmuir 25:11727–11731
38. Qian J, Wang J, Gao H (2009) Tension-induced growth of focal adhesions at cell-substrate interface. IUTAM symposium on cellular. Mol Tissue Mech 16:193–201
39. Wang J, Qian J, Gao H (2008) Stability of molecular adhesion mediated by confined polymer repellers and ligand-receptor bonds. Mol Cell Biomech 5:19–26
40. Qian J, Wang J, Gao H (2008) Lifetime and strength of adhesive molecular bond clusters between elastic media. Langmuir 24:1262–1270
41. Wang J, Gao H (2008) Clustering instability in adhesive contact between elastic solids via diffusive molecular bonds. J Mech Phys Solids 56:251–266
42. Honerkamp J (1994) Stochastic dynamic systems: concepts, numerical methods, data analysis. Wiley-VCH, New York
43. van Kampen NG (1992) Stochastic processes in physics and chemistry. Elsevier, Amsterdam
44. Chan P-Y, Lawrence MB, Dustin ML, Ferguson LM, Golan DE, Springer TA (1991) Influence of receptor lateral mobility on adhesion strengthening between membranes containing LFA-3 and CD2. J Cell Biol 115:245–255
45. Kloboucek A, Behrisch A, Faix J, Sackmann E (1999) Adhesion-induced receptor segregation and adhesion plaque formation: a model membrane study. Biophys J 77:2311–2328
46. Doi M, Edwards SF (1986) The theory of polymer dynamics. Oxford University Press, New York
47. Zuckerman DM, Bruinsma RF (1998) Vesicle-vesicle adhesion by mobile. Phys Rev E 57:964–977
48. Rief MF, Oesterhelt F, Heymann B, Gaub HE (1997) Single molecule force spectroscopy on polysaccharides by atomic force microscopy. Science 275:1295–1297
49. Torney DC, Dembo M, Bell GI (1986) Thermodynamics of cell adhesion. II. Freely mobile repellers. Biophys J 49:501–507
50. de Gennes PG (1979) Scaling concepts in polymer physics. Cornell University Press, Ithaca, New York
51. Erdmann T, Schwartz US (2006) Bistability of cell-matrix adhesions resulting from nonlinear receptor-ligand dynamics. Biophys J 91:L60–L62
52. Lulevich V, Zink T, Chen H-Y, Liu F-T, Liu G-Y (2006) Cell mechanics using atomic force microscopy-based single-cell compression. Langmuir 22:81151–81155
53. Trickey WR, Baaijens FPT, Laursen TA, Alexopoulos LG, Guilak F (2006) Determination of the Poisson's ratio of the cell: recovery properties of chondrocytes after release from complete micropipette aspiration. J Biomech 39:78–87
54. Tzlil S, Deserno M, Gelbart WM, Ben-Shaul A (2004) A statistical-thermodynamic model of viral budding. Biophys J 86:2037–2048
55. Briggs JAG, Wilk T, Fuller SD (2003) Do lipid rafts mediate virus assembly and pseudotyping? J Gen Virol 84:757–768
56. Quinn P, Griffiths G, Warren G (1984) Density of newly synthesized plasma membrane proteins in intracellular membranes II biochemical studies. J Cell Biol 98:2142–2147
57. Adams JC (2001) Cell-matrix contact structures. Cell Mol Life Sci 58:371–392
58. Bell GI (1978) Models for specific adhesion of cells to cells. Science 200:618–627
59. Johnson KL (1985) Contact mechanics. Cambridge University Press, Cambridge
60. Tada H, Paris PC, Irwin GR (2000) The stress analysis of cracks handbook. ASME, New York

61. Arnold M, Cavalcanti-Adam E, Glass R, Bluemmel J, Eck W, Kantlehner M, Kessler H, Spatz JP (2004) Activation of integrin function by nanopatterned adhesive interfaces. Chemphyschem 5:383–388
62. Spatz JP, Mossmer S, Hartmann C, Moller M, Herzog T, Krieger M, Boyen HG, Ziemann P, Kabius B (2000) Ordered deposition of inorganic clusters from micellar block copolymer films. Langmuir 16:407–415
63. Lin Y, Inamdar M, Freund LB (2008) The competition between Brownian motion and adhesion in soft materials. J Mech Phys Solids 56:241–250
64. Vitte J, Benoliel A, Pierres A, Bongrand P (2005) Regulation of cell adhesion. Clin Hemorheol Microcirc 33:167–188
65. Mulivor AW, Lipowsky HH (2004) Inflammation- and ischemia-induced shedding of venular glycocalyx. Am J Physiol Heart Circ Physiol 286:H1672–H1680
66. Sabri S, Soler M, Foa C, Pierres A, Benoliel A, Bongrand P (2000) Glycocalyx modulation is a physiological means of regulating cell adhesion. J Cell Sci 113:1589–1600
67. Yamakawa H (1997) Helical wormlike chains in polymer solutions. Springer, Berlin
68. Chen JZY, Sullivan DE (2006) Free energy of a wormlike polymer chain confined in a slit: crossover between two scaling regimes. Macromolecules 39:7769–7773
69. Marko JF, Siggia ED (1995) Stretching DNA. Macromolecules 28:8759–8770
70. Goodman SL, Sims PA, Albrecht RM (1996) Three-dimensional extracellular matrix textured biomaterials. Biomaterials 17:2087–2095
71. Abrams GA, Goodman SL, Nealey PF, Franco M, Murphy CJ (2000) Nanoscale topography of the basement membrane underlying the corneal epithelium of the rhesus macaque. Cell Tissue Res 299:39–46
72. Bozec L, Horton M (2005) Topography and mechanical properties of single molecules of type I collagen using atomic force microscopy. Biophys J 88:4223–4231
73. Bettinger CJ, Langer R, Borenstein JT (2009) Engineering substrate topography at the micro- and nanoscale to control cell function. Angew Chem Int Edit 48:5406–5415
74. Sykaras N, Iacopino AM, Marker VA (2000) Implant materials, designs, and surface topographies: their effect on osseointegration. A literature review. Int J Oral Maxillofac Implants 15:675–690
75. Eisenbarth E, Meyle J, Nachtigall W, Breme J (1996) Influence of the surface structure of titanium materials on the adhesion of fibroblasts. Biomaterials 17:1399–1403
76. Gao H, Ji B, Jaeger IL, Arzt E, Fratzl P (2003) Materials become insensitive to flaws at nanoscale: lessons from nature. Proc Natl Acad Sci USA 100:5597–5600
77. Alberts B, Bray D, Lewis J, Raff M, Roberts K, Watson JD (2002) Molecular biology of the cell. Taylor & Francis, New York
78. Gardel ML, Shin JH, MacKintosh FC, Mahadevan L, Matsudaira P, Weitz DA (2004) Elastic behavior of cross-linked and bundled actin networks. Science 304:1301–1305
79. Wagner B, Tharmann R, Haase I, Fischer M, Bausch AR (2006) Cytoskeletal polymer networks: the molecular structure of cross-linkers determines macroscopic properties. Proc Natl Acad Sci USA 103:13974–13978
80. Hinner B, Tempel M, Sackmann E, Kroy K, Frey E (1998) Entanglement, elasticity, and viscous relaxation of actin solutions. Phys Rev Lett 81:2614–2617
81. Odijk T (1998) Microfibrillar buckling within fibers under compression. J Chem Phys 108:6923–6928
82. Wang J, Gao H (2007) Stretching a stiff polymer in a tube. J Mater Sci 42:8838–8843

Chapter 9
Diversified Material Designs in Biological Underwater Adhesives

Kei Kamino

9.1 Introduction

In nature there exists a variety of diversified adhesives to meet the individual demands of many organisms. These adhesives have been artificially designed for use in medicine, yet are fragile in water and thus are limited to air. Because adhesive mechanisms that allow attachment under water are much more complex than those that allow attachment in the air, we continue to study them, particularly to characterize the adhesive's native proteins. In this chapter, we compare biological material designs for similarities and differences from the macroscopic to molecular levels to potentially provide clues for designing new artificial adhesives. Specifically, we present information about how the mussel, barnacle, and tubeworm inform us about how underwater "firm" adhesives work.

Many organisms prefer to attach to various interfaces such as gas-solid or liquid-solid, since these attachments enable them to inhabit a fixed environment. These attachments can actually become a part of the organism's physiological function, and specialized processes have evolutionally developed to accomplish this. An attachment could occur under water or in the air, with fixation or locomotion, with the animal's body part attached to foreign materials or by joining different foreign materials together. There may be differences in the attachment area's size and surface cleanness, different time lengths needed to attain a full strength of attachment, and differences of foreign stresses in the strength and direction (tensile or shear) to be loaded.

Adhesives have been developed for commercial use in product manufacturing, thanks to the assiduous efforts and experiences of material scientists and engineers. However, their use in general remains limited to air, since attaching materials in water remains a troublesome and undeveloped technology.

K. Kamino (✉)
Biotechnology Center, National Institute of Technology and Evaluation, Kisarazu, Chiba, Japan
e-mail: kamino-kei@nite.go.jp

S. Thomopoulos et al. (eds.), *Structural Interfaces and Attachments in Biology*, 175
DOI 10.1007/978-1-4614-3317-0_9,

Typical processes to obtain attachment in the air may include the following steps. First, material surfaces are cleaned (pre-cleaning) and kept dry by removing the water layer. Adhesives are then uniformly and thinly spread onto the material surfaces (spreading or wetting). Materials are joined together and are compressed to make the adhesive layer as thin as possible. Following the hand-processing, the adhesive molecules form several bonds with molecules on the material's surface (surface coupling) and are allowed to sit for minutes to hours until the bonding strength reaches a sufficient level (curing). To summarize, attachment in the air may simply be achieved by coping with two minimal requirements: surface coupling and curing.

In water, the requirements for attachment are much more challenging [1]. First, it is very difficult to remove the water layer and spread the adhesive on the material's surface. A much higher dielectric constant of water [2] also makes it difficult to keep the surface coupling for a longer period (e.g., more than a year). And because of fouling of organic materials and/or microbial cells, the underwater surface quickly becomes dirty. The fouled layer makes coupling of the adhesive to the material surface difficult. In addition, the bulk layer of the adhesive becomes swollen from excess hydration, resulting in weaker adhesive strength.

To achieve this troublesome underwater attachment, sessile organisms ranging from microbes to hard and soft animals and plants have developed diversified ways to tightly and continuously attach to several material surfaces. These biological adhesives are excellent models from which to learn how to artificially attach materials in water and to obtain information that will be useful to develop general theories in the interface sciences.

9.2 Basic Differences Between Commercial Adhesives and Biological Adhesives

The basic differences between commercially available and biological adhesives can be summarized as follows (Table 9.1). Biological adhesives consist of biomolecular materials that, typically, are protein complexes involved in firm underwater attachment. The protein molecules have several functional groups on their side chains, including carboxyl, amino, aromatic, imidazole, guanidino, alkyl, and hydroxyl groups. Additionally, posttranslational modifications of proteins produce further functional groups (e.g., phosphate). In contrast, synthetic polymers used in commercially available adhesives have limited functional groups on their side chains, mainly due to constraints of the simpler synthetic processes, which is directly related to the cost of mass production. The protein molecules have, in general, defined conformations wherein each functional group of side chains is given an individual orientation. The orientation of each functional group is essential to function, keeping the molecular conformation or the interaction with another molecule. Specificity and/or higher efficiency of protein functions are generally defined by the molecular

Table 9.1 Distinction between biological adhesives and artificial synthetic adhesives

	Synthetic (in air)	Biological (in water)
Molecular species	Synthetic polymer	Protein
Diversity of functional group	1 to a few	Several
Molecular heterogeneity (Mol. Weight, branched)	High	Low
Solvents	Non-aqueous	Aqueous
Number of molecular species	1 to a few	More than 3
Molecular localization	Non	Exist
Stratified structure	Non	Exist
Material to be attached	Clean	Dirty

design. On the other hand, fine control of orientation in the side chains is unusual in the designs of synthetic polymers. Biomolecular materials are, of course, biosynthesized in water, and the molecules have bound waters inside and on the surface of the protein molecules. Molecular interfaces among self-assembled proteins also have bound water molecules. In other words, the water molecule is an essential component in biological underwater adhesives. This is another distinct feature of biomolecular materials compared to synthetic polymers. The latter is usually synthesized in an organic solvent and is devoid of water molecules. However, it must be used in water if it is an underwater adhesive. Different conditions between production and usage may be essential obstacles for material scientists who are designing underwater adhesives or wet materials from typical synthetic polymers [3]. Thus, nature may serve as a subtle teacher [4]. However, peptide- or protein-based materials should be considered transitional products from which to learn how to achieve firm attachment in water. Information obtained by the challenge to create peptide- or protein-based underwater adhesives may lead to following cheaper and simpler polymer mimics. Elucidation of the natural system, practice in peptide/protein-based materials, and design of simpler polymer mimics should be separately addressed but tightly intertwined so that we may develop a roadmap to perform innovative and successful material science.

9.3 Models of Underwater Attachment

There are diversified sessile organisms that attach onto foreign materials in water. These organisms include hard and soft coral, sponges, seaweed, tubeworms, mussels, barnacles, sea squirts, starfish, oysters, limpets, microbes, and invertebrate larvae. Some of these organisms attach to foreign materials during nearly all of their life cycle, whereas others attach during a given life cycle or just occasionally. Among these, mussels, barnacles, and tubeworms are model organisms from which we may learn the nature of underwater "firm" adhesives (Fig. 9.1). All are biologically classified in different taxa and provide multi-protein complexes for underwater attachment. The complex nature of their adhesives implies a multi-functionality of the underwater attachment process that may be required to

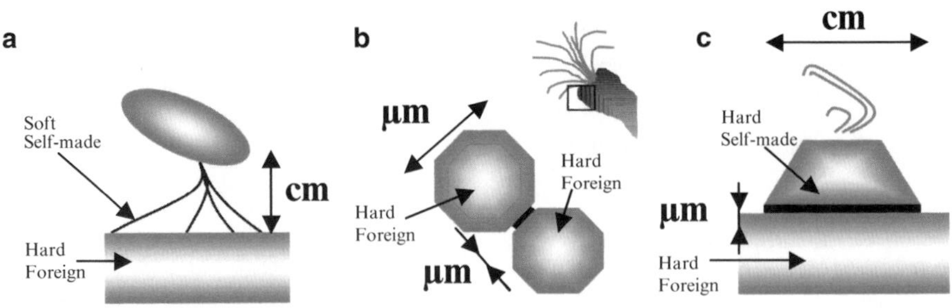

Fig. 9.1 Different modes of attachment among different sessile organisms: (**a**) mussel, (**b**) tubeworm, and (**c**) barnacle

Table 9.2 Comparison of biological adhesives among three model organisms

	Mussel	Barnacle	Tube worm
Taxonomy	Mollusk	Crustacean	Annelida
Role of attachment	Holdfast	Holdfast	Tube building
Sort of components	Protein/Fe^{3+}/Ca^{2+}	Protein	Protein/Ca^{2+}/Mg^{2+}
Number of proteins	6 in the disk	>6	3
Protein-modification	DOPA/PhoSer/HyArg/Hyp etc.	Glycosylation	DOPA/PhoSer
Cross-linking	Involved	Unknown	Involved
Macro-structure	Thread/disk	Homogenous	Homogenous
Microstructure	Solid foam, granular cuticle	Fused granule	Solid foam
Protein localization	Functional localization	Unknown	Unknown
Distance of attachment	2–4 cm	>1 μm	10–20 μm
Fresh start of adhesive	Possible	Impossible	Possible
Adherends	Foreign/end of thread	Foreign/base shell	Foreign/foreign

overcome difficulties in firm and durable underwater attachment. There are differences and similarities in macroscopic and molecular levels of the underwater adhesives (Table 9.2). Studying them could reveal essential functionalities in underwater attachment, clarify reasons for diversified ways to overcome obstacles for underwater attachment, and provide hints for potential best combinations that we can use. The individual adhesive systems used by the three organisms are summarized in the following three sections.

9.4 Overview of the Mussel Byssal Holdfast

The mussel is a bivalve and attaches to material surfaces by forming several byssal threads [5]. The animal hangs down by its byssus or sits on a trampoline made by byssus (Fig. 9.1). Occasionally, a mussel will move its habitat by cutting off its byssus at the proximal stem, thus the thread is disposable. Simply, their main body is a few centimeters away from foreign material surface separated by the

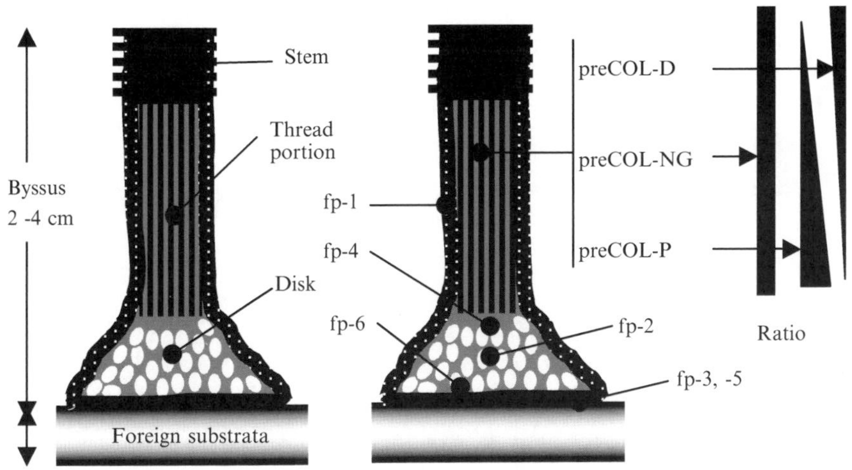

Fig. 9.2 Mussel byssus as complex and hierarchical material from the macroscopic to molecular levels

biomolecular threads, byssus. Because the animal is tossed about by the sweeping action of turbulent waves, this mode of holdfast with a centimeter distance from substratum would latently include several breakpoints. The mussel, however, overcomes this obstacle due to the fine design of its byssal thread structure from the meso-/microscopic level to the molecular level [6].

The byssal thread has a macroscopically modular structure that includes a thread portion and an adhesive disk (Fig. 9.2). The byssal thread overall has an outer coating in its microscopic level. The adhesive disk is microscopically separated by a bulk layer and a tip layer, wherein the latter is directly coupled with foreign materials [7]. The coating layer [8] and bulk of adhesive disk [7] have individual meso-scopic structures, respectively. Specific localizations of the individual components in the molecular level also seem to occur. Bulk of the disk [9], surface coupling layers at the tip of the disk [2], and outer coating layer [10] are actually formed by individual specific proteins. The thread portion has remarkably distinct physical characteristics proximally and distally, each of which has different protein compositions [11]. Linking proteins may also occur at junctions of the surface coupling layer and bulk of the disk [12], or between the bulk of the disk and distal end of the thread portion [13]. Overall, these fine, delicate designs support mussel attachment in water.

9.4.1 Unique Proteins in the Byssal Thread

Byssal thread consists of proteins to an extent of 95% in weight, which includes nine unique proteins, five of which are found at the adhesive disk, three at the thread portion, and one at the overall outer coating (Fig. 9.3). Two proteins directly bind to foreign materials and have molecular weights less than 10 kDa, which are the lowest ones among all of the proteins. A protein in the bulk of the disk has a

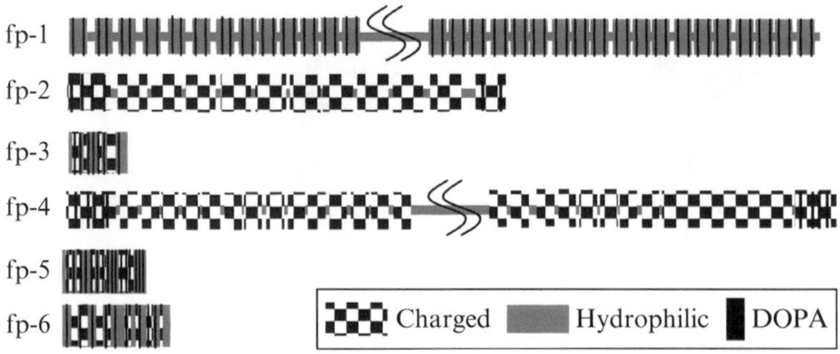

Fig. 9.3 Schematic illustration of proteins in the disk of mussel byssal thread and the coating layer. All proteins contain DOPA, with its content ranging from a few to 20 mol%. Each relative length of illustration roughly corresponds to the molecular weight of the respective proteins. Primary structures of larger proteins are composed of tandem repetitions. Although those of smaller proteins are not composed of clear repetition, their complexities are actually lower. No hydrophobic component is found

molecular weight of 50 kDa. A 11 kDa-protein is assumed to link two portions of the disk, i.e. the coupling layer and the bulk. Another 90 kDa-protein hypothetically links the bulk of the disk with the distal end of the thread portion. A protein in the coating layer has a molecular weight of 110 kDa.

The primary structures of two surface coupling proteins [14, 15] appear to be simple and do not possess clear tandem repetitions. Both proteins have the highest 3, 4-dihydroxy phenylalanine (DOPA)-contents (10–30 mol%) and have additional residues that are posttranslationally modified, namely 4-hydroxyarginine [16] and *O*-phosphoserine. On the other hand, the bulk protein in the disk is composed of 11 tandem repetitions of epidermal growth factor (EGF)-like motif flanked by negatively charged units in both ends of the primary structure [14]. The protein has a relatively lower content of DOPA (3–5 mol%). The primary structure of the linking 11 kDa-protein [12] is simpler and has no clear tandem repetitions. The protein also has a lower content of DOPA (2 mol%), whereas a high Cys content of 11 mol% was found. The linking 90 kDa-protein [13] is rich in His with its content reaching to 22 mol%, and its primary structure is composed of two domains, namely a His-rich decapeptide repeat and an Asp-rich undecapeptide repeat. The protein also has a lower content of DOPA (2 mol%). The primary structure of the coating protein [17, 18] is composed of 80 tandem repetitions of a decapeptide with a DOPA content of 10–15 mol%.

On the whole, proteins in the byssal thread, except for the bulk protein, have a lower level of complexity in their primary structures because they have biased amino acid compositions. Each protein therefore appears to have their specific amino acid (s) with respect to the dominance or posttranslational modifications. Based on this, the specific amino acid(s) has been considered important for the respective function(s) rather than conformations or primary structures of the proteins. Among them, DOPA has been well characterized and shown to be versatile in terms of its roles in surface coupling and the potential to form cross-linkages.

9.4.2 Versatile DOPA

Several studies on model peptides, proteins, or single amino acids indicate that DOPA strongly couples to metal/metal oxide with the strength nearly comparable to that of covalent bonding [19]. The highest content of DOPA in the two surface coupling proteins of the adhesive disk is in agreement with a significant role of DOPA for coupling to foreign metal/metal oxide surfaces in the natural system.

Results of *in vitro* studies have indicated the potential of DOPA to form several cross-linkages, including nucleophilic addition of thiolate of Cys to form Cys-DOPA [20], Michael addition via DOPA quinone [21, 22] to form di-DOPA and Lys-DOPA, and coordination bonding via metal ion, mostly Fe^{3+} [23]. Molecular assembly and curing are considered to be essential functions to form the bulk of the disk, the coating layer, and linking between separate microstructures, thus intermolecular cross-linkage is assumed to be crucial for function. The occurrence of cross-links was indicated by the results of *in vivo* analyses, which include spectroscopic evidence [24] and the finding of co-localization of Fe^{3+} with DOPA (a suggestion for their coordination bonding) [25], the detection of 1 mol% 5-*S*-Cys-DOPA out of all of the DOPA in the hydrolysate of foot-print remained onto glass substratum [2], and the detection of 5, 5′-diDOPA at a ratio of 1 per 1,800 total amino acids of the disk by rotational echo double resonance [26]. For instance, surface force apparatus (SFA)-measurement indicated that the bulk protein with a low concentration of Fe^{3+} (μM) have homo-protein interaction with a strength of 2.2 mJ/m^2 that approaches the 10 mJ/m^2 energy measured for the strongest known non-covalent protein-ligand interaction (biotin-avidin) [25]. Thus, several intermolecular cross-linkages via DOPA-residues have practical responsibility to form the bulk of the disk.

The curing not only forms the bulk of the adhesive, but is also responsible for mechanical properties such as tensile strength at loading and recovery at unloading. The metal-coordination bonding is actually reversible [27], thus it may be a good design for durable bulk-formation.

The coating layer of byssal thread is dual-functional, since coating is known to be essential for both extensibility and stiffness of the whole byssal thread [28, 29] in addition to protection from microbial degradation. The protein at the coating layer has the third highest level of DOPA at 10–15 mol% among nine byssal proteins. The co-localization of a metal ion, Fe^{3+}, implies the significance of metal-coordination bonding via DOPA. EDTA-treatment reduced the coating hardness by 50%, indicating that the coordination bonding is, at least, involved in the stiffness.

Both possible linking proteins contain lesser amounts of DOPA and are rich in His/Asp and Cys, respectively. The abundant His and Asp residues in a linking protein [13] are considered to form coordination bonding with metal ions Cu^{2+} and Ca^{2+}, respectively, thus the protein is suggested to link other proteins via intermolecular metal-coordination bonding. The other possible linking protein with abundant Cys is considered to form Cys-DOPA cross-linkage intermolecularly [12]. More recently, SFA-measurements suggested that one of the surface coupling proteins directly interacts with the bulk protein of the disk, with the strength of 1.3 mJ/m^2 by a yet unknown mechanism [25]. It is intriguing to know how nature links distinct microscopic domains because this mechanism is important for the design of artificial adhesives. Another important question to be addressed is the molecular mechanism to localize the proteins at the specific localization(s) of the joint.

9.4.3 Molecular Design Beyond DOPA

Almost all of the chemistry employed by the mussel adhesive has been interpreted based on the versatile single amino acid DOPA or the functional group catechol. There is no doubt about the significance of this amino acid and functional group in the natural system. The mussel, however, employs several DOPA-proteins for different portions of its byssal thread. The proteins have different characters and thus other amino acids and primary structures should have several roles in cooperation with the functionalities of DOPA. This was noticed by a study using SFA-measurement on both a surface coupling protein and the coating protein [30], which have similar DOPA-contents. The measurement indicated different properties between them, thus it was suggested that amino acids other than DOPA or primary structures may also play essential roles for the individual functions of each protein in underwater attachment. Moreover, coupling to hydrophobic surfaces such as synthetic polymers cannot be interpreted by the functioning of DOPA alone. The principles employed for fine design of the underwater attachment need to be further unraveled.

An EGF-like sequence motif [14] typically found in proteins with a cellular function, as illustrated by its name, was also found in the bulk protein of the disk. Because amino acids essential for cellular function are lacking in the byssal bulk protein, the sequence motif is considered to serve as a structure unit for possible protein-protein interactions in curing of the bulk. Similar alternative use of the structure has been known in cases such as the bio-silicification protein in the marine sponge [31]. The EGF-motif in proteins with a cellular function usually has a defined conformation, which is essential for the function. In extension, bulk-formation of the byssal disk may also depend on the conformation of the EGF-like motif, though no reports on the significance of the conformation have appeared.

The thread portion of the mussel byssus is composed of three related proteins [32]. The proteinaceous thread is among the most well-known biomolecular materials. Silks of insects and fibrous proteins in extracellular matrix are typical examples. The proteins in the thread portion of byssus are chimera of different known fibrous proteins such as in collagen, spider silk, and elastin. Each protein domain is assumed to have individual mechanical properties, thus the chimeras

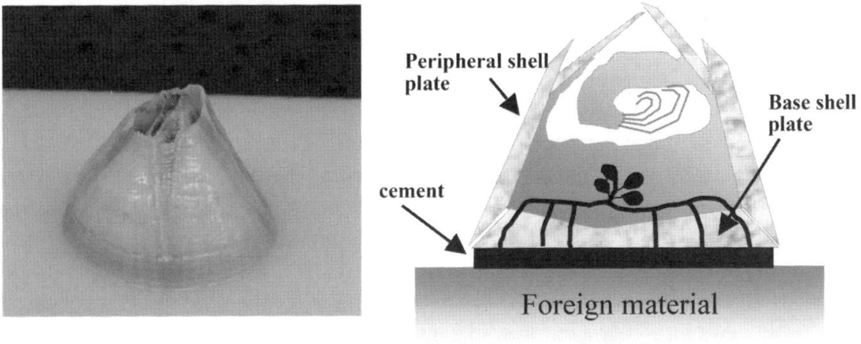

Fig. 9.4 Cross-section of a unique crustacean, the barnacle. The animal firmly fixes its base shell to a foreign material surface in water via an underwater adhesive called "cement," whose adhesive layer has a thickness of a few microns

might have complex properties beyond those of the original proteins. A gradient of ratio among the amount of the three proteins was found to exist along the longitudinal line of the byssal thread, which may contribute to formation of the gradient in the mechanical property of the whole byssal thread.

9.5 Overview of the Barnacle Cement

The barnacle is a unique sessile crustacean and attaches two materials together in water using a thin adhesive layer (Fig. 9.1). Its soft body is covered by a full armor of calcareous shell plates, which are generally composed of four to six peripheral plates, four opercular valves, and a base plate (Fig. 9.4). The animal firmly fixes its calcareous base shell to a foreign material in water via an underwater adhesive called "cement" [33] that has an adhesive layer a few microns in thickness [34]. When the barnacle grows, its base reaches a few centimeters in diameter, thus the barnacle cement fixes the calcareous base with an area of several cm^2 by an adhesive layer with a few microns in thickness. In other words, barnacle cement could support a much larger area of distinctly different materials with a thinner adhesive layer than tubeworm cement, described in the next section.

9.5.1 Unique Barnacle Adhesive

In this section, the adhesive cement formed on general hard materials is discussed with a focus on how the barnacle successfully attaches to materials in water.

The barnacle tightly attaches its calcareous shell to naturally occurring rocks and wood, artificial concrete structures, steel ship hulls, tortoise shell surfaces, and even whale epidermis. It also attaches to synthetic polymers, including fluoropolymer, and other metals/metal oxides, in water [35]. Because a barnacle's attachment causes serious damage to ship services and water uptake in power and industrial plant cooling systems, extensive research regarding barnacle adhesive has been motivated by the need to develop anti-fouling technology [36–38]. Conspicuous foul-release coatings, typically silicone, have promoted studies on the mechanism of lowering the adhesive strength produced by the barnacle cement, which would be useful to improve the performance of coatings [39, 40]. Interestingly, the adhesive joint produced by the barnacle in foul-release silicone coatings is macroscopically and microscopically different from that produced on general materials; in other words, the joint on the foul-release coating is thicker, swollen, and weaker in adhesive strength [41–44]. It is unclear whether the barnacle just fails to attach to the man-made coating or it somehow adapts to the surface with a softer adhesive to balance the stiffness.

The cement is biosynthesized in the soft tissue of the animal in a fluid form and appears to be secreted to the site of attachment. The cement is a protein complex whose proteins are unique among all of the proteins found in public databases [3]. Neither sequence homology to mussel byssal proteins/tubeworm cement proteins nor modification of an amino acid residue of tyrosine to DOPA, which is a typical and essential one in adhesives of mussel and tubeworm, was found in the barnacle cement proteins [45, 46]. Furthermore, no indication of protein modification has been found in the barnacle cement proteins. The exception is glycosylation in one of the proteins [47], which is in contrast to the mussel byssal thread and tubeworm cement where all proteins were found to undergo multiple posttranslational modifications in a number of amino acid residues. Thus, among the model organisms, the barnacle cement is unique in its molecular mechanism of attachment.

The adhesive layer of the animal is macroscopically uniform, whereas a microscopic structure seems to be present in the cement. The microscopic structures might be fibrous or sponge-like [43, 48, 49], which seem to be different depending on the materials to be attached [50]. It is unclear whether specific localization of some components in the molecular level occurs in the adhesive joint, although the cement is actually composed of distinct proteins, as mentioned below.

9.5.2 The Cement Proteins

Five proteins are identified to be components of the cement (Fig. 9.5), which are different from each other in terms of their chemical structures/physicochemical properties [33]. Among them, two bulk proteins are larger molecules with molecular weights of 100 kDa [51] and 52 kDa [47], whereas two other proteins possibly

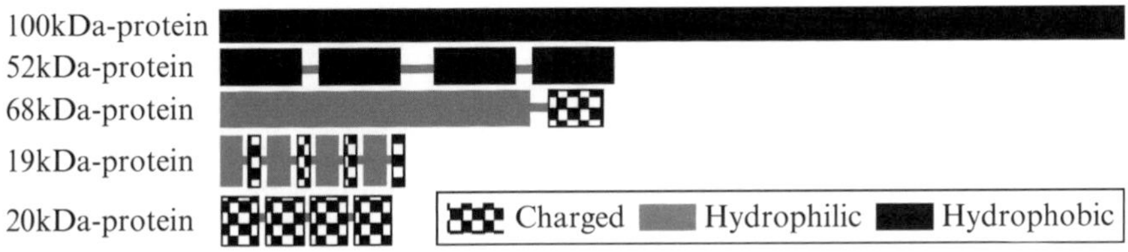

Fig. 9.5 Schematic illustration of proteins in barnacle cement. Each relative length of illustration roughly corresponds to the molecular weight of respective proteins. Hydrophobic proteins occur only in the barnacle cement

functioning at the coupling surface are smaller ones with molecular weights of 20 kDa [52] and 19 kDa [53]. The last one is a 68 kDa-protein [46] whose function in underwater attachment is not yet clear. The primary structures of the two bulk proteins are highly complex and not as simple as those found in mussel byssal proteins and tubeworm cement proteins. The amino acid compositions and primary structures roughly look like those of typical cellular proteins such as enzymes, whose hydrophobic amino acids form the core of the molecule and hydrophilic amino acids largely occur in the external area of the molecule. The primary structure of the 52 kDa-protein is composed of four long degenerated repeats, whereas no clear repetitions are found in the 100 kDa-protein. The two proteins with possible surface functions are simpler in the amino acid compositions than those of the two bulk cement proteins. The 20 kDa-protein is rich in charged amino acids such as His and Asp/Glu, and Cys, whereas the content of hydrophobic amino acids is limited. The primary structure is composed of six degenerated repeats. The 19 kDa-protein also has a simple amino acid composition in which six amino acids, Ser, Thr, Gly, Ala, Lys, and Val, occupy more than 60% of the total amino acids, though no clear repetitions in the primary structure is found. The 68 kDa-protein is composed of two domains whose longer N-terminal domain has somewhat similar amino acid composition to that of the 19 kDa-protein. The two surface functional proteins are found not to be posttranslationally modified, whereas the 52 kDa-bulk protein is glycosylated. It is unclear whether the other proteins are posttranslationally modified or not; however, no DOPA is found in all of the barnacle cement proteins.

9.5.3 *Bulk of the Cement*

Though the bulk of the cement is generally insoluble in most solvents and by any treatments, two methods have been found to render almost all of it soluble [46, 51]. This is remarkably different from what is seen in the two other model organisms, where very limited amounts of protein are rendered soluble from the byssal thread and the tubeworm cement. Investigation of the processes that rendered a bulk protein soluble from the barnacle cement indicated that conformation of the molecule as a building block and molecular interactions such as hydrophobic interactions and hydrogen bonding are essential for curing. Molecular interactions among the bulk proteins seem to be optimized in a manner similar to that found in the process of amyloid-beta self-assembly [54]. Amyloid-beta is well-known for its characteristics of forming ordered peptide self-assembly with beta-sheets. The amyloid formation is different from a simple process of nonspecific aggregation because the fibrils show ordered structures. This suggests the presence of a specific pattern of molecular interactions, rather than nonspecific hydrophobic interactions, that lead to such an ordered process. One of the bulk proteins of the barnacle cement actually contains an amyloid-like sequence, thus a similar manner of protein-protein interactions may partly occur in the bulk of the cement. Though a few studies have produced speculation about the occurrence of intermolecular covalent cross-linkage [55], no direct evidence for its involvement in the formation of the bulk is yet known [56].

9.5.4 Interface of the Cement

Barnacles seem to employ two different types of proteins for surface functions: Among all biological underwater adhesive proteins, the 20 kDa-protein is the only one that has been shown to have a defined conformation [57, 58]. The abundant Cys-residues in the protein form intramolecular disulfide bonding, which appears to be essential in keeping the conformation. The protein is adsorbed to specified materials, and among these, calcified material is best. Calcified shell is at least one of two foreign materials that the barnacle cement must attach to, thus the protein is assumed to be a specific coupling agent for the most-encountered calcareous material.

Since barnacles attach to diversified foreign materials, a function for surface coupling to unspecified materials is required. This has been suggested to be fulfilled by the 19 kDa-protein [53]. The protein actually adsorbs to various materials with almost a monolayer amount [59]. Materials to be coupled include metals/metal oxides and synthetic polymers. The protein might not exhibit a defined secondary structure. Thus, the barnacle employs different types of surface coupling proteins, one with a defined 3D-structure for coupling to a specific surface, and the other with a more flexible structure for coupling to unspecified materials. Although the function of the 68 kDa-protein is unknown, it is intriguing that it has an abundant number of amino acids similar to the 19 kDa-protein. Since underwater attachment is a multi-functional process [1], it may not be accomplished by a simple addition of two functions, such as surface coupling and setting. It is possible that in-depth characterization of each component might make the obscure multi-functional underwater attachment process more clear.

9.6 Overview of Tubeworm Cement

The tube that the tubeworm inhabits is made of natural particulates that are bonded together with tubeworm cement [60]. The cement attaches two hard materials together in water using a thin adhesive layer (Fig. 9.1). The process is as follows: The animal grasps an environmental particulate that is several hundred microns in diameter, puckers to put the cement onto the particulate, and presses it against a tip of building tube for attachment [61]. The cement, which is several tens of microns in thickness, attaches to two hard particulates in water. Thus, it attaches particulates with an area of several hundreds of μm^2 by a cement layer of several tens of μm in thickness.

The cement is uniform in structure at the macroscopic level, while the bulk has a similar microscopic structure with that of the mussel byssal disk, i.e., a solid foam-like structure. It is unclear whether a specific localization of different components at the molecular level occurs.

The cement is a proteinaceous material that contains three proteins (Fig. 9.6). Among the model organisms reviewed in this chapter, the tubeworm's cement has the fewest components. Two proteins with basic pIs [62] have apparent molecular weights of 21 and 18 kDa, and the third protein has an acidic pI [63] of nearly 1 and an apparent molecular weight of about 10–30 kDa. Both basic proteins are rich in Gly with its content at 42 and 30 mol%, respectively, and also contain a high content of DOPA at 10 and 7 mol%, respectively. The acidic protein has at least seven variants and is comprised of Ser at 60–90 mol%, with a very limited number of Tyr. The Ser residues in the protein seem to be almost phosphorylated. Although the occurrence of DOPA in the acidic protein has not yet been shown, sporadic Tyr in the deduced sequence from cDNA may be converted to DOPA. The primary structure of the basic 21 kDa-protein contains 15 tandem repetitive sequences of a decapeptide with a consensus sequence, which are mostly composed of three amino

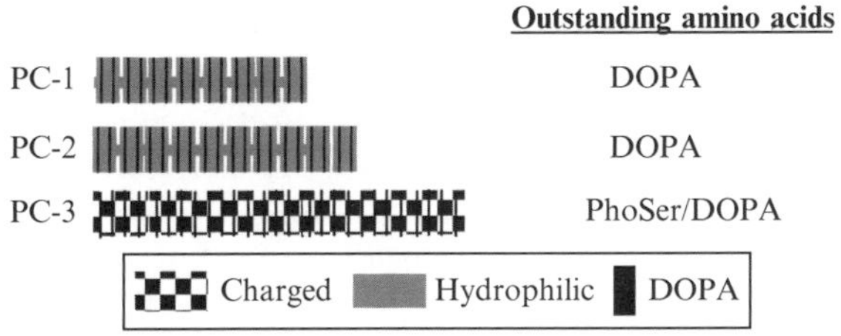

Fig. 9.6 Schematic illustration of the proteins in tubeworm cement. Each relative length of illustration roughly corresponds to the molecular weight of respective proteins. Tubeworm cement is composed of three proteins, which is the minimum number among underwater adhesives of the three model sessile organisms. Primary structures of PC-1 and PC-2 are composed of tandem repetitions, and that of PC-3 is a very simplified one due to a high content of Ser ranging from 60 to 90 mol%

acids: Gly, Lys, and DOPA. The primary structure of the other basic protein (18 kDa) contains degenerate copies of a consensus repeat with a large variation in the individual sequences. The acidic protein is almost completely occupied by Ser, with a sporadic insertion of Tyr. Only one variant is found in the C-terminal basic sequence, which contains six Cys.

It is presumed that the function of the tubeworm's cement surface coupling to foreign materials is due to DOPA and Pho-Ser, analagous to the mussel byssal system. Metal-coordination bonding and Cys-DOPA cross-linkage are suggested to be involved with setting the cement [64]. The cement contains Mg^{2+} and Ca^{2+} in an extractable form in the EDTA solution, and EDTA-treatment actually reduces adhesive force and compressive characteristics [65]. The detection of Cys-DOPA in the whole cement [63] also suggests the occurrence of intermolecular cross-linkage.

The components found in the tubeworm cement look like water-soluble polyelectrolyte solutes. It diffuses into the surrounding water if a specific mechanism is not provided. However, the physicochemical properties of the cement proteins, occurrence of divalent cation species, and pH-shift in the secretory gland and seawater might fulfill conditions for complex coacervation [64]. Complex coacervate seems to have good properties for removing the water boundary layer and spreading onto material surfaces.

9.7 Impacts to Artificial Material Design

Most research aimed at learning about biological adhesives (Fig. 9.7) has been focused on amino acids, DOPA, or the side chain, catechol group. In three decades of challenges, it has been shown that intermolecular cross-linking with several styles and surface coupling to metal/metal oxide are practical for materials design with DOPA. Numerous forms of gel and coating materials have been made from synthetic peptide mimics, protein extracts from the mussel foot, recombinant forms of proteins, and DOPA/catechol-incorporated synthetic polymers.

There are two main ways to introduce DOPA into a backbone of material. These are: post-conversion of Tyr to DOPA by the enzyme or oxidants, and the direct incorporation of DOPA. The former style has been used for synthetic peptides [22] and the recombinant forms [66, 67], while the latter has been principally possible in chemical synthesis [68–70] and protein extracts from the animal [71]. Recently, *in vivo* conversion of Tyr to DOPA in the recombinant form of a eukaryotic host was also reported as an additional case of the latter [72].

Prior studies have primarily focused on a covalent cross-linkage, and post-conversions from Tyr have been used to produce some materials. The post-conversion not only includes conversion to DOPA, but also the subsequent conversion to the quinone and the immediate formation of any covalent cross-linking at an elevated pH. Initial research has increased our experience for controlling the

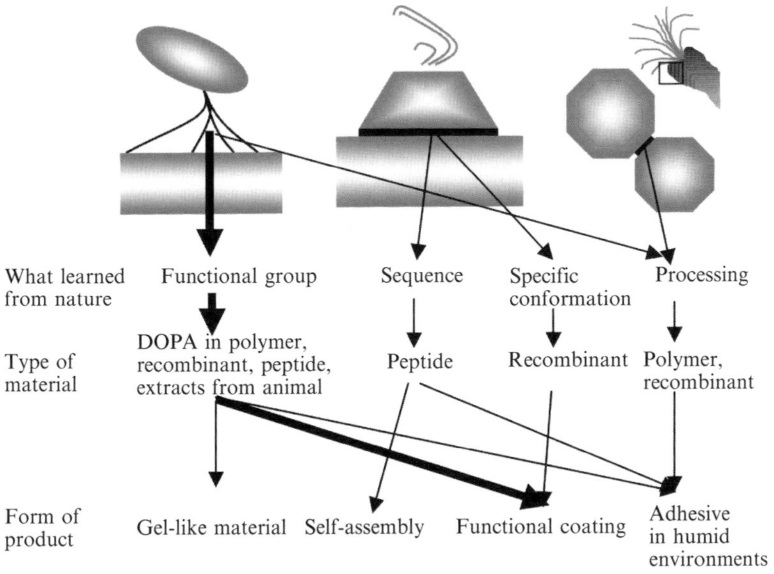

Fig. 9.7 Impacts to artificial material designs

troublesome reaction [73, 74]. Recently, metal-coordination bonding via DOPA is a further trend to form intermolecular cross-linking [75, 76]. The bonding is possibly reversible, thus self-healing and tough mechanical properties are expected. In the case of metal-coordination bonding, the free catechol group instead of the quinone is essential. The chemical incorporation of DOPA seems to have priority in those cases of metal-coordination bonding due to easy control of the chemistry. The gel-like materials formed by DOPA cross-linkage may be available for tissue sealants and drug delivery systems in medical applications, although it is not known how good the properties of the materials will be. Moreover, the addition of tyrosinase or harmful oxidants and metals to form the gel may be unwelcome for medical applications. The current process for using the material is also not yet practical.

Great impacts of DOPA/catechol have been found in the area of coating/surface functionalization of materials. Incorporation of DOPA into a polyethylene glycol (PEG) backbone was the first applicable case of a coating material [77]. The material, adsorbed onto titanium, prevented the fouling of the surface by mammalian cells for 6 months. DOPA-structure in the material was employed as the anchor and the anti-fouling property was given by the PEG-structure. After the initial report, adaptation of DOPA/catechol as a surface anchoring structure was investigated extensively and is now a platform for materials design. Materials with DOPA/catechol-anchor structure include anti-fouling coatings against proteins [78], cells [79], and animals [80], functionalizing surfaces [81, 82], and gels [83].

Apart from DOPA, protein-based materials are another choice to anchor foreign functional proteins to material surfaces. Two barnacle proteins with surface

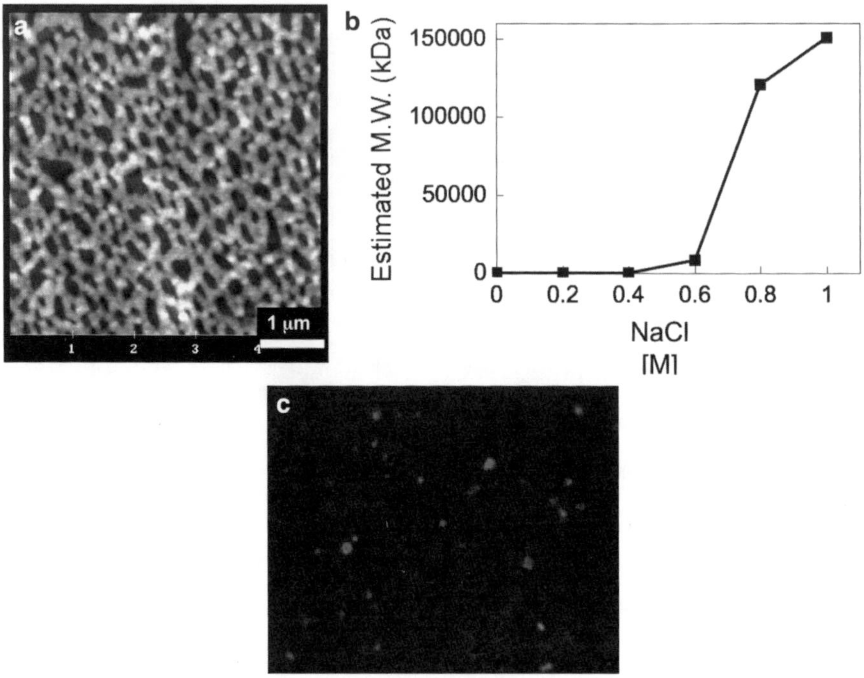

Fig. 9.8 Peptide- and protein-based materials from biological underwater adhesives. (**a**) Salt concentration-dependent peptide self-assembly designed from cp-20k. (**b**) Self-assembly has a threshold level close to the salt concentration of seawater. (**c**) The cp-19k protein as a multi-surface coupling tag. The polymer particles were quickly covered with the bacterial recombinant protein of Mrcp19k fused with green fluorescent protein and emitted fluorescence (reproduced, with permission, from [84])

function [53, 57] might be useful as multi-anchoring or specific anchoring tags to deposit functional proteins onto a solid material (Fig. 9.8) [84]. The protein would be ready to use immediately after the bio-process production fusing it with a foreign functional protein without post-modification, which is usually required in materials with DOPA. Such tools would be useful for depositing functional proteins onto any surface by genetic design.

Needless to say, researchers have long been interested in learning from nature how to develop an adhesive to be used in humid conditions and in water. In one study, a DOPA-containing polydecapeptide mimic was synthesized from the sequence of the byssal coating protein. The aqueous solution of the peptide mimics was spread onto pieces of iron, combined with air, and placed for 3 days in 60% relative humidity. Without the addition of tyrosinase or oxidant, a tensile strength of 28 kg/cm^2 was obtained [68]. A co-polypeptide of Tyr and Lys with the addition of tyrosinase showed limited success, with a tensile strength of 30 kg/cm^2 in the same conditions [85]. Adhesive strength of a co-polypeptide of DOPA and Lys was also measured on strips of porcine bone and skin [86]. The co-polypeptide with an oxidant, citrate ferric, was applied to the adherents, and the strips were combined together, fixed for 30 min in air, and then placed into water for 12 h. The conditions gave an adhesive strength of 0.16 MPa for the bone specimen, while the skin specimen failed to attach. In the experiment, because the bone specimen has a porous surface, the mechanical locking by the permeating and setting of the co-polypeptide via the covalent cross-linkage, rather than the chemisorption to the surface, might occur. Excess formation of covalent cross-linking via DOPA might lose another side of function in the free catechol group. Application of simple DOPA-peptides via covalent cross-linkage might depend on controlled amounts of the counterpart; although the free catechol group remains, control using tyrosinase or oxidant is difficult. This might be the reason for the limited success in studies on humid attachment. In air, a co-polypeptide of Tyr and Lys with oxidant or tyrosinase gave the tensile strength of a maximal 4 MPa on steel [69]. Much lower adhesive strengths of simplified peptides in humid conditions than those in the air imply that other amino acids may be significant for composition/sequence in practical attachment under humid conditions or in water.

Protein extracts from the mussel foot were applied for attachment of porcine skin without adding an oxidant or enzyme [71]. A paste of the protein extracts with water was applied onto the specimens, and then they were combined together in air and placed in 80% relative humidity for 24 h for curing. This resulted in 1 MPa for the failure stress, which is comparable to that of fibrin measured under the same conditions. The material is actually a mixture of several proteins and is assumed to mainly contain the bulk protein in the disk and the coating protein of whole byssus, both of which are probably posttranslationally modified to DOPA. The proteins are actually denatured in the preparation, thus they act as a random polymer. Adhesive shear strength of mussel protein extracts for porcine intestinal submucosa was also measured with the addition of metal ions as a curing agent [87]. In a similar manner as the sample preparation mentioned above, 0.2–0.5 MPa of adhesive strength resulted from 1 h-curing with metal ions in the air. The values were, however, much lower than those of a commercial ethyl cyanoacrylate.

Combining natural processing with DOPA-functionality is a recent challenge. A simple polymer mimic of the tubeworm cement system was attempted for bonding materials in wet conditions with a preparation of the coacervation complex [88]. The complex coacervate was prepared from two acrylic copolymer mimics: one with a phosphate group and catechol group and another with primary amine [89]. An oxidant in water was first placed on the surfaces of bovine bone specimens, and the coacervate was subsequently added to the surfaces. The two specimens were joined together, were covered with wet gauze, and were placed for more than 24 h into a container containing a wet sponge to maintain humidity. This produced about 0.1 MPa for the failure stress, which is one-third the value of commercial cyanoacrylate glue under the same conditions. A hybrid recombinant protein with modification by tyrosinase was also applied to the formation of complex coacervation, and it seemed to have increased the adhesive strength by nearly twofold [90]. Though this research is in its initial steps, the approaches cited combined with natural processing are essential to develop practical materials.

Another way to design a humid adhesive may be found in a report in which DOPA was introduced into a hydrophobic polymer unit [91]. The design principle of the material may be interpreted based on a combination of surface coupling used by the mussel with the bulk curing employed by the barnacle, because the curing of the barnacle cement is maintained by hydrophobic interactions. In the study, polymer scientists used an organic solvent to control the hydrophobic interactions, while the barnacle introduced conformational changes of the proteins to control the hydrophobic interactions in water. Further evidence to design a humid adhesive may be found in peptide self-assemblies. The structures of the barnacle cement proteins include units for self-assembly, because the cement proteins are fated to tightly interact with homo-/hetero-cement proteins for self-assembly to form the adhesive bulk. Simple peptides designed from the barnacle cement proteins [54, 92] gave the peptide self-assembly capability upon increment of ionic strength or shift of pH (Fig. 9.8). Therefore combinations of self-assembly structures with surface coupling structures may be another choice for developing practical adhesives in wet conditions or in water. On the other hand, how to control the hydrophobic interactions in an aqueous solution remains a challenging task.

Mimetic or inspired materials aimed at humid adhesives or underwater adhesives from sessile organisms are fragile and seem to be far from practical use in water or humid conditions, though we have extensively learned the way to coat/functionalize material surfaces. This suggests that we still have not learned from nature how to attach materials in water. This may be due to our too-simplified ideas on how underwater attachments function: designing only from two simple functions, strong surface coupling and curing of bulk. Researchers have tended to interpret the role of the components by assuming a single function for each component. Since underwater attachment appears to be a process much more complex than air attachment, it is essential to further study the functions required in nature to accomplish underwater attachment. Perhaps, protein- and peptide-based materials might be the keys to understanding natural design. It is intriguing that there are two barnacle proteins with surface functions because at least one of the recombinant proteins prepared under physiological conditions has the native conformation. An in-depth understanding to characterize the native proteins is essential to learning about underwater attachment.

9.8 Comparison of Biological Material Designs

As previously stated, the three model organisms have similarities and differences in their adhesive abilities that occur at the macroscopic to molecular levels [3]. Similarities in their principles of design may indicate a specific role for underwater attachment, whereas differences in their designs might be related to the particular conditions that individual adhesive requirements must meet. In this last section, similarities and differences are addressed to consider future technology.

All of the adhesives used by the three model organisms involve a protein complex. Proteins would be the suitable choice among biological molecules due to the availability of several functional groups and control of the orientation based on conformation of the molecules. Therefore, there are several available choices of molecular interactions and chemistries. Protein is known to be one of the best components for making hierarchical materials with varied mechanical properties. A complex of different types of proteins is also a common design among the three model organisms. The complex nature of the protein compositions might be a result of the multi-functionality of the underwater attachment and implies that each component might have its own function(s) in forming a firm and durable adhesive joint in water. Surface coupling and curing of bulk are essential functions in adhesives in air or underwater. Specific proteins appear to be provided for the respective function in the mussel byssal disk and barnacle cement. The occurrence of specific surface coupling proteins in the mussel and barnacle may be similar to cases where engineers pre-treat a surface with so-called primer to improve surface coupling of an adhesive. However, natural designed systems seem to have additional molecular mechanisms to link the surface coupling layer with the bulk of the adhesive.

Involvement of smaller and hydrophilic proteins in surface coupling might be a common design in the mussel and barnacle, though molecular designs for curing are different. Tubeworm cement is composed of only three proteins, the minimum number among the three organisms, and all of the three proteins seem to contribute to curing the bulk of the cement together. It is unclear whether all three proteins are involved in surface coupling or whether one of them is specifically involved. In either case, surface coupling seems to depend on dominant chemisorption via the side chain of amino acid(s) in the three model organisms.

Underwater attachment should have additional function(s) beyond those of air attachment. We should explore not only the structural designs for the known functions for attachment in air, but also functions that are not yet clearly understood in underwater attachment. For instance, spreading onto the underwater surface should be another essential function in underwater attachment. The biological underwater adhesives may include specific component(s) for this function. Alternatively, the function may rely on a part of the structure(s) of protein(s). The abundance of hydroxyl groups in adhesive proteins is noticed as a common feature among the three model organisms. Residues abundant in hydroxyl groups such as Ser, Thr, hydroxy-Arg, and hydroxy-Pro are found in proteins with the surface coupling and the curing. It might be a common molecular design that is essential in a function not clearly understood yet, such as wetting on wet surfaces or keeping adhesives stable in water for a longer period. In this respect, introduction of PEG by Dalsin et al. [77], as mentioned in the previous section, may be one of appropriate manners for the artificial design.

The bulks of biological adhesives are not homogeneous and have microscopic structures. This seems to be a common design, which probably contributes to the mechanical properties of the adhesives, although the detailed structures are not the same among the three model organisms. A technology to add a filler to improve the bulk properties of materials may yield improvements as seen in the natural design. The three model organisms were studied at different stages, complicating interpretation, and further investigations should reveal both the essential functions and universal designs.

Differences in the designs of the adhesives may be easier to find than universal design principles, as discussed above. Microscopic as well as molecular structures might be much more involved in the modes of adhesives in the organisms, especially with respect to the quality of resulting attachment.

Mussels evolutionally developed their holdfast with an order of centimeter-distance between the animal and its foreign materials. This mode of attachment indicates that a multi-angle environmental stress is given to the adhesive joint of the mussel, and the stress would be remarkably higher among the three model organisms. Therefore, the mussel might need the multiplex mechanism in the holdfast. The solid foam-like microstructure in the disk, gradient of mechanical properties in the thread portion, the durable coating of the whole byssus, and combination of the reversible and irreversible molecular cross-linking will scatter a given multi-angle and repetitive stress. On the other hand, the barnacle adhesive joint might receive a stress from a limited angle, mainly from a horizontal direction. The thinner and larger adhesive joint of the barnacle also makes that attachment more secure than the other two model organisms. Thus, barnacle cement may simply rely on molecular interactions for curing rather than a polymerization via cross-linkage. The molecular mechanism may also be involved in the fact that the cement attaches to its enlarged marginal area, and thus, the central adhesive joint already formed would provide the supporting layer [3]. However, attachment of the calcareous shell and a foreign hard material by using the softer proteinaceous cement with the thinner joint may require a further-specialized mechanism. The fact that the microscopic structure of the cement differs depending on the materials to be attached [50] may indicate that the microscopic structure may be also involved in the balance of different stiffnesses. The adhesive joint of the tubeworm cement may be exposed to a multi-angle stress because surfaces of foreign materials to be attached to are not flat and the area of the joint is smaller than the areas of materials to be attached. It may be the reason why tubeworm cement needs to employ similar solid foam- like microstructure to that of the mussel disk. The combination of irreversible and reversible molecular cross-linking may be suitable for mechanical properties required by the adhesive joint. Both the mussel byssus and dwelling tube of the tubeworm are disposable. This fact may indicate how high the strength is in their modes of attachment.

Mussels and tubeworms employ hydrophilic components as specialized mechanisms to avoid dispersion and keep the components condensed after secretion might be required. The complex coacervation might be suitable to the mechanism, which might simultaneously result in a solid foam-like microscopic structure. Self-assembly of the barnacle cement bulk, which is composed of hydrophobic proteins, may be triggered by conformational changes of the proteins after secretion, although this hypothesis needs to be tested.

Mussels and barnacles provide two proteins each for the surface function in underwater attachment. The mussel employs the proteins with the highest post-translational modifications among the components. The amino acid compositions and thereby sequences have lower complexity, and the proteins seem to owe their functions to the character of their side chains. The barnacle also has two proteins with surface function that have no posttranslational modifications. One has lower complexity and may have less ordered structure, whereas the other one has a defined conformation. Thus, the barnacle provides two distinct molecular designs for surface functions: side chain-dependent and conformation-dependent. Although the three models all encounter the same obstacles in underwater attachment, they have diversified ways to overcome them. They will therefore give different insights on material designs for engineering and medical applications.

Acknowledgments I greatly appreciate Prof. Jian-Ren Shen of Okayama University for his careful correction of the manuscript.

References

1. Waite JH (1987) Nature's underwater adhesive specialist. Int J Adhes 7:9–14
2. Zhao H, Robertson NB, Jewhurst SA, Waite JH (2006) Probing the adhesive footprints of Mytilus californianus byssus. J Biol Chem 281:11090–11096
3. Kamino K (2010) Molecular design of barnacle cement in comparison with those of mussel and tubeworm. J Adhesion 86:96–110
4. Ball P (2003) Does nature know best? Nat Mater 2:510
5. Waite JH (1992) The formation of mussel byssus: anatomy of a natural manufacturing process. In: Case ST (ed) Results and problems in cell differentiation 19, Biopolymers. Springer, Berlin, pp 27–54
6. Waite JH, Andersen NH, Jewhurst S, Sun C (2005) Mussel adhesion: finding the tricks worth mimicking. J Adhesion 81:297–317
7. Benedict CV, Waite JH (1986) Composition and ultrastrcuture of the Byssus of *Mytilus edulis*. J Morphol 189:261–270
8. Holten-Andersen N, Fantner GE, Hohlbauch S, Waite JH, Zok FW (2007) Protective coatings on extensible biofibers. Nat Mater 6:669–672
9. Rzepecki LM, Hansen KM, Waite JH (1992) Characterization of a cystine-rich polyphenolic protein family from the Blue Mussel *Mytilus edulis* L. Biol Bull 183:123–137
10. Sun CJ, Waite JH (2005) Mapping chemical gradients within and along a fibrous structural tissue, mussel byssal threads. J Biol Chem 280:39332–39336
11. Harrington MJ, Waite JH (2007) Holdfast heroics: comparing the molecular and mechanical properties of *Mytilus californianus* byssal threads. J Exp Biol 210:4307–4318
12. Zhao H, Waite JH (2006) Linking adhesive and structural proteins in the attachment plaque of Mytilus californianus. J Biol Chem 281:26150–26158
13. Zhao H, Waite JH (2006) Proteins in load-bearing junctions: the histidine-rich metal-binding protein of mussel byssus. Biochemistry 45:14223–14231
14. Inoue K, Takeuchi Y, Miki D, Odo S (1995) Mussel adhesive plaque protein gene is a novel member of epidermal growth factor-like gene family. J Biol Chem 270:6698–6701
15. Waite JH, Qin XX (2001) Polyphosphoprotein from the adhesive pads of *Mytilus edulis*. Biochemistry 40:2887–2893

16. Papov VV, Diamond TV, Biemann K, Waite JH (1995) Hydroxyarginine-containing polyphenolic proteins in the adhesive plaques of the marine mussel *Mytilus edulis*. J Biol Chem 270:20183–20192
17. Waite JH (1983) Evidence for a repeating 3,4-dihydroxyphenylalanine- and hydroxyproline-containing decapeptide in the adhesive protein of the mussel, *Mytilus edulis* L. J Biol Chem 258:2911–2915
18. Inoue K, Odo S (1994) The adhesive protein cDNA of *Mytilus galloprovincialis* encodes decapeptide repeats but no hexapeptide motif. Biol Bull 186:349–355
19. Lee H, Scherer NF, Messersmith PB (2006) Single-molecule mechanics of mussel adhesion. Pro Natl Acad Sci USA 103:12999–13003
20. Sagert J, Sun C, Waite JH (2006) Chemical subtleties of mussel and polychaete holdfasts. In: Smith AM, Callow JA (eds) Biological adhesives. Springer, Berlin, pp 125–140
21. Yu M, Hwang J, Deming TJ (1999) Role of L-3,4-dihydroxyphenylalanine in mussel adhesive proteins. J Am Chem Soc 121:5825–5826
22. Nagai A, Yamamoto H (1989) Insolubilizing studies of water-soluble poly(Lys Tyr) by tyrosinase. Bull Chem Soc Jpn 62:2410–2412
23. Taylor SW, Chase DB, Emptage MH, Nelson MH, Waite JH (1996) Ferric ion complexes of a DOPA-containing adhesive protein from *Mytillus edulis*. Inorg Chem 35:7572–7577
24. Sever MJ, Weisser JT, Monahan J, Srinivasan S, Wilker JJ (2004) Metal-mediated cross-linking in the generation of a marine-mussel adhesive. Ang Chem Int Ed 43:448–450
25. Hwang DS, Zeng H, Masic A, Harrington MJ, Israelachvili JN, Waite JH (2010) Protein- and metal-dependent interactions of a prominent protein in mussel adhesive plaque. J Biol Chem 285:25850–25858
26. McDowell LM, Burzio LA, Waite JH, Schaefer J (1999) Rotational echo double resonance detection of cross-links formed in mussel byssus under high-flow stress. J Biol Chem 274:20293–20295
27. Holten-Andersen N, Harrington MJ, Birkedal H, Lee BP, Messersmith PB, Lee KYC, Waite JH (2011) pH-induced metal-ligand cross-links inspired by mussel yield self-healing polymer networks with near-covalent elastic moduli. Proc Natl Acad Sci USA 108:2651–2655
28. Holten-Andersen N, Mates TE, Toprak MS, Stucky GD, Zok FW, Waite JH (2009) Metals and the integrity of a biological coating: the cuticle of mussel byssus. Langmuir 25:3323–3326
29. Harrington MJ, Masic A, Holten-Andersen N, Waite JH, Fratzl P (2010) Iron-clad fibers: a metal-based biological strategy for hard flexible coatings. Science 328:216–220
30. Lin Q, Gourdon D, Sun C, Holten-Andersen N, Anderson TH, Waite JH, Israelachvili JN (2007) Adhesion mechanisms of the mussel foot proteins mfp-1 and mfp-3. Proc Natl Acad Sci USA 104:3782–3786
31. Shimizu K, Cha J, Stucky GD, Morse DE (1998) Silicatein alpha: cathepsin L-like protein in sponge biosilica. Proc Natl Acad Sci USA 95:6234–6238
32. Waite JH, Lichtenegger HC, Stucky GD, Hansma P (2004) Exploring molecular and mechanical gradients in structural bioscaffolds. Biochemistry 43:7653–7662
33. Kamino K (2006) Barnacle underwater attachment. In: Smith AM, Callow JA (eds) Biological adhesives. Springer, Berlin, pp 145–166
34. Saroyan JR, Lindner E, Dooley CA (1970) Repair and reattachment in the balanidae as related to their cementing mechanism. Biol Bull 139:333–350
35. Becka A, Loeb G (1984) Ease of removal of barnacles from various polymeric materials. Biotechnol Bioeng 26:1245–1251
36. Alberte RS, Shyder S, Zahuranec BJ, Whetstone M (1992) Biofouling research need for the united states NAVY: program history and goals. Biofouling 6:91–95
37. Clare AS, Fusetani N, Jones MB (1998) Introduction: settlement and metamorphosis of marine invertebrate. Biofouling 12:1–2
38. Sommer S, Ekin A, Webster DC, Stafslien SJ, Daniels J, VanderWal LJ, Thompson SEM, Callow ME, Callow JA (2010) A preliminary study on the properties and fouling-release

performance of siloxane-polyurethane coatings prepared from poly(dimethylsiloxane)(PDMS) macromers. Biofouling 26:961–972
39. Swain G, Schultz MP (1996) The testing and evaluation of non-toxic antifouling coatings. Biofouling 10:187–197
40. Swain G, Anil A, Baier RE, Chia F, Conte E, Cook A, Hadfield M, Haslbeck E, Holm E et al (2000) Biofouling and barnacle adhesion data for fouling-release coatings subjected to static immersion at seven marine sites. Biofouling 16:331–344
41. Wendt DE, Kowalke GL, Kim J, Singer IL (2006) Factors that influence elastomeric coating performance: the effect of coating thickness on basal plate morphology, growth and critical removal stress of the barnacle *Balanus amphitrite*. Biofouling 22:1–9
42. Berglin M, Gatenholm P (2003) The barnacle adhesive plaque: morphological and chemical differences as a response to substrate properties. Colloids Surf B 28:107–117
43. Wiegemann M, Watermann B (2003) Peculiarities of barnacle adhesive cured on non-stick surfaces. J Adhesion Sci Technol 14:1957–1977
44. Ramsay DB, Dickinson GH, Orihuela B, Rittschof D, Wahl KJ (2008) Base plate mechanics of the barnacle *Balanus Amphitrite*. Biofouling 24:109–118
45. Naldrett MJ (1993) The importance of sulphur cross-links and hydrophobic interactions in the polymerization of barnacle cement. J Mar Bio Ass UK 73:689–702
46. Kamino K, Odo S, Maruyama T (1996) Cement proteins of the acorn barnacle, *Megabalanus rosa*. Biol Bull 190:403–409
47. Kamino K, Nakano M, Kanai S (2012) Significance of the conformation of building blocks in curing of barnacle underwater adhesive. FEBS J 279:1750–1760
48. Sullan RMA, Gunari N, Tanur AE, Chan Y, Dickinson GH, Orihuela B, Rittschoff D, Walker GC (2009) Nanoscale structures and mechanics of barnacle cement. Biofouling 25:263–275
49. Barlow DE, Dickinson GH, Orihuela B, Kulp JL III, Rittschof D, Wahl KJ (2010) Characterization of the adhesive plaque of the barnacle Balanus amhpitrite: amyloid-like nanofibrils are a major component. Langmuir 26:6549–6556
50. Raman S, Kumar R (2011) Interfacial morphology and nanomechanics of cement of the barnacle, *Amphibalanus reticulatus* on metallic and non-metalic substrata. Biofouling 27:569–577
51. Kamino K, Inoue K, Maruyama T, Takamatsu N, Harayama S, Shizuri Y (2000) Barnacle cement proteins: importance of disulfide bonds in their insolubility. J Biol Chem 275:27360–27365
52. Kamino K (2001) Novel barnacle underwater adhesive protein is a charged amino acid-rich protein constituted by a Cys-rich repetitive sequence. Biochem J 356:503–507
53. Urushida Y, Nakano M, Matsuda S, Inoue N, Kanai S, Kitamura N, Nishino T, Kamino K (2007) Identification and functional characterization of a novel barnacle cement protein. FEBS J 274:4336–4346
54. Nakano M, Kamino K Amyloid-like structure in barnacle cement. Unpublished
55. Dickinson G, Vega IE, Wahl KJ, Orihuela B, Beyley V, Rodriguez EN, Everett RK, Bonaventura J, Rittschof D (2009) Barnacle cement: a polymerization model based on evolutionary concepts. J Exp Biol 212:3499–3510
56. Kamino K (2010) Absence of cross-linking via trans-glutaminase in the barnacle cement and redefinition of the cement. Biofouling 26:755–760
57. Mori Y, Urushida Y, Nakano M, Uchiyama S, Kamino K (2007) Calcite-specific coupling protein in barnacle underwater cement. FEBS J 274:6436–6446
58. Suzuki R, Mori Y, Kamino K, Yamazaki T (2006) 3D-structure of barnacle cement protein, Mrcp-20k. Pept Sci 2005:257–258
59. Urushida Y, Mori Y, Sano K, Kotera M, Hirose Y, Kanai S, Inoue N, Shimoura Y, Shiba K, Nishino T, Nakasuga A, Shen J-R, Kamino K Identification and characterization of a multi-surface coupling protein in barnacle underwater cement. Unpublished
60. Jensen RA, Morse DE (1988) The bioadhesive of *Phragmatopoma californica* tubes: a silk-like cement containing–DOPA. J Comp Physiol B 158:317–324

61. Stevens MJ, Steren RE, Hlady V, Stewart RJ (2007) Multiscale structure of the underwater adhesive of *Phragmatopoma californica*: a nanostructured latex with a steep microporosity gradient. Langmuir 23:5045–5049
62. Waite JH, Jensen RA, Morse DE (1992) Cement precursor proteins of the reef-bilding polychaete *Phragmatopoma californica* (Fewkes). Biochemistry 31:5733–5738
63. Zhao H, Sun C, Stewart RL, Waite JH (2005) Cement proteins of the tube-building polychaete *Phragtopoma californica*. J Biol Chem 280:42938–42944
64. Stewart RJ, Weaver JC, Morse DE, Waite JH (2004) The tube cement of *Phrgmatopoma californica*: a solid foam. J Exp Biol 207:4727–4734
65. Sun C, Fantner GE, Adams J, Hansma PK, Waite JH (2007) The role of calcium and magnesium in the concrete tubes of the sandacastle worm. J Exp Biol 210:1481–1488
66. Filpula DR, Lee S-M, Link RP, Strusberg SL, Strausberg RL (1990) Structural and functional repetition in a marine mussel adhesive proteins. Biotechnol Prog 6:171–177
67. Hwang DS, Yoo HJ, Jun JH, Moon WK, Cha HJ (2004) Expression of functional recombinant mussel adhesive protein Mgfp-5 in *Escherichia coli*. Appl Environ Microbiol 70:3352–3359
68. Yamamoto H (1987) Synthesis and adhesive studies of marine polypeptides. J Chem Perkin Trans 1:613–618
69. Yu M, Deming TJ (1998) Synthetic polypeptide mimics of marine adhesives. Macromolecules 31:4739–4745
70. Lee BP, Dalsin JL, Messersmith BP (2002) Synthesis and gelation of DOPA-modified poly (ethylene glycol) hydrogels. Biomacromology 3:1038–1047
71. Ninan L, Monahan J, Stroshine RL, Wilker JJ, Shi R (2003) Adhesive strength of marine mussel extracts on porcine skin. Biomaterials 24:4091–4099
72. Lim S, Kim KR, Choi YS, Kim DK, Hwang D, Cha HJ (2011) *In vivo* post-translational modifications of recombinant mussel adhesive protein in insect cells. Biotechnol Prog 27:1390–1396
73. Taylor SW (2002) Chemoenzymatic synthesis of peptidyl 3,4-dihydroxyphenylalanins for structure-activity relationships in marine invertebrate polypeptides. Anal Biochem 302:70–74
74. Marumo K, Waite JH (1986) Optimization of hydroxylation of tyrosinase and tyrosinase-containing peptides by mushroom tyrosinase. Biochim Biophys Acta 872:98–103
75. Zeng H, Hwang DS, Israelachvili JN, Waite JH (2010) Strong reversible Fe3+-mediated bridging between dopa-containing protein films in water. Proc Natl Acad Sci 107:12850–12853
76. Holten-Andersen N, Harrington MJ, Birkedal H, Lee BP, Messersmith PB, Lee KYC, Waite JH (2011) pH-induced metal-ligand cross-links inspired by mussel yield-healing polymer networks with near-covalent elastic moduli. Proc Natl Acad Sci 108:2651–2655
77. Dalsin JL, Hu BH, Lee BP, Messersmith PB (2003) Mussel adhesive protein mimetic polymers for the preparation of nonfouling surfaces. J Am Chem Soc 125:4253–4258
78. Dalsin JL, Lin L, Tosatti S, Voros J, Textor M, Messersmith PB (2005) Protein resistance of titanium oxide surfaces modified by biologically inspired mPEG-DOPA. Langmuir 21:640–646
79. Statz AR, Meagher RJ, Barron AE, Messersmith PB (2005) New peptidemimetic polymers for antifouling surfaces. J Am Chem Soc 127:7972–7973
80. Statz A, Finlay J, Dalsin J, Callow M, Callow JA, Messersmith PB (2006) Algal antifouling and fouling-release properties of metal surfaces coated with a polymer inspired by marine mussels. Biofouling 22:391–399
81. Lee H, Dellatore SM, Miller WM, Messersmith PB (2007) Mussel-inspred surface chemistry for multi-functional coatings. Science 318:426–430
82. Fan X, Lin L, Dalsin JL, Messersmith PB (2005) Biomimetic anchor for surface-initiated polymerization from metal substrates. J Am Chem Soc 127:15843–15847
83. Su J, Chen F, Messersmith PB (2011) Catechol polymers for pH-responsive, targeted drug delivery to cancer cells. J Am Chem Soc 133:11850–11853

84. Kamino K (2008) The underwater adhesive of marine organisms as the vital link between biological science and material science. Mar Biotechnol 10:111–121
85. Yamamoto H, Kuno S, Nagai A, Nishida A, Yamauchi S, Ikeda K (1990) Insolubiliing and adhesive studies of water-soluble synthetic model proteins. Int J Biol Macromol 12:305–310
86. Wang J, Liu C, Lu X, Yin M (2007) Co-polypeptides of 3,4-dihydroxyphenylalanine and L-lysine to mimic marine adhesive protein. Biomaterials 28:3456–3468
87. Ninan L, Stroshine RL, Wilker JJ, Shi R (2007) Adhesive strength and curing rate of marine mussel protein extracts on porcine small intestinal submucosa. Acta Biomater 3:687–694
88. Stewart RJ (2011) Protein-based underwater adhesives and the prospects for their biotechnological production. Appl Microbiol Biotechnol 89:27–33
89. Shao H, Bachus KN, Stewart RJ (2009) A water-borne adhesive modeled after the sandcastle glue of *P. californica*. Macromol Biosci 9:464–471
90. Lim S, Choi YS, Kang DG, Song YH, Cha HJ (2010) The adhesive properties of coacervated recombinant hybrid mussel adhesive proteins. Biomaterials 31:3715–3722
91. Guvendiren M, Messersmith PB, Shull KR (2008) Self-assembly and adhesion of DOPA-modified methacrylic triblock hydrogels. Biomacromology 9:122–128
92. Nakano M, Shen JR, Kamino K (2007) Self-assembling peptide inspired by a barnacle adhesive protein. Biomacromology 8:1830–1835

Chapter 10
Mechanics of Self-Similar Hierarchical Adhesive Structures Inspired by Gecko Feet

Haimin Yao and Huajian Gao

10.1 Introduction

Geckos and many insects have evolved specialized adhesive tissues with hierarchical structures that allow them to maneuver on vertical walls and ceilings. The adhesion mechanisms of gecko must be robust enough to function on unknown rough surfaces and easily releasable upon animal movement. How does nature design such robust and releasable adhesion devices? How can an adhesion system designed for robust attachment simultaneously allow easy detachment? These questions are discussed in this chapter from the point of view of contact mechanics and fracture mechanics. On the question of robust adhesion, a fractal gecko hairs model shows that structural hierarchy plays a key role in robust adhesion: it allows the work of adhesion to be exponentially enhanced with each added level of hierarchy. Barring fiber fracture, the fractal gecko hairs can be designed to achieve flaw tolerant adhesion at any length scale. However, consideration of crack-like flaws in the hairs themselves results in an upper size limit for flaw tolerant design. On the question of releasable adhesion, the asymmetrically aligned seta hairs of gecko form a strongly anisotropic material with adhesion strength that can significantly vary with the direction of pulling. It is shown that a strongly anisotropic elastic solid indeed exhibits a strongly anisotropic adhesion strength when sticking on a rough surface. Therefore, the switch between attachment and detachment can be achieved through direction control. These findings not only provide a theoretical foundation to understand adhesion mechanisms in biology, but

H. Yao
Department of Mechanical Engineering, The Hong Kong Polytechnic University, Hung Hom, Kowloon, Hong Kong
e-mail: mmhyao@polyu.edu.hk

H. Gao (✉)
School of Engineering, Brown University, Providence, RI, USA
e-mail: huajian_gao@brown.edu

S. Thomopoulos et al. (eds.), *Structural Interfaces and Attachments in Biology*,
DOI 10.1007/978-1-4614-3317-0_10, © Springer Science+Business Media New York 2013

also suggest possible strategies to develop novel adhesive materials for engineering applications.

10.2 Hierarchical Attachment Structures of Gecko

Among hundreds of animal species for which adhesion plays an important role for survival, the gecko stands out in terms of body weight and its extraordinary ability to maneuver on vertical walls and ceilings [1]. Recent experimental measurements [2–5] have provided evidence that the adhesion ability of gecko is primarily due to van der Waals adhesion [6] between the contact surfaces (e.g., walls or ceilings) and the gecko's feet, which are equipped with hundreds of thousands of keratinous hairs called setae (Fig. 10.1). Each seta is about 110 μm long and branches near its tip region into hundreds of thinner fibrils called spatulae, arranged in a fractal-like hierarchical pattern (Fig. 10.1c). While it is remarkable that gecko can make use of the relatively weak van der Waals interactions to maneuver on unpredictable rough surfaces under harsh environmental conditions, it may be even more impressive that such robust adhesion appears to be easily releasable during animal locomotion. What are the mechanics principles behind such robust and releasable adhesion in biology?

Contact mechanics theories have been used to understand adhesion mechanisms in both engineering and biology. The classical Hertz theory [8] assumes no adhesive interactions between contacting objects. Johnson et al. [9] extended the Hertz theory to contact between adhesive elastic spheres and developed the JKR (Johnson-Kendall-Roberts) model in which the contact area is determined via a balance

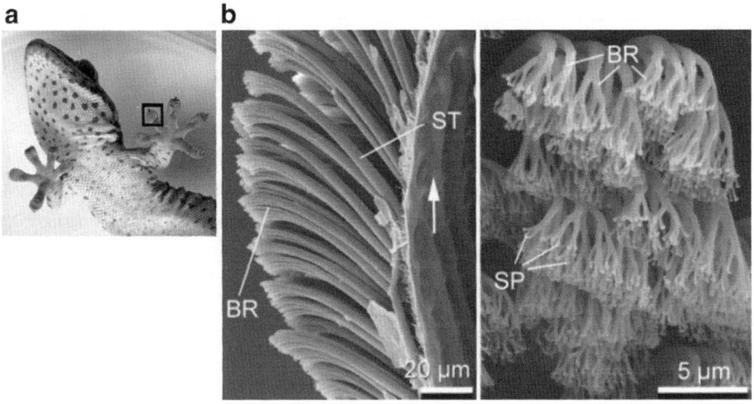

Fig. 10.1 The hierarchical adhesion structures of *Gekko gecko*. A toe of gecko contains hundreds of thousands of setae and each seta branches near its tip region into hundreds of spatulae. (**a**) Scanning electron micrographs of setae. (**b**) Spatulae, the finest terminal branches of seta. *ST* seta; *SP* spatula; *BR* branch (adapted, with permission, from: [7])

between elastic and surface energies similar to Griffith's [10] criterion for crack growth in an elastic solid. The JKR theory introduces into the Hertz solution an additional crack-like singular term which satisfies the Griffith condition near the contact edge. While the JKR theory is quite appropriate for modeling contact between large and soft materials, the assumption of a crack-like singular field becomes increasingly inaccurate for small and stiff materials, in which case different assumptions on the elastic deformation of contacting objects have led to the models of DMT (Derjaguin-Muller-Toporov) [11] and Bradley [12]. Maugis [13] generalized the Dugdale model of a crack in a plastic sheet [14] to adhesive contact and developed a more general model (Maugis-Dugdale model) that includes the JKR and DMT models as two limiting cases. More recent studies have further extended these theories to viscoelastic materials [15, 16], coupled normal and shear loads [17] and biological attachments [4, 5, 18–21].

For contact between single smooth asperities, one can define *adhesion strength* as the tensile force per unit contact area at pull-off. It has been shown that the adhesion strength can be enhanced up to the *theoretical adhesion strength* via size reduction [7, 22–24]. In this respect, it is interesting to note that the existing contact mechanics theories, including JKR, DMT, and Maugis-Dugdale models, all predicted infinite adhesion strength as the size of contacting objects is reduced to zero. This behavior seems contradictory to the physics that adhesion strength would never exceed the theoretical strength of adhesive interaction. The fact that this behavior also occurs in the Maugis-Dugdale model is especially surprising since the original Dugdale model correctly predicted that the fracture strength is bounded by the yield strength of the material. Gao et al. [7] found that the root of this illogical behavior of the classical contact models can be attributed to the original Hertz approximation of contact surfaces as parabolas, which is strictly valid only if the size of the contact area is much smaller than the overall dimension of the contacting objects; the lack of strength saturation in these models is thus explained from the fact that the parabolic approximation fails in the limit of very small contacting bodies. As an example, Gao et al. [7] showed that, if the exact geometry of a sphere is taken into account, the adhesion strength indeed saturates at the theoretical strength as the diameter of the sphere is reduced to zero. On the other hand, Gao and Yao [23] showed that the adhesion strength can in principle approach the theoretical strength for any contact size via shape optimization. In practice, interfacial crack-like flaws due to surface roughness or contaminants inevitably weaken the actual adhesion strength. Gao et al. [7] performed finite element calculations to show that the adhesion strength of a flat-ended cylindrical punch in partial contact with a rigid substrate saturates at the theoretical strength below a critical radius around 200 nm for the van der Waals interaction. Similar discussions of strength saturation for small contacting objects have been made by Persson [22] for a rigid cylindrical punch on an elastic half-space and by Glassmaker et al. [24] for an elastic cylindrical punch in perfect bonding with a rigid substrate. Gao and Yao [25] showed that the theoretical strength can be achieved by either optimizing the shape of the contact surfaces or by reducing the size of the contact area; the smaller the size, the less important the shape. A shape-insensitive optimal adhesion can be realized below a critical contact size, which can be related to the intrinsic capability of a small scale material to tolerate crack-like flaws [25–28] and Glassmaker et al. [24] demonstrated that fibrillar structures with slender elastic fibrils can significantly enhance the adhesion strength. Northen and Turner [29] made use of massively parallel MEMS processing technology to produce hierarchical hairy adhesive materials containing single slender pillars coated with polymer nanorods and reported significantly improved adhesion in such multiscale systems.

In contrast to the increasing volume of research on robust adhesion, the question of how adhesion is released upon animal movement has so far received relatively little attention. Autumn et al. [2] reported experimental data that the pull-off force of an individual seta of gecko depends strongly on the pulling angle. Gao and Chen [27] numerically simulated the pull-off force of a single seta and found that the asymmetrical alignment of seta allows the pull-off force to vary strongly (more than an order of magnitude) with the direction of pulling.

Previous studies have provided significant insights into various aspects of adhesion mechanisms in biology. However, a general understanding is still lacking with respect to a number of critical issues. First, robust adhesion at the level of a single hair or fiber does not automatically address the problem of robust adhesion on rough surfaces at macroscopic scales. It has been shown that size reduction can result in optimal adhesion strength at the level of a single fiber [7, 22–24]. However, it is not clear how this size-induced optimization might work at the system level of hierarchical structures. Similarly, releasable adhesion at the level of a single seta [2, 7] does not provide full explanations on how releasable adhesion is achieved in macroscopic contact. The present chapter is aimed to address the basic mechanics principles which underline these issues.

10.3 Bottom-Up Designed Hierarchical Structures for Robust Adhesion

10.3.1 Flaw Tolerant Adhesion of a Single Fiber

Adhesive contact between elastic objects usually fails by propagation of crack-like flaws initiated at poor contact regions around surface asperities, impurities, trapped contaminants, etc. As an external load is applied to pull the contacting objects apart, stress concentration is induced near the edges of contact regions around surface asperities. With increasing load, the intensity of stress concentration at the largest interfacial flaw will first reach a critical level and the contact starts to fail by crack growth and coalescence. Under this circumstance, the adhesion strength is not optimal because only a small fraction of material is highly stressed at any instant of loading. From the robustness point of view, it would be best to seek a design of

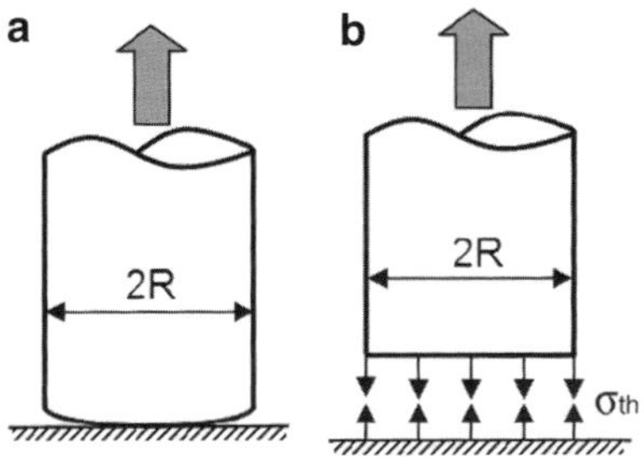

Fig. 10.2 A fiber is brought into contact with a substrate. Depending upon the shape of the fiber tip, the detachment process can occur either by (**a**) crack propagation (*singular shapes*) equivalent to an infinite crack external to the contact area or by (**b**) uniform detachment (*optimal shapes*) in which the stress at pull-off is uniformly distributed and equal to the theoretical adhesion strength σ_{th}. The difference between the adhesive strength of these two failure modes vanishes as the size of the fibril is reduced to below a threshold $R_{\text{cr}} = \frac{8E^*\Delta\gamma}{\pi\sigma_{\text{th}}^2}$, which is taken as the condition for flaw tolerant adhesion

material that allows the contact to fail not by crack propagation, but always by uniform detachment at the theoretical strength of adhesion, a concept termed as *flaw tolerance* [7, 25, 26]. According to this concept, in an ideal flaw tolerant adhesion system, there should be no crack propagation and coalescence as the contact interface is pulled apart by uniform detachment.

For a single fiber on substrate, Gao and Yao [23] investigated the condition for flaw tolerant adhesion from the point of view of variations in contact shape. It was shown that there exist two extreme classes of contact shapes: one class (singular shapes) gives rise to a singular stress field at pull-off similar to that of an external crack (Fig. 10.2a) and the other class (optimal shapes) leads to a uniform stress at pull-off (Fig. 10.2b). For singular shapes, the pull-off force can be calculated according to the Griffith condition [10] as

$$P^f_{\text{crack}} = \pi R^2 \sqrt{\frac{8}{\pi}} \left(\frac{E^* W_{\text{ad}}}{R} \right)^{1/2} \tag{10.1}$$

where W_{ad} denotes the work of adhesion and $E^* = \left[(1 - \nu_f^2)/E_f + (1 - \nu_s^2)/E_s\right]^{-1}$, E_f, E_s, ν_f, ν_s being the Young's moduli and Poisson's ratios of the fiber and the substrate, respectively. For a gecko sticking to a solid surface, we assume $E_s \gg E_f$, therefore $E^* \cong E_f/(1 - \nu_f^2)$. On the other hand, the pull-off force for optimal contact shapes (Fig. 10.2b) is

$$P^f_{\text{th}} = \pi R^2 \sigma_{\text{th}} \tag{10.2}$$

where σ_{th} is the theoretical adhesion strength. Generally, P^f_{crack} is much smaller than P^f_{th}. However, as the size of the fiber is reduced, the value of P^f_{crack} increases towards P^f_{th}. At the critical size

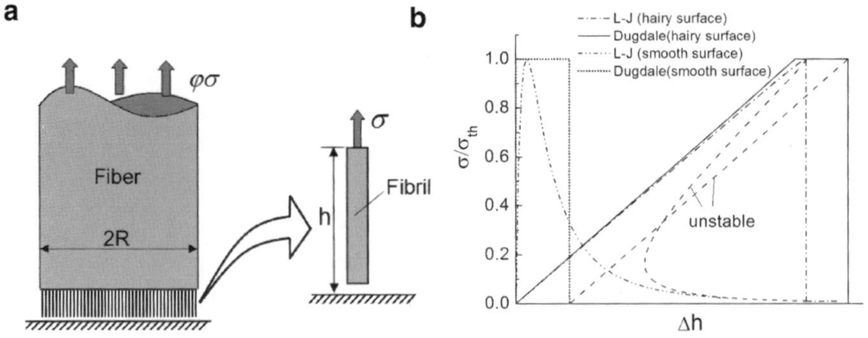

Fig. 10.3 Work of adhesion of a hairy surface. (**a**) Schematic of a hairy surface containing arrays of fibrillar protrusions contacting a substrate. (**b**) Effective stress-separation law for the hairy surface on substrate vs. that for two smooth surfaces

$$R_{\mathrm{cr}} = \frac{8}{\pi} \frac{E_f W_{\mathrm{ad}}}{(1 - \nu_f^2)\sigma_{\mathrm{th}}^2} \tag{10.3}$$

the pull-off force for the singular shapes predicted by the Griffith condition in (10.1) reaches that of the optimal shapes in (10.2). Alternative derivations based on partial contact [7] or perfectly bonded contact [24] lead to similar, but more relaxed, conditions on the fiber size. In this chapter, we shall adopt (10.3) as the basic flaw tolerant condition for adhesion of a single fiber.

10.3.2 Energy Dissipation in Fibrillar Structures

It can be seen from (10.3) that R_{cr} is proportional to the work of adhesion W_{ad} which is commonly taken as the differential surface energy $\Delta\gamma = \gamma_f + \gamma_s - \gamma_{fs}$, where γ_f, γ_s, γ_{fs} denote the surface energies of fiber, substrate, and fiber-substrate interface, respectively. However, this interpretation is correct only in the absence of other dissipation mechanisms. For slender elastic hairs in strong, flaw tolerant adhesion with a solid surface, additional energy dissipation terms should be taken into account.

Consider the adhesion between a larger fiber with a hairy tip surface in contact with a substrate, as shown in Fig. 10.3a. Compared to the case shown in Fig. 10.2, the larger fiber in Fig. 10.3a consists of a number of finer fibrils on its tip, resulting in a two-leveled structure: an array of smaller fibrils on the tip surface of a larger fiber. For this structure, the effective work of adhesion for the larger fiber is no longer equal to $\Delta\gamma$ even though the small fibrils interact with the substrate only via van der Waals forces. To estimate the work of adhesion of the large fiber, we assume that the fibrils are thin enough to meet the condition for flaw tolerant adhesion. Figure 10.3b plots the effective stress-separation relationship for the hairy surface, assuming Lennard-Jones (e.g., [30]) or Dugdale [14] interaction law. While the stress-separation curves for two smooth surfaces are described by the van der Waals or Dugdale interaction laws at the atomic scale, the separation at the level of the larger fiber is strongly influenced by the elastic properties and geometry of the fibrils. For sufficiently long fibrils, the elastic deformation of the fibrils will make significant contributions to the separation process and adhesion failure occurs by an abrupt drop in stress near the theoretical strength of surface interaction. In this way, the strain energy stored in the fiber becomes part of the cohesive energy to be dissipated through dynamic snapping of the thin fibrils. In other words, the thin fibrils behave effectively as cohesive bonds for the larger fiber. The work of adhesion for the large fiber should therefore include the elastic energy stored in the fibrils when they are stretched to failure, i.e.,

$$W_{\mathrm{ad}} = (\Delta\gamma + \sigma_{\mathrm{th}}^2 L/2E_f)\varphi \tag{10.4}$$

where L is the length of the fibrils and φ is the area fraction of the fibril array. The first term within the bracket represents the original van der Waals interaction energy and the second term is the elastic energy lost during dynamic snapping of the fibrils as they are detached from the substrate near the theoretical strength of van der Waals interaction. Equation (4) also shows why it is important to optimize the strength of the lower level fibril structure via size reduction: the strength of the lower scale fibrils directly contributes to the work of adhesion of the larger scale fiber. Taking $\Delta\gamma = 0.01\ \mathrm{J/m^2}$, $\sigma_{\mathrm{th}} = 20$ MPa, $L = 100\ \mu\mathrm{m}$, $E_f = 1$ GPa, $\varphi = 0.5$, the work of adhesion for the hairy tipped fiber is calculated to be $W_{\mathrm{ad}} \approx 10\ \mathrm{J/m^2}$, a value much larger than $\Delta\gamma$. Such enhancement in work of adhesion by fibrillar structures has also been reported or discussed by Jagota and Bennison [31], Persson [20], Gao et al. [25], and Tang et al. [32]. Hence, slender hairs with large aspect ratios can significantly increase the work of adhesion and contribute to the robustness of adhesion at larger scales. However, the length of the fibrils cannot be too long, as there is an instability leading to fiber bunching as the aspect ratio of the fibrils increases.

10.3.3 Anti-Bunching Condition of Fibrillar Array

In an array of slender hairs planted on a solid surface, the van der Waals interaction between neighboring fibers will cause them to bundle together [7, 20, 33–36]. The anti-bunching condition is an important factor in the design of hairy adhesion structures. The exact form of the anti-bunching condition depends on the geometry of the fiber. For example, the anti-bunching condition for fibers of square cross section has been discussed by Hui et al. [35] and Gao et al. [7]. Here, we focus on cylindrical fibers that have been considered by Glassmaker et al. [33].

Consider two neighboring identical cylindrical fibers with circular cross sections. When the separation $2w$ becomes small, the surface adhesive forces may

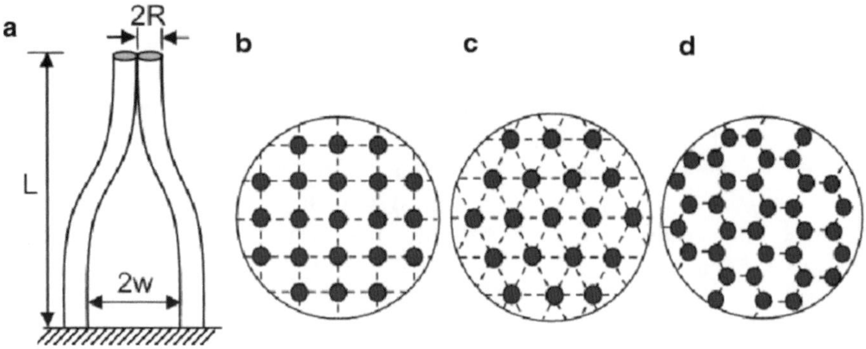

Fig. 10.4 Anti-bunching condition of a fibrillar structure. (**a**) Configuration of self-bunching in an array of fibers distributed in (**b**) *square*, (**c**) *triangular*, or (**d**) *hexagonal* patterns

cause them to bundle together, as shown in Fig. 10.4a. The stability condition can be derived from the point of view of a maximum fiber length for spontaneous separation of two fibers sticking together (e.g., [7]). In other words, given fiber separation w and radius R, there exists a critical length L_{cr} beyond which lateral bunching of neighboring fibers becomes stable configurations. Glassmaker et al. [33] have derived the critical length for bunching of cylindrical fibers as

$$L_{cr} = \left[\frac{\pi^4 E_f R}{2^{11}\gamma_f(1-v_f^2)}\right]^{1/12}\left[\frac{12E_f R^3 w^2}{\gamma_f}\right]^{1/4} \tag{10.5}$$

Assuming that the fibers are distributed in a regular lattice pattern, one can relate the fiber separation w, radius R to the area fraction φ of a fiber array by

$$w = \left(\sqrt{\varphi_{max}/\varphi} - 1\right)R \cdots\cdots\cdots (0 < \varphi < \varphi_{max}) \tag{10.6}$$

where φ_{max} stands for the maximum area fraction of the given hair pattern. It can be shown that $\varphi_{max} = \pi/2\sqrt{3}$ for a triangular lattice (Fig. 10.4b), $\varphi_{max} = \pi/4$ for a square lattice (Fig. 10.4c), and $\pi/3\sqrt{3}$ for a hexagonal lattice (Fig. 10.4d). Inserting (10.6) into (10.5) leads to

$$L_{cr} = R\alpha\left(\frac{E_f R}{\gamma_f}\right)^{1/3}\left(\sqrt{\varphi_{max}/\varphi} - 1\right)^{1/2} \tag{10.7}$$

where $\alpha = \left[\frac{3^3\pi^4}{2^5(1-v_f^2)}\right]^{1/12}$.

Equation (10.7) has been derived for the lateral sticking between two neighboring fibrils. Similar analysis can also be carried out for other possible bunching configurations involving multiple neighboring fibers. We find that the critical fiber

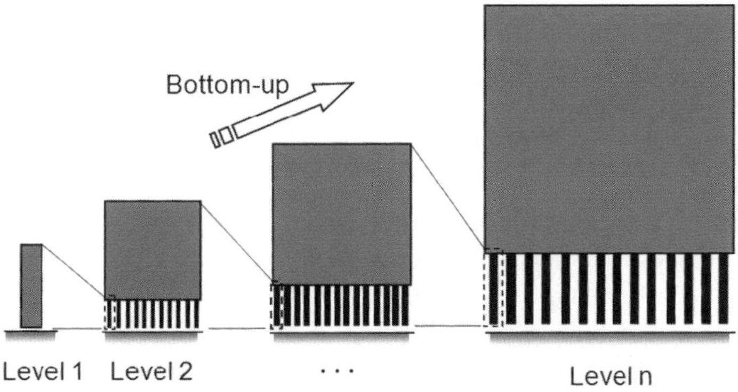

Fig. 10.5 Bottom-up design scheme of a hierarchical fibrillar structure. At each level, the fibers depend on smaller fibrils from the lower hierarchical levels as effective "adhesive bonds" with a surface. Interestingly, the fibers themselves act as "adhesive bonds" for larger fibers from higher hierarchical levels

length for multiple fiber bunching is no less than that given by (10.7). It seems that the anti-bunching condition between two fibers is the most critical condition against bunching involving multiple fibers.

10.3.4 "Fractal Gecko Hairs": Bottom-Up Designed Hierarchical Fibrillar Structures

Given that the work of adhesion can be increased to a larger value by adopting a "hairy" structure [20, 25, 31, 32], the critical length for flaw tolerant adhesion can also be extended to a larger scale, according to (10.3). Meanwhile, the increase in work of adhesion with each level of added hierarchy should be limited by the maximum length of the fibers allowed by the anti-bunching condition. In other words, bunching between fibers provides an upper limit on how much the flaw tolerant length scale can be extended by one level of hierarchy. In order to achieve flaw tolerant adhesion at macroscopic length scales, multiple levels of hierarchy may be needed. To demonstrate the principle of flaw tolerance via structure hierarchy, we propose a "fractal gecko hairs" model, in which a hierarchical fibrillar structure is made from multiple levels of self-affine "brush" structures, as shown in Fig. 10.5. In this fractal structure, the tips of fibers at each level of hierarchy are assumed to be coated with a "brush" structure consisting of smaller fibrils from one level below. The flaw tolerance and anti-bunching conditions are applied to all hierarchical levels from bottom and up to ensure robustness and stability at all levels. That is, the robustness principle of flaw tolerance and the stability principle of anti-bunching are used to determine the fiber geometry at different scales. The bottom-up construction of the desired hierarchical structure is described in some detail below.

At the lowest level of hierarchy, the failure process is governed by the van der Waals interaction between the smallest fibers (ultrastructure) and a solid surface. In this case, the maximum fiber radius ensuring flaw tolerant adhesion is given by

$$R_1 = \frac{8\Delta\gamma E_f}{\pi(1 - v_f^2)\sigma_{\mathrm{th}}^2} \tag{10.8}$$

where the work of adhesion is simply equal to the surface energy $\Delta\gamma$ due to van der Waals interaction and σ_{th} is the theoretical strength of van der Waals forces.

In light of the anti-bunching condition of (10.7), the maximum fiber length of the bottom level can be expressed as a function of the area fraction φ_1 of this level as

$$L_1(\varphi_1) = R_1\alpha\left(\frac{E_f R_1}{\gamma_f}\right)^{1/3}\left(\sqrt{\varphi_{\max}/\varphi_1} - 1\right)^{1/2} \tag{10.9}$$

With these parameters, the work of adhesion associated with the next (second) level is given by

$$W_2^{\mathrm{ad}}(\varphi_1) = \left(\frac{\sigma_{\mathrm{th}}^2 L_1}{2E_f} + \Delta\gamma\right)\varphi_1 \tag{10.10}$$

which is a function of the area fraction φ_1. This function exhibits a maximum at a specific value of φ_1 due to the opposing trends of variation of the parameters L_1 and φ_1: denser fibers with larger φ_1 require smaller L_1 for stability against bunching. Therefore, we can choose the fiber area fraction φ_1 to maximize the work of adhesion at the next level according to (10.10). After φ_1 is calculated, the fiber length L_1 is immediately determined by (10.9). In this way, all the structural parameters characterizing the first level R_1, L_1, φ_1 have been determined. Then, by using (10.10), the work of adhesion for the second level W_2^{ad} is obtained as well.

We now advance further to design the second (next) level. The fiber radius is again chosen to ensure flaw tolerant adhesion,

$$R_2 = \frac{8W_2^{\mathrm{ad}}E_f}{\pi(1 - v_f^2)(S_2)^2} = \frac{8W_2^{\mathrm{ad}}E_f}{\pi(1 - v_f^2)(\varphi_1\sigma_{\mathrm{th}})^2} \tag{10.11}$$

where $S_2 = \varphi_1\sigma_{\mathrm{th}}$ is the effective adhesion strength of the second level. Similarly, the anti-bunching condition allows the fiber length to be determined as a function of the area fraction φ_2 as

$$L_2(\varphi_2) = R_2\alpha\left(\frac{E_f R_2}{\gamma_f}\right)^{1/3}\left(\sqrt{\varphi_{\max}/\varphi_2} - 1\right)^{1/2} \tag{10.12}$$

upon which the work of adhesion for the third level can be determined,

$$W_3^{\text{ad}}(\varphi_2) = \left(W_2^{\text{ad}} + \frac{(S_2)^2 L_2}{2E_f} \right) \varphi_2 = \left(W_2^{\text{ad}} + \frac{(\varphi_1 \sigma_{\text{th}})^2 L_2}{2E_f} \right) \varphi_2 \quad (10.13)$$

Next, the area fraction φ_2 is determined by maximizing $W_3^{\text{ad}}(\varphi_2)$. Once φ_2 is known, the fiber length L_2 is determined from (10.12). Hence all the structural parameters, R_2, L_2, φ_2, for the second hierarchical level, as well as the work of adhesion W_3^{ad} for the third level, have been determined.

An iterative procedure can now be described to determine the structural parameters at all hierarchical levels, starting from the lowest level. Assuming we have completed the design from the first to $(n-1)$-th levels so that $R_i, L_i, \varphi_i, W_i^{\text{ad}}$ $(i = 1, 2, \cdots, n-1)$ as well as W_n^{ad} have been determined, for the n-th level $(n > 1)$, the (maximum) fiber radius ensuring flaw tolerant adhesion is given by

$$R_n = \frac{8W_n^{\text{ad}} E_f}{(1 - v_f^2)\pi (S_n)^2} = \frac{8W_n^{\text{ad}} E_f}{(1 - v_f^2)\pi (\sigma_{\text{th}} \Phi_{n-1})^2} \quad (10.14)$$

where

$$S_n = \sigma_{\text{th}} \Phi_{n-1}, \ \Phi_{n-1} = \varphi_1 \varphi_2 \cdots \varphi_{n-1} = \prod_{i=1}^{n-1} \varphi_i \quad (10.15)$$

is the effective adhesion strength of the n-th level. The (maximum allowable) fiber length of the n-th level can then be expressed, according to the ant-bunching condition, as a function of the area fraction φ_n,

$$L_n(\varphi_n) = \alpha R_n \left(\sqrt{\varphi_{\max}/\varphi_n} - 1 \right)^{1/2} \left(\frac{E_f R_n}{\gamma_f} \right)^{1/3} \quad (10.16)$$

The work of adhesion for the $(n + 1)$-th level is

$$W_{n+1}^{\text{ad}}(\varphi_n) = \left(W_n^{\text{ad}} + \frac{(S_n)^2 L_n}{2E_f} \right) \varphi_n = \left(W_n^{\text{ad}} + \frac{(\sigma_{\text{th}} \Phi_{n-1})^2 L_n}{2E_f} \right) \varphi_n \quad (10.17)$$

The area fraction for the n-th level φ_n can now be determined by maximizing $W_{n+1}^{\text{ad}}(\varphi_n)$, upon which L_n and W_{n+1}^{ad} can be readily calculated. This iterative, bottom-up design procedure can be repeated until the desired size scale for flaw tolerant adhesion is reached. Upon the knowledge of the fiber radius and area fraction of each level, we can calculate the number of fibrils on the tip of a fiber at the next higher level,

$$N_n^f = \varphi_n (R_{n+1}/R_n)^2 \tag{10.18}$$

as well as the net pull-off force at each hierarchical level,

$$F_n = \pi R_n^2 S_n \tag{10.19}$$

Figure 10.6 shows the calculated hierarchical fibrillar structures following the bottom-up design procedure described above. In the calculations, we have taken the material properties of keratin as $E_f = 1.0$ GPa, $\nu_f = 0.3$, $\Delta\gamma = 10$ mJ/m^2, $\gamma_f = 5$ mJ/m^2, and $\sigma_{\mathrm{th}} = 20$ MPa. Three lattice patterns, triangular, square, and hexagonal, for the fiber array are considered. As shown in Fig. 10.6a, b, both the fiber radius and length increase exponentially with the hierarchy level. Under the selected parameters, the critical fiber radius of flaw tolerant adhesion is only around 100 nm at the lowest level of structure. With hierarchical design, the flaw tolerant radius increases to 1 μm with 2 levels, 1 mm with 3 levels, 1 m with 4 levels of hierarchy. With 8 levels, the dimension of flaw tolerant radius has reached 10^{26} m, which is an astronomical size! These calculations demonstrate the enormous potential of a hierarchical structure for flaw tolerant adhesion. Figure 10.6c displays the variation of the area fraction with the number of hierarchy levels. Interestingly, the area fraction converges to a constant after the third hierarchy level for each fiber layout pattern. Figure 10.6d shows the work of adhesion at different hierarchical levels. In the first 6 levels, the triangular fiber pattern exhibits higher work of adhesion than the other two patterns. With further increase in hierarchy levels, this advantage is taken over by the hexagonal fiber pattern. Figure 10.6e shows the effective adhesion strength, which decreases and asymptotically approaches zero with the increasing hierarchy level. However, the net pull-off force, as shown in Fig. 10.6f, increases exponentially with the hierarchy level. Figure 10.6g illustrates the number N_n^f of fibrils on the tip of a fiber at the next level. We see that N_n^f increases sharply with increasing hierarchy levels. Most results in Fig. 10.6 are presented in the normalized form. The quantitative estimates based on the assumed materials properties are tabulated in Table 10.1.

It is of interest to make a comparison between our calculated results with the observed hierarchical structure in nature. Under the selected parameters, our results show that the diameter and length of the first level fiber are 140 nm and 1.37 μm, respectively. These values are not inconsistent with the dimension of the topmost spatula hairs (stalk) of Tokay gecko (*Gekko gecko*), which is around 100–200 nm wide and 0.5–3 μm long [2, 37]. [Note: These values are estimated from the micrographs in the references.] The dimension of the second level of our bottom-up constructed structure is around 7.56–11.34 μm wide and 286–491 μm long, depending upon the pattern of the fiber array, while the size of a seta on gecko's feet is about 5 μm in width and 110 μm in length [37]. In addition, our calculation predicts that the number of the lowest level fibrils accommodated by a fiber of the second level is around 1,539–2,309, which is qualitatively similar to the observation of 100–1,000 spatulae/seta [3]. Furthermore, from our calculated results we

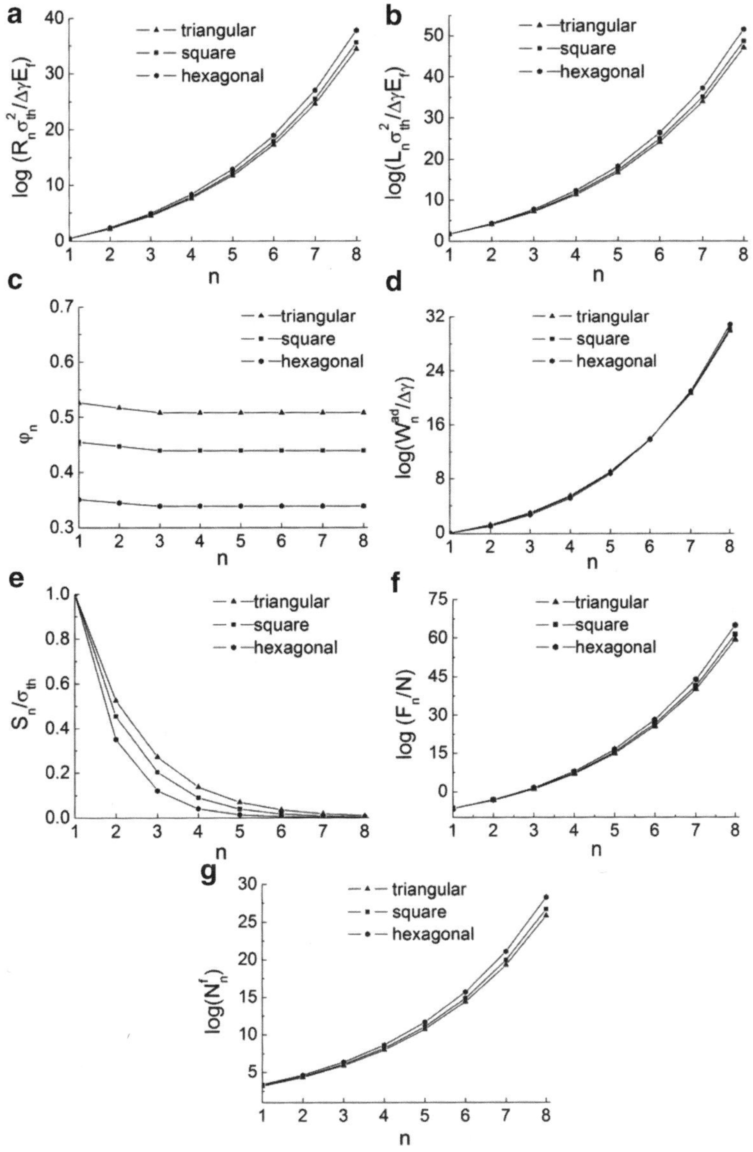

Fig. 10.6 Variations of (**a**) fiber radius R_n, (**b**) fiber length L_n, (**c**) area fraction φ_n, (**d**) work of adhesion W_n^{ad}, (**e**) adhesion strength S_n, (**f**) pull-off force F_n, and (**g**) the number of fibers N_n^f as a function of the hierarchical level n

evaluate the density $N_2^f/\pi R_3^2$ of the second level fiber to be 11,494 mm^{-2}, 7,363 mm^{-2}, 3,439 mm^{-2} for triangular, square, and hexagonal patterns, respectively. This is also comparable to the observed density of gecko's seta around 14,400 mm^{-2} [3]. Interestingly, in nature, the spatula density within single species

Table 10.1 Calculated geometrical and mechanical properties of bottom-up designed fractal gecko hair structure

n	R_n (m)	L_n (m)	φ_n	W_n^{ad}(J/m^2)	S_n(MPa)	F_n (N)	N_n^f
Triangular							
1	7.0×10^{-8}	1.37×10^{-6}	0.5260	0.01	20	3.08×10^{-7}	1.539×10^{3}
2	3.78×10^{-6}	2.86×10^{-4}	0.5169	0.15	10.52	4.73×10^{-4}	2.2032×10^{4}
3	7.81×10^{-4}	0.36	0.5079	8.26	5.44	10.43	7.9914×10^{5}
4	0.98	4.80×10^{3}	0.5079	2.67×10^{3}	2.76	8.33×10^{6}	9.2685×10^{7}
5	1.32×10^{4}	1.55×10^{9}	0.5079	9.31×10^{6}	1.4026	7.72×10^{14}	5.2558×10^{10}
6	4.26×10^{9}	3.41×10^{16}	0.5079	7.72×10^{11}	0.7123	4.06×10^{25}	2.4676×10^{14}
7	9.39×10^{16}	2.11×10^{26}	0.5079	4.39×10^{18}	0.3618	1.00×10^{40}	1.9399×10^{19}
8	5.80×10^{26}	2.39×10^{39}	0.5079	7.0×10^{27}	0.1837	1.94×10^{59}	6.5330×10^{25}
Square							
1	7.0×10^{-8}	1.37×10^{-6}	0.4555	0.01	20	3.08×10^{-7}	1.777×10^{3}
2	4.37×10^{-6}	3.46×10^{-4}	0.4477	0.13	9.11	5.47×10^{-4}	2.7977×10^{4}
3	1.10×10^{-3}	0.56	0.4398	6.49	4.08	15.50	1.1534×10^{6}
4	1.7691	1.06×10^{4}	0.4398	2.03×10^{3}	1.79	1.76×10^{7}	1.5865×10^{8}
5	3.36×10^{4}	5.35×10^{9}	0.4398	7.47×10^{6}	0.79	2.80×10^{15}	1.1291×10^{11}
6	1.70×10^{10}	2.16×10^{17}	0.4398	7.33×10^{11}	0.35	3.16×10^{26}	7.1761×10^{14}
7	6.88×10^{17}	3.0×10^{27}	0.4398	5.72×10^{18}	0.15	2.27×10^{41}	8.4482×10^{19}
8	9.53×10^{27}	9.97×10^{40}	0.4398	1.53×10^{28}	0.067	1.91×10^{61}	4.8744×10^{26}
Hexagonal							
1	7.0×10^{-8}	1.37×10^{-6}	0.3507	0.01	20	3.08×10^{-7}	2.309×10^{3}
2	5.68×10^{-6}	4.91×10^{-4}	0.3446	0.10	7.01	7.10×10^{-4}	4.3203×10^{4}
3	2.0×10^{-3}	1.25	0.3386	4.20	2.42	30.37	2.2486×10^{6}
4	5.18	4.42×10^{4}	0.3386	1.24×10^{3}	0.82	6.90×10^{7}	4.2178×10^{8}
5	1.83×10^{5}	5.12×10^{10}	0.3386	5.02×10^{6}	0.28	2.91×10^{16}	4.5376×10^{11}
6	2.12×10^{11}	6.23×10^{18}	0.3386	6.66×10^{11}	0.0938	1.32×10^{28}	5.0028×10^{15}
7	2.57×10^{19}	3.75×10^{29}	0.3386	9.27×10^{18}	0.0318	6.61×10^{43}	1.2276×10^{21}
8	1.55×10^{30}	8.85×10^{43}	0.3386	6.40×10^{28}	0.0108	8.14×10^{64}	1.8860×10^{28}

remains almost constant in spite of several orders of magnitude change in body mass [38]. How do we understand this from a mechanics point of view? Within single species, it is easier to adopt the same design for single contact element and simply multiply this strategy by increasing the adhesion pad size. This strategy is limited, since eventually the adhesion pad becomes too large and flaw sensitive. New species will have to emerge with more sophisticated structural hierarchy. It seems that gecko only adopts a few levels of hierarchical fibrillar structures to achieve robust adhesion. A question then is: why has nature not evolved more hierarchical levels, and thus larger adhesion species heavier than gecko? A possible answer to this question is addressed in the following section.

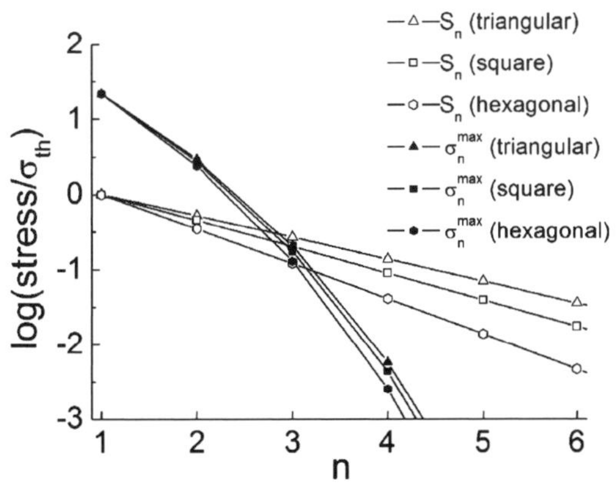

Fig. 10.7 Comparison between the fracture strength $\sigma_n^{\max}$ of a cracked fiber and the n-th level adhesion strength S_n of the bottom-up designed fractal hairs. If $\sigma_n^{\max} > S_n$, adhesion failure is regarded as the principal failure mode, otherwise ($\sigma_n^{\max} < S_n$) fiber fracture is thought of as the principal failure mode

10.3.5 Fiber Fracture: An Upper Limit on Flaw Tolerant Adhesion Design

In the preceding discussions, we have focused on failure along an adhesion interface and implicitly assumed that the fibers themselves do not fracture. In practice, as the adhesion strength is enhanced by introducing hierarchical fibrillar structures, the fracture of fibers eventually rises to become the dominant issue for failure at the system level. In other words, a robust adhesion system must be robust against not only adhesion failure, but also fiber fracture.

Consider a single fiber at hierarchy level n. A penny-shaped crack is introduced in the center of the cross section as a possible internal flaw. Other configurations of crack-like flaws, such as edge/corner cracks/singularities, can be considered without affecting the basic idea. The maximum tensile stress that this fiber can sustain can be determined from the Griffith's criterion [10] for crack growth as [39],

$$\sigma_n^{\max} = \sqrt{\frac{E_f^* \Gamma_f}{R_n}} \frac{\sqrt{\pi R_n / 2a}}{g(a/R_n)} \tag{10.20}$$

where a is the crack radius, Γ_f is the fracture energy and

$$g\left(\frac{a}{R_n}\right) = \frac{1 - 0.5a/R_n + 0.148(a/R_n)^3}{\sqrt{1 - a/R_n}} \tag{10.21}$$

is a geometrical parameter. Considering a crack half the size of the fiber, i.e., $a/R_n = 0.5$, (10.20) can be further reduced to

$$\sigma_n^{\max} = 1.63\sqrt{E_f^* \Gamma_f / R_n} \tag{10.22}$$

The relative significance of fiber fracture can be measured by a comparison between $\sigma_n^{\max}$ and the effective adhesion strength S_n at the n-th hierarchical level. If $\sigma_n^{\max} > S_n$, adhesion failure is regarded as the dominant issue and further increase in hierarchical levels can be considered. On the other hand, if $\sigma_n^{\max} < S_n$, fiber fracture is regarded as the dominant issue, hence an upper limit on the hierarchical design. Taking $\Gamma_f = 5\ \mathrm{J/m^2}$ and $E_f^* = 1$ GPa, we compare $\sigma_n^{\max}$ and S_n for the fractal hair structures constructed above. As shown in Fig. 10.7, for triangular and square fiber layout, only fibers within the first two levels satisfy the condition $\sigma_n^{\max} > S_n$; for the hexagonal layout, this condition is satisfied for the first three levels. Hence, although there is no upper bound for flaw tolerant adhesion via fractal hairs design, crack-like flaws in the hairs themselves would impose a practical limit for the usefulness of this strategy. Of course, above conclusions are based on the properties of keratin, which is the material of gecko's attachment system. Therefore, unless new structural protein is formed, gecko seems to stand near the limit of evolution.

10.4 Releasable Adhesion

For geckos and insects, robust adhesion alone is insufficient for survival as these animals also need to move swiftly on walls and ceilings; the reversibility of attachment is just as important as the attachment. A conceivable strategy for reversible adhesion is to design an orientation-controlled switch between attachment and detachment, with adhesion strength varying strongly with the direction of pulling. An ideal scenario of robust and releasable adhesion is that the adhesion strength would be maintained near the theoretical strength when pulled in some range of directions, but then dramatically reduced when pulled in another range of directions. The switch between attachment and detachment can thus be accomplished simply by changing the pulling angles (e.g., by exerting different muscles). Some known examples of anisotropic adhesion systems in which the pull-off force varies strongly with the direction of pulling include an elastic tape on substrate [5, 21, 40] and a single seta of gecko sticking on a wall [2, 7]. Here we show that such behavior can actually be generalized to three-dimensional elastic solids as long as there is sufficiently strong elastic anisotropy.

10.4.1 Directional Adhesion Strength of an Elastic Tape

For an elastic tape adhering on a substrate, as shown in Fig. 10.8a, Kendall [40] showed that the critical force required to peel the tape off the substrate can be written as

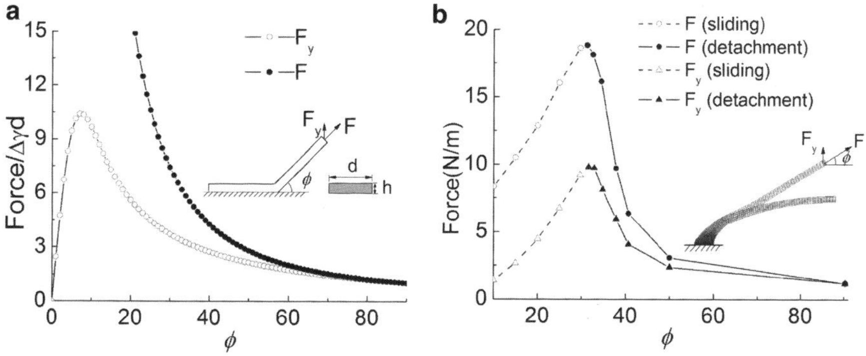

Fig. 10.8 Releasable adhesion in one-dimensional structures. Variation of the pull-off force as a function of the pulling angle for (**a**) an elastic tape and (**b**) a single seta of gecko on a surface (adapted, with permission, from [7])

$$F = E_{\mathrm{tp}}hd\left[\sqrt{(1-\cos\varphi)^2 + 2\Delta\gamma/E_{\mathrm{tp}}h} - (1-\cos\varphi)\right]$$
$$= \frac{2\Delta\gamma d}{\sqrt{(1-\cos\varphi)^2 + 2\Delta\gamma/E_{\mathrm{tp}}h} + (1-\cos\varphi)} \qquad (10.23)$$

where E_{tp} denotes the Young's modulus of the tape; h and d stand for the thickness and width of the tape, respectively. For a given elastic tape, (10.23) indicates that the peel-off force varies with the pulling angle φ. Taking $\Delta\gamma/E_{\mathrm{tp}}h = 10^{-4}$ ($\Delta\gamma = 0.01$ J/m^2, $E_{\mathrm{tp}} = 1.0$ GPa, $h = 100$ nm), Fig. 10.8a plots the variation of the normalized peel-off force and its projection normal to the contact interface as a function of the pulling angle φ. It is evident that the peel-off force varies strongly with the pulling angle. [Note: Recently, Chen and Gao [41] have generalized Kendall's model to peeling of a prestressed elastic tape on substrate, with results showing that a significantly large prestress can cause spontaneous detachment at a critical angle, independent of the magnitude of the peeling force. However, the role of prestress in reversible adhesion is beyond the scope of this chapter and will not be discussed here.] Under the selected parameter values, the normal projection of the peeling force exhibits a maximum value around $\varphi \approx 7°$.

10.4.2 Directional Adhesion Strength of a Single Seta

Autumn et al. [2] reported experimental data that the detachment force of a single seta of gecko on a surface strongly depends on the orientation of pulling, with the peak value achieved as the seta is pulled at an inclined angle of $\varphi = 30°$ with respect to the tangent of the surface. Motivated by this experiment, Gao et al. [7] performed finite element calculations of the pull-off force of a single seta and, as shown in their results plotted in Fig. 10.8b, confirmed theoretically that the pull-off force of gecko's seta strongly varies with the pulling orientation, with the maximum value achieved around $\varphi = 30°$.

In the case of single contact by an elastic tape or seta, the anisotropic behavior of the pull-off force can be attributed to the asymmetric alignment and slender structure of the contacting object. While this behavior suggests that the pull-off force of a single hair in contact can be controlled by pulling in different directions, an open question is whether the adhesive strength of a large array of fibers or a macroscopic attachment pad in contact with a rough surface would show similar behaviors. To address this question, we shall consider the issue of releasable adhesion from the point of view of continuum interfacial failure mechanics. We use theoretical modeling and numerical simulations to show that strong elastic anisotropy on the continuum level, achieved via fibrillar microstructures or some other means, plays a key role in releasable adhesion: a strongly anisotropic elastic solid also exhibits a strong orientational dependence of the pull-off force, similar to the behavior of a single seta studied by Gao et al. [7].

10.4.3 Directional Adhesion Strength of an Anisotropic Elastic Material

To illustrate the intrinsic orientation-dependence of adhesion strength of an anisotropic elastic material in contact with a rough surface, we consider the linear elastic plane-strain problem shown in Fig. 10.9a where a transversely isotropic elastic half-space ($y \geq 0$) is brought to contact with a rigid substrate. A plane-strain interfacial

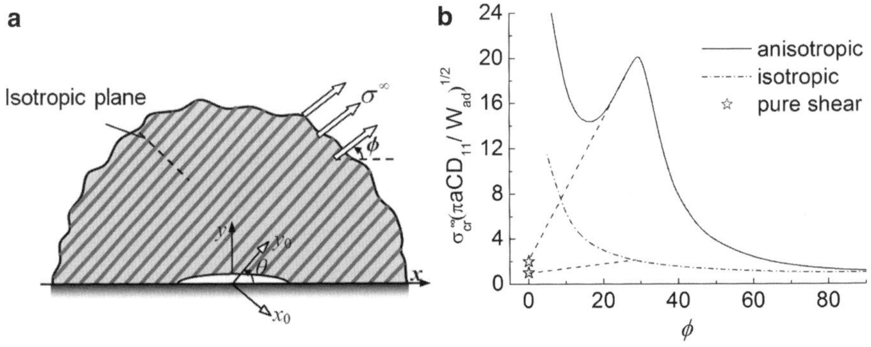

Fig. 10.9 Releasable adhesion in three dimension. The pull-off stress of a strongly anisotropic (transversely isotropic) elastic half-space sticking to a substrate. (**a**) An interfacial crack-like flaw with width $2a$ is introduced as a representative contact flaw due to surface roughness or contaminants. (**b**) Variation of the adhesion stress as a function of the pulling angle for the anisotropic material in comparison with that for an isotropic material

crack of size $2a$ is used to represent random contact flaws due to surface roughness or contaminants. Although the actual adhesion strength depends on the crack size, the ratio between the maximum and minimum pull-off stresses as the pulling angle varies will be shown to be independent of the crack geometry and can be used as a measure of the releasability of adhesion.

In this interfacial crack model, the longitudinal direction of the material (y_0 axis) is tilted at an angle θ from the tangent of the substrate surface (x-axis). A remote uniaxial tensile stress σ^∞ is applied at an angle φ with respect to the x-axis. The transversely isotropic material is characterized by five independent elastic constants: E_t, E_l, v_t, v_l and μ. E_t and E_l stand for the transverse (x_0 direction) and longitudinal (y_0 direction) Young's moduli, respectively; v_t and v_l are Poisson's ratios associated with transverse (x_0 direction) and longitudinal (y_0 direction) loading, respectively; μ denotes the shear modulus in the x_0–y_0 plane.

We are interested in the pull-off stress of the above adhesion system as a function of the pulling direction. This problem can be solved as a classical interfacial crack between two dissimilar anisotropic elastic solids [42–47]. The energy release rate induced by remotely applied normal and shear stresses (σ_{xy}^∞, σ_{yy}^∞) is calculated to be [48]

$$G = \frac{\pi a(1+4\varepsilon^2)}{4\cosh^2 \pi\varepsilon}\left[D_{22}(\sigma_{xy}^\infty \cos\theta + \sigma_{yy}^\infty \sin\theta)^2 + D_{11}(\sigma_{xy}^\infty \sin\theta - \sigma_{yy}^\infty \cos\theta)^2\right] \tag{10.24}$$

where

$$\begin{aligned}
&\varepsilon = \frac{1}{2\pi}\ln\frac{1+\beta}{1-\beta}, \quad \beta = \left|W_{21}(D_{11}D_{22})^{-1/2}\right|,\\
&D_{11} = \frac{1}{E_t}\sqrt{\frac{E_t}{E_l}}(1-v_t^2)^{1/2}\left(\frac{E_l}{\mu}+2\left[\sqrt{(1-v_t^2)\left(\frac{E_l}{E_t}-v_l{}^2\right)}-v_l(1+v_t)\right]\right)^{1/2},\\
&D_{22} = \frac{1}{E_l}\left(1-\frac{v_l^2}{E_l}E_t\right)^{1/2}\left(\frac{E_l}{\mu}+2\left[\sqrt{(1-v_t^2)\left(\frac{E_l}{E_t}-v_l^2\right)}-v_l(1+v_t)\right]\right)^{1/2},\\
&W_{21} = -\sqrt{\frac{1}{E_tE_l}}\left[\sqrt{(1-v_t^2)\left(1-\frac{v_l^2E_t}{E_l}\right)}-(1+v_t)v_l\sqrt{\frac{E_t}{E_l}}\right]
\end{aligned} \tag{10.25}$$

For the uniaxial pulling stress σ^∞ applied at an inclined angle φ, as shown in Fig. 10.9a, the components σ_{xy}^∞ and σ_{yy}^∞ can be expressed as

$$\sigma_{xy}^\infty = \sigma^\infty \sin\varphi\cos\varphi, \sigma_{yy}^\infty = \sigma^\infty \sin\varphi \sin\varphi \tag{10.26}$$

Substituting (10.26) into (10.24) and then applying the Griffith's criterion for crack initiation $G = W_{\text{ad}}$ lead to the adhesion strength

$$\sigma_{\mathrm{cr}}^{\infty}(\theta,\varphi)=\frac{\sqrt{W_{\mathrm{ad}}/\pi a}}{\sin\varphi\sqrt{C[D_{22}\cos^2(\theta-\varphi)+D_{11}\sin^2(\theta-\varphi)]}} \tag{10.27}$$

where

$$C=\frac{(1+4\varepsilon^2)}{4\cosh^2\pi\varepsilon} \tag{10.28}$$

Given material constants and the anisotropy direction θ, (10.27) indicates that the adhesion strength varies as a function of the pulling angle φ. To calculate the critical (maximum and minimum) values as well as the corresponding directions, we solve equation $\frac{\partial\sigma_{\mathrm{cr}}^{\infty}(\theta,\varphi)}{\partial\varphi}=0$ and obtain

$$\frac{1+D_{22}/D_{11}}{1-D_{22}/D_{11}}\cos\varphi=\cos(3\varphi-2\theta), D_{22}/D_{11}=\sqrt{\frac{E_t(E_l-\nu_l^2E_t)}{E_l^2(1-\nu_t^2)}} \tag{10.29}$$

If the Young's modulus in the longitudinal direction (e.g., along a fiber array) is much larger than that in the transverse direction (e.g., transverse to the fiber direction), i.e., $E_l/E_t \gg 1$, (10.29) has two roots

$$\varphi_1=\theta,\ \varphi_2=\theta/2+\pi/2 \tag{10.30}$$

corresponding to the directions of the maximum and minimum pull-off stresses, respectively. The adhesion releasability thus can be measured by the ratio of the maximum to the minimum pull-off stresses:

$$\frac{(\sigma_{\mathrm{cr}}^{\infty})_{\max}}{(\sigma_{\mathrm{cr}}^{\infty})_{\min}}=\frac{(1+\cos\theta)}{2\sin\theta}\left(\frac{D_{11}}{D_{22}}\right)^{1/2}=\frac{(1+\cos\theta)}{2\sin\theta}\left[\frac{E_l^2(1-\nu_t^2)}{E_t(E_l-\nu_l^2E_t)}\right]^{1/4} \tag{10.31}$$

For small Poisson's ratios, (10.31) suggests that the releasibility of adhesion mainly depends on the stiffness ratio E_l/E_t and the anisotropy direction θ. The stronger the anisotropy, the higher the releasibility of adhesion. Assuming $\nu_t=\nu_l=0.3, \theta=30°$, and $E_l/E_t=10^4$, Fig. 10.9b plots the normalized pull-off stress as a function of the pulling angle φ. We can see that the elastic anisotropy causes about an order of magnitude change in adhesion strength as the pulling angle varies. A switch between attachment and detachment can thus be accomplished just by shifting the pulling angle between these two directions. In contrast, the adhesion strength for an isotropic material with $E_l=E_t$ and $\nu_l=\nu_t$ is much less sensitive to the pulling direction. We conclude that strong elastic anisotropy can result in an orientation-controlled switch between attachment and detachment. Similar orientation-dependent behavior can also be seen from the adhesive contact between a rigid sphere and an anisotropic elastic substrate [49].

One might note that (10.27) implies an infinite adhesion strength in the limit of $\varphi = 0$. This is caused by the uniaxial tensile stress that we have assumed. Actually, the limit $\varphi = 0$ should be characterized as sliding under an applied shear stress. If, instead of pulling, we apply a remote shear stress σ_{xy}^{∞}, the critical shear stress becomes

$$(\sigma_{xy}^{\infty})_{\mathrm{cr}} = \frac{\sqrt{W_{\mathrm{ad}}/\pi a}}{\sqrt{C(D_{22}\cos^2\theta + D_{11}\sin^2\theta)}} \tag{10.32}$$

which can be reduced to

$$(\sigma_{xy}^{\infty})_{\mathrm{cr}} = \frac{2\sqrt{W_{\mathrm{ad}}/\pi a}}{\sqrt{CD_{11}}} \tag{10.33}$$

when $D_{22} \ll D_{11}$ and $\theta = 30°$, and to

$$(\sigma_{xy}^{\infty})_{\mathrm{cr}} = \frac{\sqrt{W_{\mathrm{ad}}/\pi a}}{\sqrt{CD_{11}}} \tag{10.34}$$

when $D_{22} = D_{11}$ for the isotropic case. The results of (10.33) and (10.34) are shown by the star symbols in Fig. 10.9b.

10.4.4 Directional Adhesion Strength of an Attachment Pad: Numerical Simulation

To further verify the principle of orientation-controlled adhesion switch via strong elastic anisotropy, we have also performed numerical simulations of the adhesion of a strongly anisotropic attachment pad (mimicking the hairy structured tissue on gecko's feet) via a general-purpose finite element code Tahoe (http://tahoe.ca.sandia.gov) with specialized cohesive surface elements for modeling adhesive interactions between two surfaces. The constitutive relation for the cohesive surface elements is specified in terms of a relation between the traction and separation across the contact interface. Tahoe supports a number of traction-separation laws including the Tvergaard-Hutchinson law [50] and the Xu-Needleman law [51]. In present simulations, we adopt the Tvergaard-Hutchinson law based on the following interaction potential

$$\Phi(\lambda) = \delta_{\mathrm{cn}} \int_0^{\lambda} \bar{\varphi}(\tilde{\lambda})\mathrm{d}\tilde{\lambda} \tag{10.35}$$

where

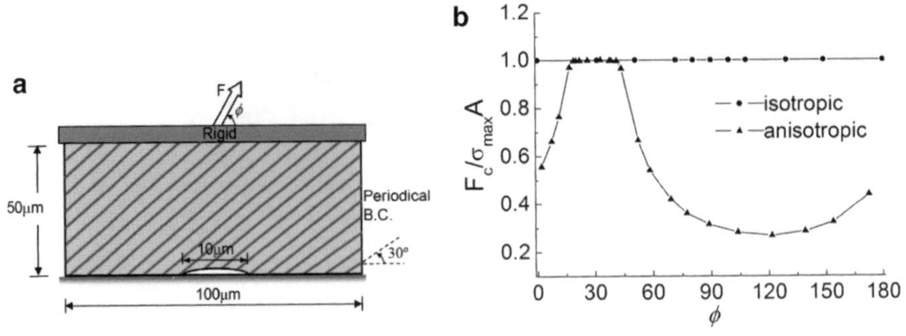

Fig. 10.10 Releasable adhesion in an attachment pad. (**a**) Geometry of the attachment pad used in FEM calculations. (**b**) Variation of normalized pull-off force with the pulling angle. Periodic B.C.: periodic boundary condition

$$\lambda = \sqrt{\left(\frac{\Delta_n}{\delta_{\text{cn}}}\right)^2 + \left(\frac{\Delta_t}{\delta_{\text{ct}}}\right)^2} \tag{10.36}$$

Here, Δ_n denotes the normal separation and Δ_t the tangential separation; δ_{cn} and δ_{ct} are the corresponding critical separations. The force function $\bar{\varphi}$ is taken to be trilinear,

$$\bar{\varphi}(\lambda) = \begin{cases} \sigma_{\max}\lambda/\Lambda_1 & (\lambda < \Lambda_1) \\ \sigma_{\max} & (\Lambda_1 < \lambda < \Lambda_2) \\ \sigma_{\max}(1-\lambda)/(1-\Lambda_2), & (\Lambda_2 < \lambda < 1) \end{cases} \tag{10.37}$$

where Λ_1 and Λ_2 define the values of λ at which the cohesive force reaches the peak. Taking the partial derivatives of the potential with respect to the normal and tangential separations gives the normal and tangential tractions as

$$T_n = \frac{\partial \Phi}{\partial \Delta_n} = \frac{\Delta_n}{\delta_{cn}} \frac{\bar{\varphi}(\lambda)}{\lambda} \tag{10.38}$$

$$T_t = \frac{\partial \Phi}{\partial \Delta_t} = \frac{\delta_{\text{cn}}}{\delta_{\text{ct}}} \frac{\Delta_t}{\delta_{\text{ct}}} \frac{\bar{\varphi}(\lambda)}{\lambda} \tag{10.39}$$

Clearly, Tvergaard-Hutchison law takes into account both normal and tangential tractions with a constant work of adhesion

$$W_{\text{ad}} = 1/2(1 + \Lambda_2 - \Lambda_1)\sigma_{\max}\delta_{\text{cn}} \tag{10.40}$$

The simulation system consists of a plane-strain anisotropic (transversely isotropic) elastic pad adhering to a rigid substrate with a crack situated at the central region of the contact interface (representing an adhesion flaw due to surface

Table 10.2 Parameters used in FEM simulation

Isotropic case	$E = 1.0$ GPa, $\nu = 0.3$
Anisotropic case	$E_t = 0.1$ MPa, $E_l = 1.0$ GPa, $\nu_t = \nu_l = 0.3$, $\mu = 10$ MPa, $\theta = 30°$
Parameters for Tvergaard-Hutchinson model	
$\Lambda_1 = 0.1$, $\Lambda_2 = 0.9$, $\sigma_{max} = 5.44$ MPa, $\delta_{cn} = \delta_{ct} = 1.687\mu$m ($W_{ad} = 8.26$J/m^2)	

roughness), as shown in Fig. 10.10a. A displacement-controlled load is applied on the upper surface to make all the nodes on the upper surface have a uniform translation. At a given translation, summation of all the nodal forces on the upper surface gives the pulling force F with components F_x and F_y. The pulling angle is then calculated via $\varphi = \tan^{-1}(F_y/F_x)$. Periodic boundary conditions are applied on left and right sides. For comparison, both the isotropic case and the anisotropic cases are considered. The material constants and potential parameters for each simulation case are listed in Table 10.2, where we adopt the calculated S_3 and W_3^{ad} of the triangular hair pattern (see Table 10.1) as the effective adhesion strength and work of adhesion, respectively, in simulating the detachment process of the pad.

To illustrate the anisotropy-induced releasability of adhesion, Fig. 10.10b plots the normalized pull-off stress $F_c(\varphi)/(A\sigma_{max})$ as a function of the pulling angle φ. In the anisotropic case, saturation of adhesion strength is observed in the vicinity of $\varphi = \theta = 30°$, corresponding to a plateau of the curve in the range of $20° < \varphi < 40°$. If the pulling angle deviates from this range in either direction, the adhesion strength decreases quickly to a lower plateau. This two-plateau adhesion strength is ideal for rapid switch between attachment and detachment during animal movement. The ratio between the maximum and minimum strengths reaches four for the given geometry, giving rise to significant releasability. In contrast, for the isotropic cases, no variation in pull-off force is observed as the pulling angle varies. Therefore, we conclude that strong elastic anisotropy leads to releasable adhesion via an orientation-controlled switch between strong and weak adhesion.

10.5 Conclusions

In this chapter, we discussed the basic principles of robust and releasable adhesion in the hierarchical structures of gecko. The work has been inspired by comparative studies of biological attachment systems in nature. For robust adhesion, we use a bottom-up designed fractal hair structure as a model to demonstrate that hierarchical fibrillar structures can lead to robust adhesion at macroscopic scales. Barring fiber fracture, we show that the fractal gecko hairs system can tolerate crack-like flaws without size limit. However, in practice, as the adhesion strength is enhanced by structural hierarchy, fiber fracture ultimately becomes the dominant failure mechanism and places an upper bound on the size scale of flaw tolerant adhesion. An optimal design is to introduce an appropriate number of hierarchical levels so that the adhesion interface and the hairs have similar strength levels. For releasable adhesion, we showed that strong elastic anisotropy allows the adhesion strength to vary strongly with the direction of pulling. This orientation-dependent pull-off force enables robust attachment in the stiff direction of the material to be released by pulling in the soft direction. This strategy can be summarized as "stiff-adhere, soft-release."

The complex hierarchical structures in biology provide a rich source of inspirations for physical sciences and industrial applications. The concepts discussed in this chapter should be of general value in understanding biological attachment devices and the design of synthetic adhesive systems in engineering (e.g., [29, 36, 52, 53]). While we usually do not expect to capture all of the bio-complexities in simple models, it is often important to break a complex problem into many comprehensible sub-problems that can be understood using mechanics principles. Here we have considered the effects of hierarchical energy dissipation and elastic anisotropy on robust and releasable adhesion. Many other important aspects of the problem, such as viscoelasticity and large nonlinear deformation, have not been taken into account. Much further work will be needed to advance our current understanding of bio-adhesion mechanisms. The studies on such problems should be of interest not only to the mechanics community but also to a variety of other disciplines, including materials science, biology, and nanotechnology.

Acknowledgements The authors gratefully acknowledge stimulating discussions on biological adhesion systems with many colleagues including K. Autumn, E. Arzt, B. Chen, Q.H. Cheng, L.M. Dai, R. Fearing, R.J. Full, S. Gorb, P. Guduru, A. Jagota, C.Y. Hui, K. Kendall, R. Spolenak, Z.L. Wang, Z.Q. Zhang, and Y.W. Zhang. HY acknowledges helpful discussions with Dr. Patrick Klein on the FEM simulations using Tahoe. Support of this work has been provided by the Max Planck Society, Brown University, the A*Star VIP Program in Singapore, the National Natural Science Foundation of China (11072273), and the Program for New Century Excellent Talents in China.

References

1. Scherge M, Gorb S (2001) Biological micro- and nanotribology. Springer, New York
2. Autumn K, Liang YA, Hsieh ST, Zesch W, Chan WP, Kenny TW, Fearing R, Full RJ (2000) Adhesive force of a single gecko foot-hair. Nature 405:681–685
3. Autumn K, Peattie AM (2002) Mechanisms of adhesion in geckos. Integr Comp Biol 42:1081–1090
4. Autumn K, Sitti M, Liang YA, Peattie AM, Hansen WR, Sponberg S, Kenny TW, Fearing R, Israelachvili JN, Full RJ (2002) Evidence for van der Waals adhesion in gecko setae. Proc Natl Acad Sci USA 99:12252–12256
5. Huber G, Gorb S, Spolenak R, Arzt E (2005) Resolving the nanoscale adhesion of individual gecko spatulae by atomic force microscopy. Biol Lett 1:2–4
6. Israelachvili JN (1992) Intermolecular and surface forces, 2nd edn. Academic, London
7. Gao H, Wang X, Yao H, Gorb S, Arzt E (2005) Mechanics of hierarchical adhesion structures of geckos. Mech Mater 37:275–285
8. Hertz H (1882) Über die Berührung fester elastischer Körper (On the Contact of Elastic Solids). J Reine Angew Math 92:156–171

9. Johnson KL, Kendall K, Roberts AD (1971) Surface energy and contact of elastic solids. Proc R Soc Lond A 324:301–313
10. Griffith AA (1921) The phenomena of rupture and flow in solids. Philos Trans R Soc Lond A 221:163–198
11. Derjaguin BV, Muller VM, Toporov YP (1975) Effect of contact deformations on the adhesion of particles. J Colloid Interface Sci 53:314–326
12. Bradley RS (1932) The cohesive force between solid surfaces and the surface energy of solids. Philos Mag 13:853–862
13. Maugis D (1992) Adhesion of spheres: the JKR-DMT transition using a Dugdale model. J Colloid Interface Sci 150:243–269
14. Dugdale DS (1960) Yielding of steel sheets containing slits. J Mech Phys Solids 8:100–104
15. Hui CY, Baney JM, Kramer EJ (1998) Contact mechanics and adhesion of viscoelastic spheres. Langmuir 14:6570–6578
16. Haiat G, Huy MCP, Barthel E (2003) The adhesive contact of viscoelastic spheres. J Mech Phys Solids 51:69–99
17. Kim KS, McMeeking RM, Johnson KL (1998) Adhesion, slip, cohesive zones and energy fluxes for elastic spheres in contact. J Mech Phys Solids 46:243–266
18. Arzt E, Enders S, Gorb S (2002) Towards a micromechanical understanding of biological surface devices. Z Metallk 93:345–351
19. Arzt E, Gorb S, Spolenak R (2003) From micro to nano contacts in biological attachment devices. Proc Natl Acad Sci USA 100:10603–10606
20. Persson BNJ (2003) On the mechanism of adhesion in biological systems. J Chem Phys 118:7614–7621
21. Spolenak R, Gorb S, Gao H, Arzt E (2005) Effects of contact shape on the scaling of biological attachments. Proc R Soc A 461:305–319
22. Persson BNJ (2003) Nanoadhesion. Wear 254:832–834
23. Gao H, Yao H (2004) Shape insensitive optimal adhesion of nanoscale fibrillar structures. Proc Natl Acad Sci USA 101:7851–7856
24. Glassmaker NJ, Jagota A, Hui CY (2005) Adhesion enhancement in a biomimetic fibrillar interface. Acta Biomater 1(4):367–375
25. Gao H, Ji B, Buehler MJ, Yao H (2004) Flaw tolerant bulk and surface nanostructures of biological systems. Mech Chem Biosys 1:37–52
26. Gao H, Ji B, Jäger IL, Arzt E, Fratzl P (2003) Materials become insensitive to flaws at nanoscale: lessons from nature. Proc Natl Acad Sci USA 100:5597–5600
27. Gao H, Chen S (2005) Flaw tolerance in a thin strip under tension. J App Mech 72:732–737
28. Hui CY, Glassmaker NJ, Tang T, Jagota A (2004) Design of biomimetic fibrillar interface: 2. Mechanics of enhanced adhesion. J R Soc Interface 1:35–48
29. Northen MT, Turner KL (2005) A batch fabricated biomimetic dry adhesive. Nanotechnology 16:1159–1166
30. Greenwood JA (1997) Adhesion of elastic spheres. Proc R Soc Lond A 453:1277–1297
31. Jagota A, Bennison SJ (2002) Mechanics of adhesion through a fibrillar microstructure. Integr Comp Biol 42:1140–1145
32. Tang T, Hui CY, Glassmaker NJ (2005) Can a fibrillar interface be stronger and tougher than a non-fibrillar one? J R Soc Interface 2:505–516
33. Glassmaker NJ, Jagota A, Hui CY, Kim J (2004) Design of biomimetic fibrillar interfaces: 1. Making contact. J R Soc Lond Interface 1:23–33
34. Sitti M, Fearing RS (2003) Synthetic gecko foot-hair micro/nano-structures as dry adhesives. J Adhesion Sci Technol 17:1055–1073
35. Hui CY, Jagota A, Lin YY, Kramer EJ (2002) Constraints on microcontact printing imposed by stamp deformation. Langmuir 18:1394–1407
36. Geim AK, Dubonos SV, Grigorieva IV, Novoselov KS, Zhukov AA, Shapoval SY (2003) Microfabricated adhesive mimicking gecko foot-hair. Nat Mater 2:461–463

37. Williams EE, Peterson JA (1982) Convergent and alternative designs in the digital adhesive pads of scincid lizards. Science 215:1509–1511
38. Peattie AM, Full RJ (2007) Phylogenetic analysis of the scaling of wet and dry biological fibrillar adhesives. Proc Natl Acad Sci USA 104(47):18595–18600
39. Tada J, Paris PC, Irwin GR (2000) The stress analysis of cracks handbook, 3rd edn. ASME Press, New York
40. Kendall K (1975) Thin-film peeling-elastic term. J Phys D: Appl Phys 8:1449–1452
41. Chen B, Wu P, Gao H (2009) Pre-tension generates strongly reversible adhesion of a spatula pad on substrate. J R Soc Interface 6:529–537
42. Gotoh M (1967) Some problems of bonded anisotropic plates with cracks along the bond. Int J Fract Mech 3:253–265
43. Willis JR (1971) Fracture mechanics of interfacial cracks. J Mech Phys Solids 19:353–368
44. Ting TCT (1986) Explicit solution and invariance of the singularities at an interface crack in anisotropic composites. Int J Solids Struct 22:965–983
45. Suo Z (1990) Singularities, interfaces and cracks in dissimilar anisotropic media. Proc R Soc Lond A 427:331–358
46. Gao H, Abbudi M, Barnett DM (1992) On interfacial crack-tip field in anisotropic elastic solids. J Mech Phys Solids 40:393–416
47. Hwu C (1993) Fracture parameters for the orthotropic bimaterial interface cracks. Engr Fract Mech 45:89–97
48. Yao H, Gao H (2006) Mechanics of robust and releasable adhesion in biology: bottom-up designed hierarchical structures of gecko. J Mech Phys Solids 54:1120–1146
49. Yao H, Chen S, Guduru PR, Gao H (2009) Orientation-dependent adhesion strength of a rigid cylinder in non-slipping contact with a transversely isotropic half-space. Int J Solids Struct 46:1167–1175
50. Tvergaard V, Hutchinson JW (1992) The relation between crack growth resistance and fracture process parameters in elastic–plastic solids. J Mech Phys Solids 40:1377–1397
51. Xu XP, Needleman A (1994) Numerical simulations of fast crack growth in brittle solids. J Mech Phys Solids 42:1397–1434
52. Northen MT, Greiner C, Arzt E, Turner KL (2008) A gecko-inspired reversible adhesive. Adv Mater 20:3905–3909
53. Qu L, Dai L, Stone M, Xia Z, Wang ZL (2008) Carbon nanotube arrays with strong shear binding-on and easy normal lifting-off. Science 322:238–242

Part III
Regeneration of Interfaces: Development, Healing, and Tissue Engineering

Chapter 11
The Role of Mechanobiology in the Attachment of Tendon to Bone

Andrea Schwartz and Stavros Thomopoulos

11.1 Introduction

The attachment of dissimilar materials is a major engineering challenge. Stress concentrations would arise at the interface of two disparate materials unless the interface was tuned to the mechanical mismatch. An effective biologic solution to this problem can be seen at the attachment of a relatively compliant tendon to a relatively stiff and brittle bone. A functionally graded tissue develops between tendon and bone to provide a robust attachment (the "enthesis") that alleviates potential stress concentrations. The development and maintenance of this tissue is driven by mechanobiology; muscle loading is necessary for the formation of a transitional tissue between tendon and bone and a loss of loading in the adult enthesis leads to rapid loss of mechanical integrity. This unique transitional tissue is not recreated during healing, so surgical reattachment of these two tissues often fails. This chapter describes structure–function relationships at the tendon enthesis and the role of mechanobiology for the development and healing of the enthesis. Studies have demonstrated that the tendon-to-bone insertion is a functionally graded material with regard to its extracellular matrix (ECM) composition, its structural organization, its mineral content, and its mechanical properties. The fetal and postnatal development of a functionally graded enthesis requires muscle loading. The role of loading during tendon-to-bone healing is more nuanced; low levels of load are beneficial to healing while high levels of load are detrimental to healing. A better understanding of mechanobiology at the insertion may help guide rehabilitation strategies (e.g., protective immobilization followed by active motion) and tissue engineering protocols (e.g., tissue-specific bioreactor designs) for enhancing tendon-to-bone healing.

A. Schwartz • S. Thomopoulos (✉)
Department of Orthopaedic Surgery, Washington University, 660 South Euclid, Box 8233, St. Louis, MO 63110, USA
e-mail: anniegitomer@gmail.com; thomopouloss@wudosis.wustl.edu

S. Thomopoulos et al. (eds.), *Structural Interfaces and Attachments in Biology*,
DOI 10.1007/978-1-4614-3317-0_11,

11.2 Structure–Function Relationships at the Attachment of Tendon to Bone

The attachment of tendon to bone represents a fundamental engineering challenge. Relative to tendon, bone is a stiff, brittle material with an elastic modulus near 20 GPa in both tension and compression [1]. Conversely, tendon is relatively tough and extensible with an elastic modulus of 450 MPa in tension, while buckling in compression [2]. The attachment of two dissimilar materials lends itself to stress singularities at the interface and an increased risk of fracture. In order to overcome these challenges, the tendon-to-bone insertion is uniquely adapted to provide a smooth transfer of stress between two dissimilar tissues. To accomplish this, the insertion has transitional tissue characterized by structural and compositional gradients over a range of length scales that give rise to graded tissue mechanical properties.

The risk of elevated stresses leading to failure has important implications for orthopaedic interfaces, which have high rates of rupture and tearing. Two examples of interfaces prone to injury are the rotator cuff in the shoulder and the anterior cruciate ligament (ACL) in the knee. Surgical repair of these tissues is particularly difficult because the surgeon must overcome the challenge of attaching two materials with vastly different mechanical properties. This contributes to documented rates of re-rupture as high as 20% for minor rotator cuff tears and up to 94% for massive rotator cuff tears [3, 4]. Of note is that the functionally graded transitional tissue of uninjured insertion is typically not recreated after surgical reattachment and healing [5–7].

11.2.1 Functionally Graded Morphology of the Mature Tendon-to-Bone Insertion

From an anatomic perspective, two major types of attachments have been described for tendon and bone [8]. The first type of attachment is termed "fibrous"; these attachments insert into bone across a wide footprint, presumably to distribute loads over a large area and reduce stresses. These insertions may include perforating mineral fibers ("Sharpey's fibers") that interdigitate into the underlying bone [9]. This type of attachment is found at the insertion of the deltoid tendon and at the tibial insertion of the medial collateral ligament. The second type of attachment is termed "fibrocartilaginous"; these attachments are found at the bony insertions of the rotator cuff and Achilles tendons (Fig. 11.1) [8, 10]. Fibrocartilaginous attachments, which contain a unique transitional tissue adapted to withstand a complex stress environment, will be the primary focus of this chapter.

Fibrocartilaginous insertions are typically characterized by the presence of multiple distinct zones easily identified under the light microscope (Fig. 11.1) [8]. The first zone is tendon proper, the middle zones are un-mineralized and mineralized fibrocartilage, and the final zone is bone [8, 10]. Each zone is characterized by a unique profile of cell morphology and ECM composition. Tendon consists of fibroblast cells with a matrix rich in type I collagen and the

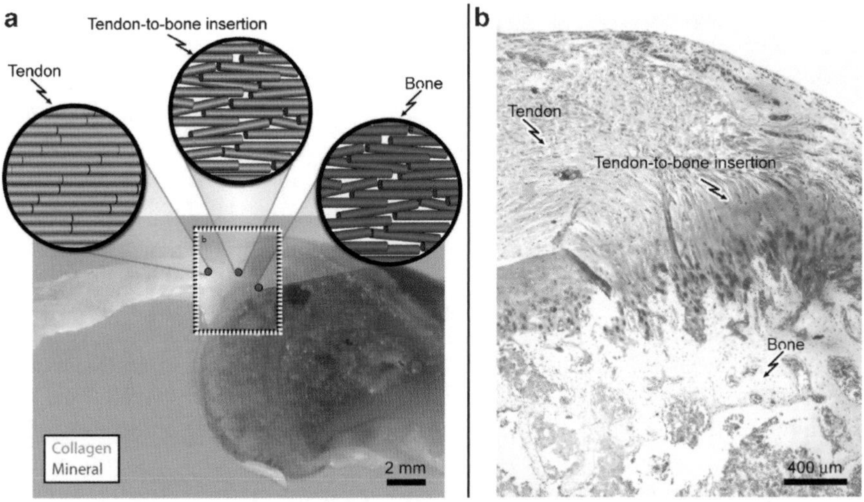

Fig. 11.1 Tendon attaches to bone across a functionally graded fibrocartilaginous transition site. A schematic of the enthesis is shown in (**a**) and a toluidine blue-stained section from a rat supraspinatus tendon-to-bone insertion is shown in (**b**)

proteoglycans decorin and biglycan [2, 11]. The tissue then transitions to a more fibrocartilaginous morphology with rounder cell morphologies. The most abundant collagens are types II and III, but collagen types I, IX, and X are also present along with the proteoglycans decorin and aggrecan [11–15]. The mineralized fibrocartilage zone is characterized by the onset of mineralization, but it is distinct from the underlying bone. The matrix is still characteristic of cartilage; rich in types II and X collagen and aggrecan [12–16]. The final zone, the underlying bone, consists of highly mineralized type I collagen.

While useful for making qualitative comparisons, this description of the insertion as consisting of discrete "zones" is likely an oversimplification. Rather than discrete zones with abrupt transitions, the insertion consists of a graded morphology that is critical to transferring muscle forces from tendon to bone without large elevations in stress at the interface. Instead of an abrupt transition at the interface between the unmineralized fibrocartilage and mineralized fibrocartilage regions, there is a gradual increase in mineral content. This mineral gradient was first described in a rat rotator cuff model as a nearly linear increase over a narrow region within the insertion [17]. A graded interface has also been identified at the cartilage-bone interface [18], suggesting that this strategy of using mineral gradients to dissipate stress at bone-soft tissue interfaces is also a feature common to other types of orthopaedic interfaces.

Microstructural variation in collagen fiber alignment is also a feature of the mature insertion. Using a rat rotator cuff model, collagen fiber alignment was measured with quantitative polarized light microscopy [12]. This experiment demonstrated that collagen fiber alignment varies across the insertion from well aligned in tendon through an increasingly disordered region of fibrocartilage before becoming again more aligned in the underlying bone.

The structure of the mature insertion shares some similar features to the growth plates of developing bone [19]. The growth plate is commonly divided into regions based on mineralization state and cell morphology [20, 21]. The reserve zone consists of small chondrocytes with little organization that are induced to proliferate in response to growth inducing stimuli. Cells of the proliferative zone are organized into columns parallel to the long axis of the bone. Near the top of the columns, cells become flattened in morphology while cells closer to the metaphysis become hypertrophied and more spherical in morphology. In this hypertrophic zone, cells become filled with calcium that begins to mineralize the matrix surrounding the cells. The late hypertrophic zone is characterized by chondrocytes undergoing cell death, interspersed with newly formed vascular channels that allow osteoclasts and osteoblasts to remodel the mineralized matrix to form bone. The fibrocartilage at the tendon enthesis also contains cells with a more rounded chondrocyte-like morphology that are arranged into stacks perpendicular to and spanning the mineralized interface [22]. Similar to the insertion, the growth plate hypertrophic zone is characterized by graded variations of cell morphology, structure, and ECM composition, including mineralization.

The mature tendon-to-bone insertion has unique characteristics that contribute to the mechanical performance of the interface. The transitional tissue within a tendon enthesis utilizes a range of structural and compositional variations across a number of length scales to effectively transfer muscle loads for joint motion. Strategies for reducing stress concentrations at the insertion include a shallow tendon attachment angle at the bone interface, shaping of transitional tissue morphology (i.e., splaying), interdigitation of transitional tissue into bone, a compliant region, and functional grading of the transitional tissue [12, 23–25]. These factors alone or in concert are all capable of reducing stress singularities at the tendon-to-bone interface.

11.2.2 The Mechanical Consequences of Morphological Gradients

The structural and compositional variations described above have mechanical consequences. The microstructural arrangement of collagen fibers across the enthesis reduces stress and strain concentrations at the attachment [25]. Using a finite element model, it was demonstrated that the pattern of fiber alignment at the rotator cuff enthesis reduces stresses at the interface via a disorganized compliant region. Whereas engineering practice would be to interpolate between the mechanical properties of dissimilar materials such as tendon and bone, experimental evidence indicates that natural insertions contain a region that is more compliant than either the soft tissue or bone. The existence of this compliant region has been verified in several orthopaedic tissues. Biomechanical tensile tests on rat supraspinatus tendons indicated that the tissue near the insertion had a lower stiffness than the tendon midsubstance [12]. Stouffer et al. measured increased

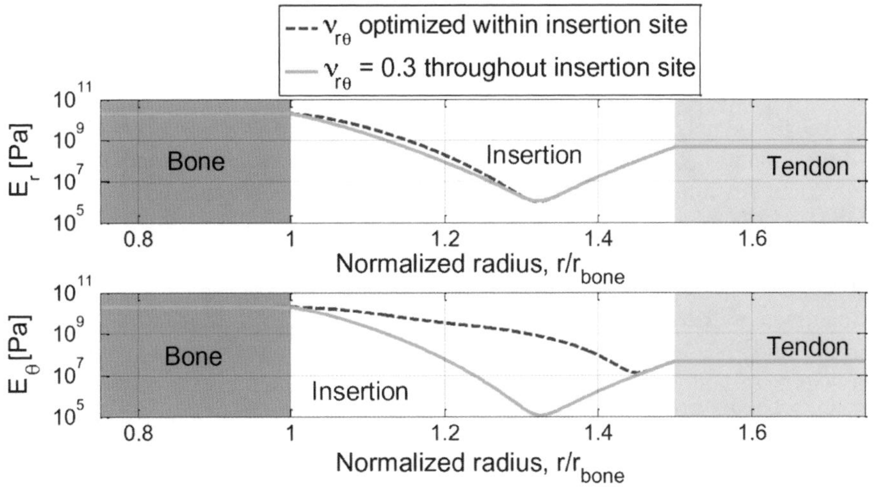

Fig. 11.2 The distribution of material properties for minimization of radial stress concentration factor contains a biomimetic compliant band between tendon and bone (reproduced, with permission, from ref. [24])

tensile strain in human patellar tendon-to-bone insertions compared to the tendon midsubstance [26]. Micro-compression experiments in the ACL insertion and meniscal attachments demonstrated that regions of uncalcified cartilage had lower compressive moduli than calcified regions [27–29]. A recent optimization study has provided some rationale for a compliant region between tendon and bone, a seemingly illogical interfacial system [24]. Through numerical optimization of a mathematical model of an insertion site, it was shown that stress concentrations can be reduced by a biomimetic grading of material properties (i.e., a compliant zone between tendon and bone) (Fig. 11.2).

The growth plate hypertrophic zone contains similar structural, compositional, and morphological gradients to the tendon-to-bone insertion. These gradients also contribute to variations in mechanical behavior that likely influence the tissue response to mechanical loading. In rat growth plates, higher compressive strains were detected in the hypertrophic region compared to the resting/proliferative region [30, 31]. The resting zone is also stiffer than the combined proliferative and hypertrophic zones [32, 33]. This result is consistent with the more compliant region detected at the tendon- and ligament-to-bone interfaces.

The presence of a gradient in mineral content at the insertion also serves to modulate the mechanical behavior of the tissue. Partially mineralized collagen fibers result in a stiffness increase only for mineral concentrations above a "percolation threshold" that corresponds to the formation of a continuous mineral network. Modeling results demonstrate that an effective mechanical attachment is created by combining the effects of a gradual increase in mineral content with variations in collagen organization [34].

11.3 Mechanobiology in Musculoskeletal Tissue Homeostasis and Development

A complex synergy between biophysical cues and biological processes gives rise to the gradations in structure and composition observed at the tendon-to-bone insertion. An improved understanding of the mechanotransduction mechanisms by which the loading environment is linked to ECM production and ultimately to tissue functional behavior will help guide the development of novel repair strategies. Based primarily on mechanical cues, musculoskeletal tissues are continually remodeled throughout the lifespan. This enables tissues to heal after injury and to adapt to environmental stimuli. The ability of musculoskeletal tissues to remodel in response to the loading environment is critical, not only to maintain mature tissue homeostasis, but also to direct the complex patterning necessary for fetal and postnatal development.

Abnormal loading conditions that result from muscle paralysis, prolonged bed rest, or overuse lead to pathological changes in the musculoskeletal system. Examples of these conditions include repetitive loading-induced tendinopathies, unloading-induced osteoporosis, joint instability-induced osteoarthritis, and paralysis-induced developmental defects. For example, neonatal brachial plexus palsy often occurs during difficult childbirth, resulting in paralysis and muscle imbalance in the shoulder [35, 36]. This paralysis leads to defects in glenohumeral joint development leading to severe functional impairments [37–39].

11.3.1 Mechanobiology in Adult Musculoskeletal Tissue Homeostasis

It is well established that musculoskeletal tissues are sensitive to changes in the mechanical loading environment. This is apparent for all tissues (bone, fibrocartilage, and tendon) and cell types (osteoblasts, chondrocytes, and fibroblasts) at the tendon-to-bone insertion. Bone is in a constant state of remodeling. Old bone is resorbed by osteoclasts and new bone is deposited by osteoblasts. Control of the relative rates of bone formation and resorption determines whether bone mass is maintained, gained, or lost. The idea that bones respond to biomechanical stimuli is attributed to what is now referred to as Wolff's Law of bone remodeling [40]. Bone structure adapts in response to the loading environment; regions of lower stress are resorbed, leading to a net bone loss, and regions of higher stresses are reinforced, leading to a net increase in bone. This results in bone trabeculae that are aligned with the direction of principal stresses. Studies in bone demonstrated that cortical thickness and trabecular architecture are both modulated by the loading environment [41, 42]. For example, astronauts lose 2% of hip bone density per month in space and tennis players have increased bone density in their dominant arm [43, 44]. While it is clear that mechanical forces are critical to bone maintenance, the exact biological mechanisms that transduce changes in the loading environment to changes in the rate of tissue formation, which ultimately affects tissue mechanical behavior, are less well understood. Moreover, extremes of unloading and overloading of musculoskeletal tissues lead to pathological conditions.

Articular cartilage serves to cushion the ends of bones and to reduce friction during movement. Mature articular cartilage has a zonal structure through its depth and is essentially an arrested bone growth front at the ends of long bones. The morphology is classified into surface, middle, and deep zones, with variations in structure, composition, and mechanical properties. The tensile modulus of the superficial zone is higher than the deep zone, while the deep zone has a greater compressive modulus [45, 46]. The two primary loading modes experienced by chondrocytes in articular cartilage due to joint loading are hydrostatic stress and shear stress. Chondrocytes subjected to high levels of compressive hydrostatic stress produce type II collagen and aggrecan while suppressing vascularization; all characteristics of a stable chondrocyte phenotype [47]. Shear stresses in cartilage promote fibrillar collagen production. Tensile stress promotes vascular invasion and ossification that result in advancement of the growth front [48]. Cyclic compressive forces induced by joint loading are required to maintain the properties of articular cartilage. Joint immobilization eliminates cyclic compressive stress, activating the subchondral growth front and inducing degradation of the cartilage layer, a characteristic of osteoarthritis [49]. This also occurs in regions of joints that experience low levels of loading.

Tendons and ligaments are responsible for transmitting forces from muscle to bone in the case of tendons and from bone to bone in the case of ligaments. Both are essential for joint stabilization and movement. Like bone, tendon and ligaments are remodeled in response to mechanical stimuli. Changes in tendon due to exercise include an increase in the cross-sectional area and an increase in collagen turnover [50]. Immobilization leads to a decrease in collagen synthesis and a decrease in stiffness and tensile strength [51, 52]. Unloading of ligaments results in changes to the composition and mechanical behavior of the tissue [51–54]. Moreover, localized changes in the tendon loading mode (e.g., tension vs. compression) due to wrapping around a bone pulley in a joint induces a more chondrogenic phenotype, with increases in the local proteoglycan content and downregulation of angiogenic factors [55–60]. Based on these observations, it is clear that mechanical stimuli are critical to the maintenance of skeletal tissues.

11.3.2 Mechanobiology in Fetal and Postnatal Development

Biophysical cues also drive developmental patterning and growth in the fetal and postnatal musculoskeletal system [61]. Bones, tendons, muscles, and joints are patterned *in utero* but development continues through postnatal stages. During

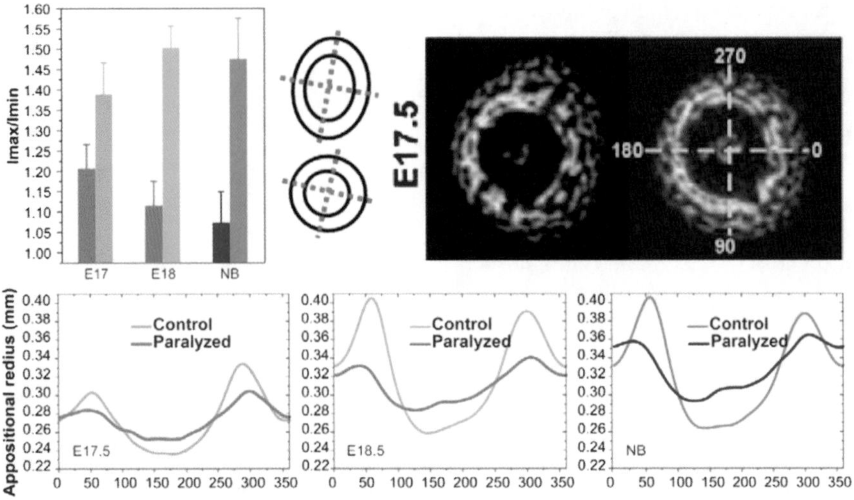

Fig. 11.3 (*Top left*) The ratio of the maximum and minimum second moment of inertia was lower for paralyzed (*darker shade*) compared to control (*lighter shade*) femora (schematics of the maximum and minimum cross-sectional moment of inertias are shown to the right of the plot for control (*top*) and paralyzed (*bottom*) mice). (*Top right*) Micro-CT cross-sectional images are shown for bones from paralyzed (*right*) and control (*left*) mice. (*Bottom*) The appositional radius, as a function of angular coordinate, is shown for paralyzed and control mice (reproduced, with permission, from ref. [66])

the embryonic stage of development, loss of muscle loading leads to severe musculoskeletal defects [62]. The Huetter-Volkmann law states that in developing bone, compressive stress reduces the bone growth rate, while tensile loads accelerate it.

The impact of muscle loading on embryonic development has been examined in several animal models. Chicken embryos have the advantage of an externally laid egg and are thus particularly easy to manipulate with chemical paralysis agents [63]. Mice are the most common model of mammalian development and are well established for genetic manipulations. Mice originally developed to examine the role of specific genes in development provide useful models of muscle-less mice. Examples of this include mutations in Pax3 or a combination of Myf5 and MyoD1, which both result in limbs without skeletal muscle [64, 65]. Muscle contractions *in utero* begin early in embryonic development. The magnitude of *in utero* forces increases dramatically when increases in muscle volume are coupled with the forces that result from bone elongation (Fig. 11.3) [66]. In the absence of muscle forces, there are defects in bone size, shape, and mineralization [63, 66–68]. Joint cavitation does not occur, leading to bone fusion [67]. This is the result of de-differentiation of joint progenitor cells, which return to a cartilage phenotype [69]. Bone shaping is altered in the absence of muscle loading, with defects observed in the knee joint, long bone cross-section, and the deltoid tuberosity [69].

Eliminating embryonic muscle forces also leads to defects in tendon and cartilage. Tendon development is initiated, but tendon precursors are not maintained, in the absence of muscle forces [65, 70]. Chondrocyte proliferation is decreased, altering bone growth rates and contributing to the observed bone defects [71]. Furthermore, the lack of joint cavitation results in the complete loss of articular cartilage surfaces [72]. Compositional changes occur in developing cartilage as a result of immobilization that lead to altered mechanical properties [73].

The importance of mechanical loading for development increases after birth. At this point, the effects of joint contact forces due to body weight are added to the effects of increasing muscle forces. Bone growth in postnatal chicks is significantly arrested by adding only 10% of body weight using an external harness [74, 75]. The reduction in bone length is reversed by removing the weight, but the resulting bones have impaired structural and mechanical behavior.

The rate of long bone growth by endochondral ossification is sensitive to the mechanical environment. Compression maintains the cartilage phenotype and slows bone growth, while tensile loads along the long axis of the bone increase elongation [76, 77]. Stokes and coworkers used three different animal models to demonstrate a linear relationship between the applied axial stress and the bone growth rate using externally applied loading plates pinned to the bones [76, 77]. This relationship held for both tensile and compressive loading of proximal tibial growth plates and vertebral bodies. The bone growth rate depends on the combined rates of cell division in the proliferative zone, cell volume increases in the hypertrophic zone, and the rate of chondrocyte maturation leading to mineralization [21]. The biological mechanisms that enable cells to transduce forces into cell fates, and the matrix production processes that control rates of bone growth are less well understood. It is likely that the mechanisms described above that influence endochondral ossification also drive the development of the unique transitional tissue at the enthesis.

11.3.3 Biological Molecules Critical to Skeletal Mechanotransduction

Members of many distinct families of molecules have been implicated in mechanotransduction pathways, all of which likely play roles in enthesis development. These include, but are not limited to, ECM proteins (collagens, proteoglycans, and glycosaminoglycans), growth factors (TGFβs, BMPs, FGFs), cytokines (IL1, IL6), hedgehog family members (Ihh), matrix metalloproteinases (MMP-1, MMP-13), and angiogenic factors (VEGF) [78]. Several mechanisms of cellular mechanotransduction have been identified. Strains in the ECM are coupled to cytoskeletal rearrangements through integrins in the cell membrane, which provide a direct structural connection between the ECM and the cytoskeleton [79]. Other cellular mediators of mechanotransduction include cell surface G-protein coupled receptors, receptor tyrosine kinases, and stretch activated ion channels [80].

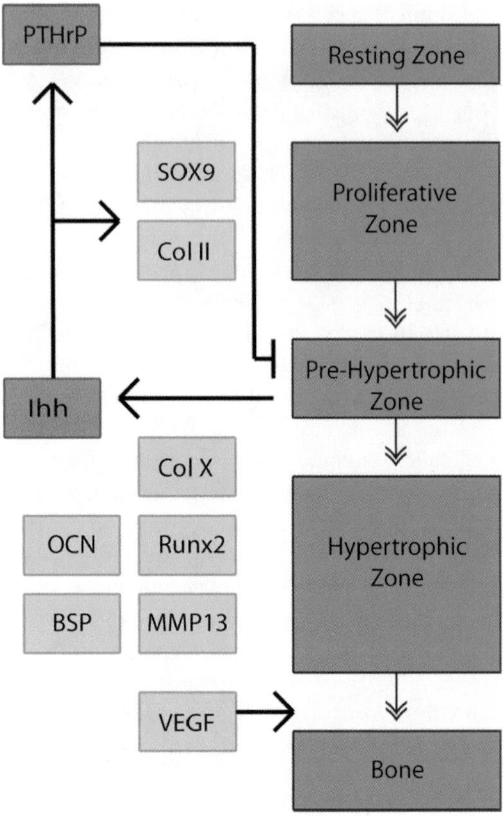

Fig. 11.4 Schematic of chondrocyte maturation at the growth plate (*blue*) showing the Ihh/PTHrP negative feedback loop and selected biomarkers. *Arrows* indicate positive regulation and bars indicate negative regulation

Endochondral bone formation is regulated by the autocrine/paracrine signaling of Indian hedgehog (Ihh) and parathyroid hormone-related protein (PTHrP) (Fig. 11.4) [81–83]. Ihh is expressed by pre-hypertrophic and early hypertrophic chondrocytes entering the early stages of terminal differentiation. This molecule stimulates the proliferating chondrocytes by binding the membrane receptor Patched (Ptch), which activates the membrane receptor Smoothened (Smo) and stimulates synthesis of PTHrP. PTHrP expression then blocks further expression of Ihh, establishing a negative feedback loop to provide fine control over the rate of chondrocyte proliferation and maturation. The transcription factor Sox9 is a target of PTHrP in the growth plate that likely influences maintenance of a stable proliferating chondrocyte phenotype [84]. Sox9 has also been implicated in later stages of chondrocyte hypertrophy [85]. Precise spatial and temporal control over these and other extracellular signaling molecules and transcription factors is critical to endochondral bone development.

Ihh expression in chondrocyte cultures is upregulated in response to tensile stretching and is required for increased proliferation [86]. This mechanoresponse gene is mediated downstream by BMP 2 and 4 and does not involve PTHrP. PTHrP has also been implicated in mechanotransduction pathways independent of interactions with Ihh [87]. In this study, when tendon insertion sites were unloaded by tail suspension or tendon transection, there was a significant decrease in PTHrP expression. This decrease was more dramatic in the transection group compared to the suspension group. Based on this, it is suggested that PTHrP might play a role in the migration of tendon insertion sites in order to accommodate increases in bone length during development. In support of this, there is increased osteoclastic activity at the leading edge of the insertion site, while more osteoblasts are observed at the trailing edge to allow bone growth.

Type X collagen is a well-described marker of chondrocyte maturation and of the early stages of mineralization in endochondral bone formation [88]. Expression of collagen X is limited to hypertrophic chondrocytes. This molecule is a response to mechanical loading. In one study, collagen X mRNA was upregulated after tensile stretch was applied to chondrocytes [89]. Other reports indicated that collagen X expression and protein levels were reduced by compressive loading in growth plate chondrocytes [90, 91]. These results are consistent with the idea that tensile loading of developing bone increases mineralization, which leads to longitudinal bone growth, while compressive loads have an arresting effect on growth.

Scleraxis (Scx) is a transcription factor noted for its role in tendon development [92–95]. Scx null mice have several defects in force transmitting tendons of the limbs and have severely compromised movement [95]. Furthermore, this mutation results in structural changes: increased disorder and decreased amounts of tendon ECM likely contribute to the noted functional losses. Recently, several studies have indicated a role for Scx in mechanotransduction. *In vitro* loading modulates Scx expression in tenocyte cultures [96]. More specifically, in tendons, mechanical force causes release of TGFβs from the ECM [97]. This activates the Smad 2 pathway through the TGFβ receptor leading to upregulation of Scx in response to mechanical loading. Loss of loading due to tendon transection or botulinum toxin-induced paralysis results in decreased Scx expression, as demonstrated using a ScxGFP reporter. In addition, Mendias et al. found that treadmill exercise upregulates Scx expression [98].

Finally, connexins are a class of gap junction forming proteins that are important to cellular mechanotransduction. Connexin 43 has been identified in bone [99, 100], cartilage, and tendon [16]. Connexin expression is upregulated in tendon fibroblasts subjected to cyclic loading [101, 102]. Connexin proteins assemble in the cell membrane to form hemichannels or gap junctions to enable direct cell-cell communication. Selective loss of connexin 43 from bone cells results in a loss of the mechanoresponsiveness of bone to both loading-induced bone formation and muscle paralysis-induced bone loss [103–106]. The mechanoresponsiveness of connexins and other molecules involved in direct cell-cell communication underlines the importance of cell-cell communication in the response to mechanical stimuli. The combined effect of the mechanotransduction mechanisms described above is to regulate ECM synthesis and degradation, ultimately affecting tissue function and development.

11.4 Mechanobiology in the Development of the Tendon-to-Bone Insertion

Muscle loading is necessary for the development of a functionally graded tendon-to-bone insertion. This complex tissue has features of bone, ossifying cartilage, and tendon and is typically subjected to a combination of compressive and tensile stresses. As described in the previous section, mechanical signals are capable of influencing the synthesis rate and composition of the ECM as well as cell fate in developing musculoskeletal tissues. It is likely that biological factors involved in mechanotransduction pathways in other orthopaedic tissues also impact enthesis development. In order to achieve the complex graded microstructure and morphological characteristics of the insertion, it follows that there must also be spatial and temporal interplay between gene expression and synthesis of ECM molecules. These expression patterns are controlled by both genetic and biophysical cues from the environment (i.e., muscle loading) and produce the complex gradients found at the mature insertion.

While neo-tendon and bone are established early in fetal development, the enthesis transitional tissue is often not evident until postnatal stages [107–110]. In an animal model, the supraspinatus neo-tendon was evident adjacent to developing humeral head bone at 15.5 days post-conception (dpc) [6]. In contrast, the mature insertion, defined by the appearance of fibrocartilaginous transitional tissue, was not identified until after birth. In mouse shoulders, an insertion region between the supraspinatus tendon and bone begins to appear 1 week after birth and mature fibrocartilage is not in evidence until 3 weeks after birth [108]. During this period, the shoulder experiences large increases in limb loading as body weight and muscle mass increase along with activity levels. It follows that large muscle forces are likely necessary to drive the development of transitional tissues in the enthesis.

The insertion develops adjacent to the mineralizing epiphyseal cartilage of the humeral head. Mineralization of the humeral head occurs through endochondral ossification, a process that proceeds by mineralization of a cartilage template followed by vascular invasion and remodeling of the mineralized cartilage template by osteoclasts and osteoblasts [20, 111]. Chondrocytes from the cartilage anlage are induced by biological and chemical factors to proliferate, resulting in an increase in size or length of the cartilage template. Cells then enter a terminal differentiation process beginning with hypertrophy, followed by mineralization of the cartilage matrix, and finally cell death and matrix resorption and remodeling by recruitment of angiogenic factors. This bone formation process is characteristic of the growth plate region of long bones during fetal development that continues into postnatal development.

In one example, Blitz et al. described the development of the deltoid tendon-humeral tuberosity attachment (Fig. 11.5) [111]. It was observed that the deltoid tuberosity formed via endochondral ossification in a two-phase process: initiation was regulated by a signal from the tendons, whereas the subsequent growth phase was muscle (i.e., load)-dependent. Specifically, Scx regulated BMP-4 production in

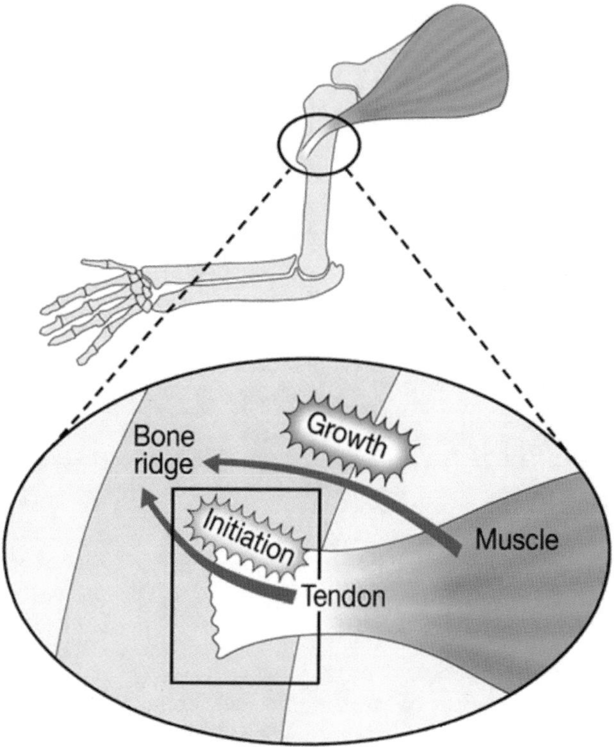

Fig. 11.5 Blitz et al. suggested the following model for the contribution of both tendons and muscles to enthesis formation. Through a biphasic process, tendons regulate enthesis initiation and muscles control its subsequent growth. Further research is necessary to determine the mechanism whereby muscle contraction regulates enthesis development (reproduced, with permission, from ref. [111])

tendon cells at their bony insertion site. When BMP-4 expression was blocked in Scx expressing cells, the enthesis (and associated bone ridges) did not form. This implicates BMP-4 as a key mediator of tendon-specific signaling for enthesis formation. The key regulators of endochondral ossification, collagen II, Ihh, PTHrP, and collagen X were expressed at the developing enthesis.

11.4.1 Development of Structural Gradients in the Enthesis

This section describes the developmental patterns that lead to the complex structure and composition of the tendon-to-bone insertion. The temporal expression of ECM molecules was described in detail using in situ hybridization experiments throughout murine fetal and postnatal development [108]. At birth, the bone side of the supraspinatus tendon-to-bone insertion was largely made up of un-mineralized

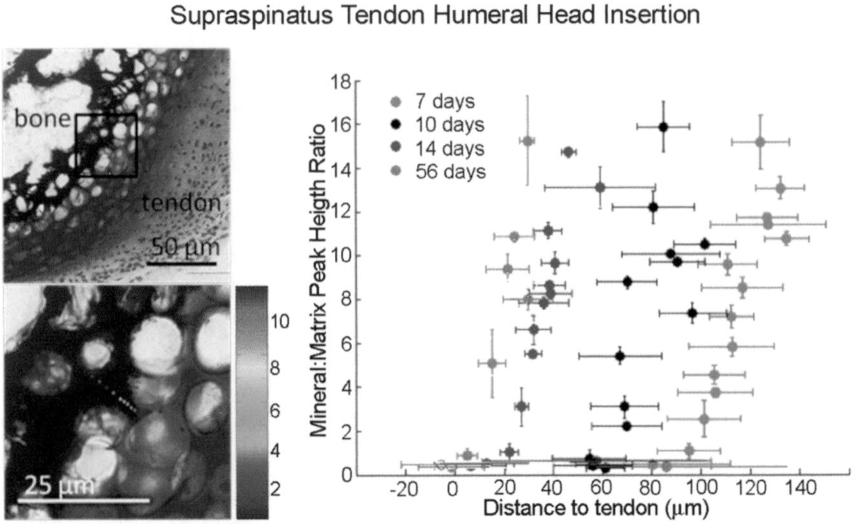

Fig. 11.6 Spatial gradients in mineral (as determined using Raman spectroscopy) form between tendon and bone at the developing entheses from the onset of endochondral ossification (7 days in the mouse supraspinatus tendon-to-bone insertion, shown here)

type II collagen, characteristic of cartilage. Neonatal collagen II gene expression was confirmed by in situ hybridization. The tendon side of the insertion expressed type I collagen, which is characteristic of tendon and bone ECM. As mineralization of the secondary ossification center proceeded over the first few weeks of postnatal development, expression of collagen II became restricted to a narrow zone in the transitional tissue of the insertion. Type I collagen was expressed by cells adjacent to the band of collagen II expressing cells on the tendon side of the insertion.

Type X collagen was evident in a band of cells on the bone side of the insertion, adjacent to the mineralizing front. Collagen X is typically localized to hypertrophic chondrocytes in the growth plate prior to mineralization. At the enthesis, expression of this marker persists after the large hypertrophic cells associated with mineralization are no longer seen, suggesting that this molecule may play a role in maintaining the mineralized interface. This result is consistent with the development of the rat Achilles tendon [107].

As previously mentioned, the appearance of a mineral gradient in the transitional tissue of the insertion likely plays an important role in mediating the transfer of muscle loads from soft tissues to bone. In the mouse, a mineral gradient is evident near the developing insertion as early as 1 week after birth (Fig. 11.6). The mineral gradient coincides with the mineralizing front of the secondary ossification center in the humeral head. The mineral gradient is first separated from the developing tendon by a region of epiphyseal cartilage yet to be mineralized. In a murine model, the gradient gradually moves into the developing transitional tissue of the tendon-bone insertion as the epiphyseal cartilage is mineralized between the first 2 weeks of postnatal growth.

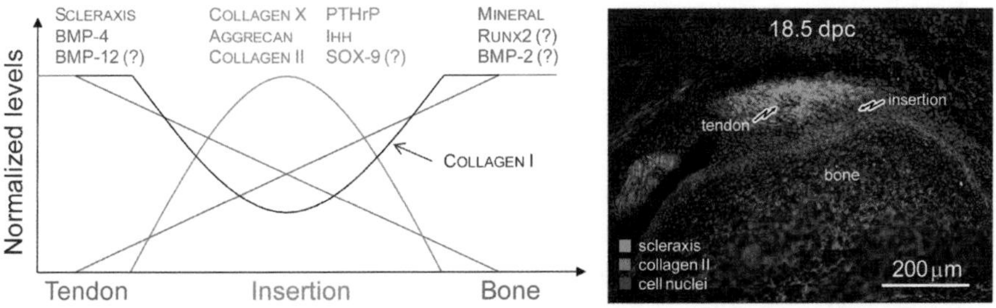

Fig. 11.7 Spatially and temporally controlled expression of a number of transcription factors, growth factors, and transcription factors likely play important roles in enthesis development

11.4.2 Biological Factors Necessary for Insertion Development

Development of the complex transitional tissue found at the tendon-to-bone insertion requires precise spatial and temporal control of a range of biological factors (Fig. 11.7). The development of transitional tissue occurs during postnatal development when tendon and bone are already established, but still actively growing and remodeling. In order for transitional tissue to develop at the interface, there must be concurrent regulation of and interaction between the biological signals of tendon, bone, and cartilage. Individually, all three tissue types are responsive to the mechanical environment. Specific biological molecules native to each tissue type have been implicated in the cellular response to the mechanical loading environment.

The mineralized side of the insertion is not yet mature bone during the early stages of enthesis development. Instead, it is an immature epiphyseal cartilage template undergoing endochondral ossification. At this stage of development, the insertion shares many features with the growth plate. Biological factors identified at precise spatial locations in the growth plate include: PTHrP, Ihh, Ptc, Sox9, and type X collagen [20, 112]. Chemical gradients of these molecules are responsible for maintaining the graded morphology of the growth plate. These factors have also been localized to the developing tendon-to-bone insertion and may also impact development of a graded insertion [107–110, 113].

PTHrP was originally described for its role in regulating the growth plate in a negative feedback loop with Ihh [81–83]. Recently, PTHrP has been localized to tendon and ligament entheses during postnatal development [87, 113]. More specifically, it is localized to a group of fibroblast-like cells in the intermediate zone between the tendon proper and the transitional tissue that inserts into the underlying cortical bone [113]. Furthermore, PTHrP has been generally localized to periosteal cells in addition to cells that will form the secondary ossification center of long bones [113]. Elevated expression of PTHrP at tendon-to-bone insertions suggests that PTHrP may be important to maintain the mineralized interface during development. In the growth plate, PTHrP maintains chondrocyte proliferation and blocks maturation and mineralization [20]. PTHrP may have a similar function for enthesis development.

Scx is a transcription factor localized to mature tendon that is necessary for tenogenesis and is found in tendon progenitor cells [92–95]. This molecule is a critical mediator of enthesis development. In a recent study, Blitz et al. demonstrated that Scx is necessary for initiation of development of the deltoid tuberosity, the attachment site of the deltoid tendon on the humerus [111]. This insertion forms by endochondral ossification and is necessary to create a stable attachment point for the deltoid tendon. Scx expression in the tendon cells mediated BMP4 expression in cells near the insertion. Subsequent growth of the insertion was dependent on muscle loading. Sox9 is a marker of a stable chondrocyte phenotype with important roles in endochondral bone formation [84, 85]. Sox9 has additional roles in embryonic development, and together with Scx helps determine chondrogenic vs. tenogenic cell lineage [114].

11.4.3 Mechanical Factors are Required for Insertion Development

In order to probe the effects of muscle loading on the postnatal development of the tendon-to-bone attachment, it is useful to employ an animal model that can be combined with biological and genetic manipulations. By injecting botulinum toxin into the rotator cuff muscles of mice throughout postnatal development, effectively paralyzing the shoulder and eliminating muscle forces, it is possible to isolate the effects of loading on the development of the supraspinatus insertion. Using mice enables this model to be combined with genetic manipulation to investigate the role of specific biological molecules implicated in mechanotransduction pathways. Botulinum toxin injections are routinely used to induce localized and reversible muscle paralysis. Botulinum toxin chemically blocks the transmission of nerve impulses through neuromuscular junctions. To study the role of muscle loading on enthesis development, mice received botulinum toxin injections in one shoulder and saline injections in the contralateral shoulder beginning within 24 h of birth [115–117]. The saline group provided an internal control for paired statistical comparisons. A third group of normal age matched mice was used as fully mobile controls.

This animal model displayed a similar phenotype to the human condition neonatal brachial plexus palsy. In order to ensure that there was no effect of botulinum toxin on shoulder development that wasn't the direct result of muscle paralysis, a group of animals received a neurotomy of the upper trunk of the brachial plexus [118]. The phenotype of the neurotomy group closely mimicked the botulinum toxin-injected group. Both groups showed a substantial decrease in muscle volume compared to controls. Decreases in muscle volume and mass correlated to decreases in muscle force generation in botulinum toxin-injected shoulders compared to saline controls after 4 and 8 weeks of paralysis [117].

The shoulder muscle paralysis induced in this animal model resulted in striking changes to tendon-to-bone insertion development (Fig. 11.8). Unloading caused severe mineralization defects in the humeral head, including reduced overall volume

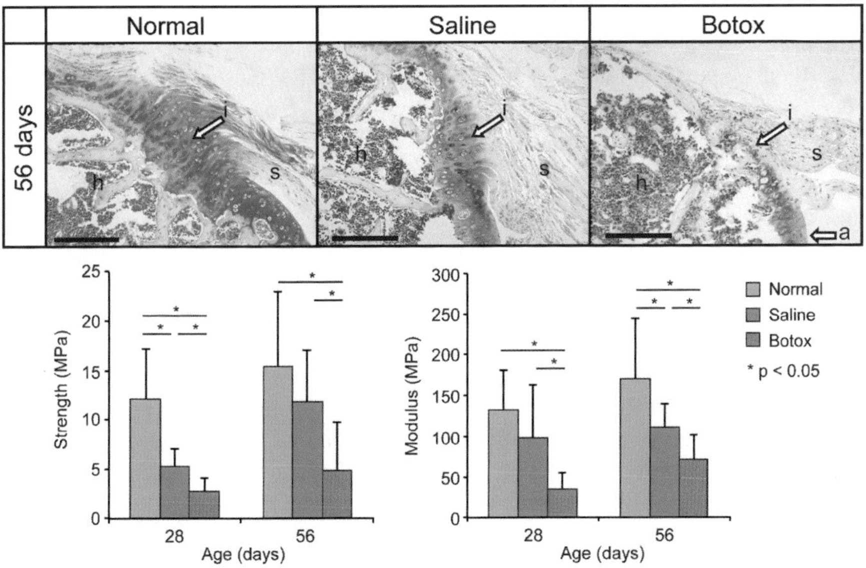

Fig. 11.8 Muscle paralysis dramatically impaired the development of the supraspinatus tendon-to-bone insertion in mice. (*Top*) A mature, compositionally graded insertion ("i") is seen by 56 days postnatally in normal mice (scale bar = 200 μm). In contrast, the enthesis in paralyzed shoulders appears disorganized, without a graded fibrocartilaginous transition between the supraspinatus tendon ("s") and the humeral head bone ("h"). (*Bottom*) Maximum stress and modulus were significantly lower in the paralyzed group compared to the normal and saline groups

and morphological changes. For example, the humeral head appeared flattened, similar to observations in children with neonatal brachial plexus palsy. This demonstrated that mechanical loading is critical for mineralization at the enthesis. The lower mineral density observed in micro-computed tomography measurements in the unloaded groups can at least in part be attributed to an increase in osteoclast activity [115]. When osteoclast activity was blocked using a bisphosphonate drug, there was a partial recovery of some bone mineralization measures [119]. Bone volume was significantly recovered in a dose-dependent manner.

Removal of muscle loading also affected the development of a fibrocartilaginous transition at the insertion (Fig. 11.8). Based on histological analysis, little to no fibrocartilage was observed in the insertion after 8 weeks of paralysis [115]. Collagen fiber alignment, investigated using quantitative polarized light microscopy, indicated fibers were more disorganized in unloaded shoulders compared to saline controls. Impaired mineralization, disordered fiber alignment, and a loss of fibrocartilage transitional tissue in the insertions likely contribute to the overall inferior mechanical properties of unloaded tendon insertions. Structural mechanical properties (e.g., maximum force, stiffness) and material mechanical properties (e.g., maximum stress, modulus) were decreased after 4 and 8 weeks of botulinum toxin injections (Fig. 11.8).

Blitz et al. used genetically modified mice with muscular defects to examine the role of muscle loading on enthesis development [111]. Consistent with the studies described above, this study demonstrated that while muscle loading was not required for initiation of enthesis formation, it was necessary for the subsequent growth and maturation of the enthesis.

11.5 Mechanobiology in Tendon-to-Bone Healing

Repair of ruptures at the tendon-to-bone insertion is a persistent problem in orthopaedic surgery. Rotator cuff tears are a common injury to the upper extremity and involve reattaching tendons to the humeral head [120]. ACL injuries are also very common and surgical reconstruction techniques use tendon grafts as ligament replacements that must heal in bone tunnels [121]. Tendon and ligament injuries can be classified as acute or chronic ruptures. Acute injuries are generally the result of extrinsic factors, while chronic injuries also involve intrinsic factors such as tissue degeneration and a predisposition toward injury. While acute tendon-to-bone ruptures usually have reasonable healing outcomes, the problem of healing in the case of a chronic injury is confounded by significant degeneration of the transitional tissue that extends to the tendon and underlying bone. Several studies have indicated that nearly all Achilles tendon ruptures have histological evidence of degeneration [122]. In contrast to acute trauma of a healthy tendon, this type of injury can result from the compounded effects of aging and overuse, often from a lifetime of repetitive motion. Increased loading from overuse disrupts the tissue homeostasis, alters tissue composition, and results in functionally inferior tissue mechanical properties leading to injury.

The role of mechanobiology in healing is less clear than the role of mechanobiology in development. Insights from development indicate that mechanical forces are critical for establishing a functional tissue. However, these forces are precisely modulated; cellular responses to physical stress lead to changes in tissue structure and function, ultimately determining tissue mechanical properties. A stress-adaptation feedback loop then leads to further remodeling of the local matrix. The same principles apply to healing, where outcomes are affected by a myriad of chemical, biological, and mechanical factors. The healing situation, however, is complicated because the ideal loading environment that leads to optimal healing is not well defined. Furthermore, the immune response to injury complicates the biological mechanotransduction outcomes. Optimization of healing will require a more precise understanding of the mechanisms of cell responses to varying loading conditions. This presents a challenge for orthopaedic surgeons attempting to optimize post-operative healing through rehabilitation-controlled loading.

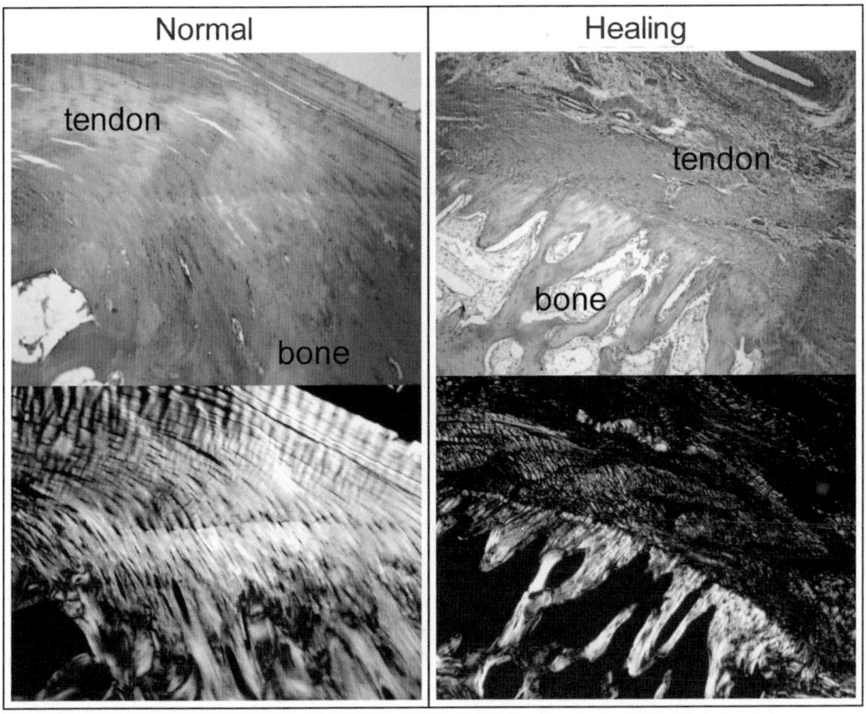

Fig. 11.9 The functionally graded transition between tendon and bone is not regenerated (hematoxylin and eosin-stained images are shown under bright-field on the *top row* and under polarized light on the *bottom row*) (reproduced, with permission, from ref. [129])

11.5.1 Injury and Repair Result in a Loss of the Functionally Graded Tendon-to-Bone Interface

Tendon-to-bone injuries are generally characterized by rupture of the tendon, requiring repair of the tissue to its original bony footprint. Tendon-to-bone healing can be roughly divided into three stages: inflammation, repair, and remodeling. The inflammation stage involves recruitment of vascular cells, such as erythrocytes and platelets, and immune cells, such as macrophages to the injury site to resorb necrotic tissues via phagocytosis. The inflammatory cells also recruit tendon fibroblasts for the repair phase, in which ECM (primarily collagen) is synthesized and deposited at the injury site. The remodeling phase begins approximately 2 months post-injury and is characterized by reduced cellularity and matrix synthesis, as the tissue becomes more fibrous and is then remodeled into scar-like tendon tissue [80].

Studies in rabbits, goats, and rats have verified that repaired interfaces have inferior mechanical behavior, presumably because the functionally graded transition between tendon and bone is not regenerated (Fig. 11.9) [5, 7, 123, 124]. The scar tissue that forms at the interface has a larger volume than the native tissue, but is functionally inferior. This may be explained by the dramatic decrease in the amount of underlying bone and the loss of collagen fiber organization [125–128]. These factors are compounded in the case of a chronic rupture, which is typically accompanied by significant degeneration prior to injury, increasing the difficulty of repair and the risk of re-rupture. While many factors contribute to the observed decrease in tissue functional behavior, the main distinction between a healing and a normal insertion is the near complete loss of transitional tissue in the enthesis.

11.5.2 Precise Control of Loading Is Needed to Improve Healing

Immobilization of the limb or joint after a repair is often utilized to prevent disruption of the recently reattached tissues during the early stages of healing. As previously described, immobilization can have undesired effects on the nearby uninjured musculoskeletal tissues, which require precisely defined loading conditions to maintain their structure and composition. Due to this, a delicate balance between periods of immobilization and controlled remobilization must be used to maximize healing while reducing unwanted damage to nearby musculoskeletal tissues.

The role of cast immobilization in tendon-to-bone healing has been investigated in a series of studies using a rat rotator cuff tendon model [7, 130–132]. Tendons were surgically transected and reattached to the bony insertion, then assigned cast immobilization, cage activity, or treadmill exercise for post-operative recovery. All interfaces healed by a fibrovascular scar without evidence of a functionally graded transitional tissue and an increased tendon cross-sectional area compared to normal uninjured controls. The exercised group had a significantly larger cross-sectional area compared to the cast immobilized group. Acute injury and repair diminished the functional biomechanical performance of the bone tendon interface for all injury groups compared to controls. The exercise group had less favorable mechanical properties, collagen fiber alignment, and matrix composition than the cast immobilized group. Furthermore, the increased joint stiffness due to post-operative immobilization was eventually resolved [132]. Finally, passive motion after surgery instead of exercise also increases joint stiffness [131]. The results of these studies suggest that exercise is detrimental to healing in a rat rotator cuff, as it results in more material accumulation at the healing interface with less desirable structural and mechanical properties.

A possible mechanism for the poor healing observed with exercise has recently been suggested by studies using a rat model of ACL reconstruction [133–135]. Cytokines produced by macrophages have been implicated in tendon-to-bone healing and reducing the number of macrophages improves the biomechanical behavior of the interface. Furthermore, immobilization seems to also block macrophage recruitment, thus contributing to improved interface healing [133].

The result is that cast immobilization leads to improved healing; this has led to further studies investigating the role of the mechanical environment in healing. Cast immobilization is difficult to enact in a clinical setting because it depends on patient compliance. Additionally, it does not completely remove all forces across the healing insertion because some motion is possible and muscle forces are still present. This led several investigators to probe the effect of complete removal of muscle loading on healing. A rat rotator cuff acute repair model used Botulinum toxin A injections to reversibly paralyze the supraspinatus muscle with and without cast immobilization [136]. Botulinum toxin and cast immobilization reduced the structural and mechanical properties of the healing insertion, indicating that complete removal of loading was unfavorable to healing. This result was corroborated by a study investigating healing of canine flexor tendon-to-bone repairs [137]. This suggests that some muscle loading is necessary for optimal healing.

A separate series of studies investigated the role of mechanical loading on ACL healing in rats. Ligaments were surgically replaced by flexor digitorum longus tendons in a bone tunnel. An *in vivo* joint loading system was used to apply controlled axial loading daily to the healing insertion [138]. In a comparison of immobilization and cyclic loading, the loaded group had increased inflammatory macrophages at the tendon-bone interface and decreased bone formation in the bone tunnel, but no differences in the biomechanical properties of the interface [139]. A separate group of animals was used to evaluate a period of immobilization followed by loading [140]. This study demonstrated an increase in bone formation and load-to-failure compared to immobilization and early cyclic loading groups. This suggests that a period of immobilization followed by loading is beneficial to healing of ACL reconstructions. A separate study investigated the effect of immobilization followed by exercise in a rat rotator cuff model. Immobilization followed by exercise reduced the desired mechanical performance of repaired tendons compared to immobilization followed by cage activity [141]. In contrast to this, a recent report using a rat Achilles tendon rupture model indicated that exercise early in the healing process combined with unloading by hindlimb suspension improved healing compared to tendons that were unloaded without exercise [142].

Taken together, the above results indicate that the healing tendon-to-bone insertion is influenced by loading environment. The conflicting results indicate that modulating the loading environment is just one factor among many that affect healing outcomes. One conclusion that may be drawn from the above studies is that complete unloading is detrimental to healing, either through chemical paralysis, hindlimb suspension, or tendon transection away from the repair site. Furthermore, excessive exercise is also harmful to the healing process. Optimal healing seems to require a precise degree of loading that is extremely difficult to accurately predict and control in laboratory or clinical settings (Fig. 11.10).

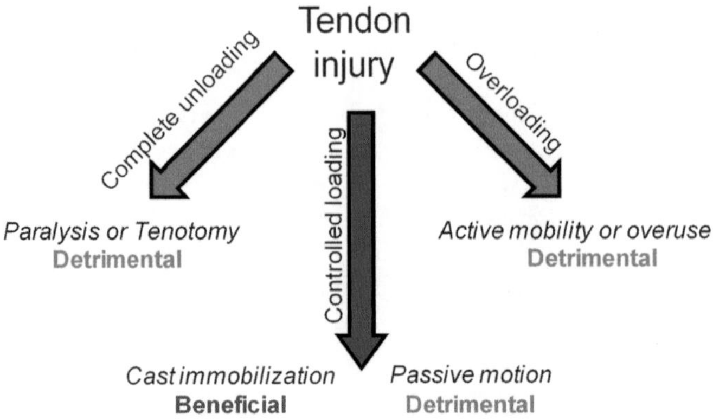

Fig. 11.10 Precise control of loading is necessary for optimal tendon-to-bone healing after surgical repair

11.6 Conclusions

The tendon-to-bone insertion is an example of a biological solution to the fundamental problem of attaching two dissimilar materials. The enthesis possesses gradients in structure and composition that help limit stress concentrations at the tendon-bone interface. The development of the functional gradient requires muscle loading. The healing insertion is also sensitive to its mechanical environment. However, a fine balance must be reached between too much load (which can lead to damage) and too little load (which can lead to a catabolic environment) to maximize tendon-to-bone healing. Approaches for improving tendon-to-bone healing must focus on recreation of a functionally graded transition between tendon and bone, either through manipulation of the loading environment or though an engineered construct.

Acknowledgments This work was supported in part by the National Institutes of Health (AR055580 and AR057836) and the National Science Foundation (CAREER 844607).

References

1. Bostrom MPG, Boskey A, Kauffman JK, Einhorn TA (2000) Form and function of bone. In: Buckwalter JA, Einhorn T, Simon SR (eds) Orthopaedic basic science, 2nd edn. American Academy of Orthopaedic Surgeons, Rosemont, IL, pp 319–370
2. Woo SLAK, Frank CB, Livesay GA, Ma CB, Zeminski JA, Wayne JS, Myers BS (2000) Anatomy, biology, and biomechanics of tendon and ligament. In: Buckwalter JA, Einhorn T, Simon SR (eds) Orthopaedic basic science, 2nd edn. American Academy of Orthopaedic Surgeons, Rosemont, IL, pp 581–616
3. Harryman DT II, Mack LA, Wang KY, Jackins SE, Richardson ML, Matsen FA III (1991) Repairs of the rotator cuff. Correlation of functional results with integrity of the cuff. J Bone Joint Surg Am 73(7):982–989

4. Galatz LM, Ball CM, Teefey SA, Middleton WD, Yamaguchi K (2004) The outcome and repair integrity of completely arthroscopically repaired large and massive rotator cuff tears. J Bone Joint Surg Am 86A(2):219–224
5. Galatz LM, Sandell LJ, Rothermich SY, Das R, Mastny A, Havlioglu N, Silva MJ, Thomopoulos S (2006) Characteristics of the rat supraspinatus tendon during tendon-to-bone healing after acute injury. J Orthop Res 24(3):541–550
6. Thomopoulos S, Hattersley G, Rosen V, Mertens M, Galatz L, Williams GR, Soslowsky LJ (2002) The localized expression of extracellular matrix components in healing tendon insertion sites: an in situ hybridization study. J Orthop Res 20(3):454–463
7. Thomopoulos S, Williams GR, Soslowsky LJ (2003) Tendon to bone healing: differences in biomechanical, structural, and compositional properties due to a range of activity levels. J Biomech Eng 125(1):106–113
8. Benjamin M, Kumai T, Milz S, Boszczyk BM, Boszczyk AA, Ralphs JR (2002) The skeletal attachment of tendons–tendon "entheses". Comp Biochem Physiol A Mol Integr Physiol 133 (4):931–945
9. Quain J (1856) Elements of anatomy, 6th edn. Walton and Maberly, London
10. Benjamin M, Toumi H, Ralphs JR, Bydder G, Best TM, Milz S (2006) Where tendons and ligaments meet bone: attachment sites ('entheses') in relation to exercise and/or mechanical load. J Anat 208(4):471–490
11. Waggett AD, Ralphs JR, Kwan AP, Woodnutt D, Benjamin M (1998) Characterization of collagens and proteoglycans at the insertion of the human Achilles tendon. Matrix Biol 16 (8):457–470
12. Thomopoulos S, Williams GR, Gimbel JA, Favata M, Soslowsky LJ (2003) Variation of biomechanical, structural, and compositional properties along the tendon to bone insertion site. J Orthop Res 21(3):413–419
13. Kumagai J, Sarkar K, Uhthoff HK, Okawara Y, Ooshima A (1994) Immunohistochemical distribution of type I, II and III collagens in the rabbit supraspinatus tendon insertion. J Anat 185(pt 2):279–284
14. Fukuta S, Oyama M, Kavalkovich K, Fu FH, Niyibizi C (1998) Identification of types II, IX and X collagens at the insertion site of the bovine achilles tendon. Matrix Biol 17(1):65–73
15. Visconti CS, Kavalkovich K, Wu J-J, Niyibizi C (1996) Biochemical analysis of collagens at the ligament-bone interface reveals presence of cartilage-specific collagens. Arch Biochem Biophys 328(1):135–142
16. Ralphs JR, Benjamin M, Waggett AD, Russell DC, Messner K, Gao J (1998) Regional differences in cell shape and gap junction expression in rat Achilles tendon: relation to fibrocartilage differentiation. J Anat 193(pt 2):215–222
17. Wopenka B, Kent A, Pasteris JD, Yoon Y, Thomopoulos S (2008) The tendon-to-bone transition of the rotator cuff: a preliminary Raman spectroscopic study documenting the gradual mineralization across the insertion in rat tissue samples. Appl Spectrosc 62 (12):1285–1294
18. Gupta HS, Schratter S, Tesch W, Roschger P, Berzlanovich A, Schoeberl T, Klaushofer K, Fratzl P (2005) Two different correlations between nanoindentation modulus and mineral content in the bone-cartilage interface. J Struct Biol 149(2):138–148
19. Gao J, Messner K, Ralphs JR, Benjamin M (1996) An immunohistochemical study of enthesis development in the medial collateral ligament of the rat knee joint. Anat Embryol 194(4):399–406
20. Provot S, Schipani E (2005) Molecular mechanisms of endochondral bone development. Biochem Biophys Res Commun 328(3):658–665
21. Villemure I, Stokes IA (2009) Growth plate mechanics and mechanobiology. A survey of present understanding. J Biomech 42(12):1793–1803
22. Benjamin M, Ralphs JR (2004) Biology of fibrocartilage cells. Int Rev Cytol 233:1–45
23. Liu Y, Birman V, Chen C, Thomopoulos S, Genin GM (2011) Mechanisms of bimaterial attachment at the interface of tendon to bone. J Eng Mater Technol 133(011006):281–288

24. Liu YX, Thomopoulos S, Birman V, Li JS, Genin GM (2012) Bi-material attachment through a compliant interfacial system at the tendon-to-bone insertion site. Mech Mater 44:83–92
25. Thomopoulos S, Marquez JP, Weinberger B, Birman V, Genin GM (2006) Collagen fiber orientation at the tendon to bone insertion and its influence on stress concentrations. J Biomech 39(10):1842–1851
26. Stouffer DC, Butler DL, Hosny D (1985) The relationship between crimp pattern and mechanical response of human patellar tendon-bone units. J Biomech Eng 107(2):158–165
27. Hauch KN, Oyen ML, Odegard GM, Haut Donahue TL (2009) Nanoindentation of the insertional zones of human meniscal attachments into underlying bone. J Mech Behav Biomed Mater 2(4):339–347
28. Villegas DF, Maes JA, Magee SD, Donahue TL (2007) Failure properties and strain distribution analysis of meniscal attachments. J Biomech 40(12):2655–2662
29. Moffat KL, Sun WH, Pena PE, Chahine NO, Doty SB, Ateshian GA, Hung CT, Lu HH (2008) Characterization of the structure-function relationship at the ligament-to-bone interface. Proc Natl Acad Sci U S A 105(23):7947–7952
30. Amini S, Veilleux D, Villemure I (2010) Tissue and cellular morphological changes in growth plate explants under compression. J Biomech 43(13):2582–2588
31. Villemure I, Cloutier L, Matyas JR, Duncan NA (2007) Non-uniform strain distribution within rat cartilaginous growth plate under uniaxial compression. J Biomech 40(1):149–156
32. Cohen B, Lai WM, Mow VC (1998) A transversely isotropic biphasic model for unconfined compression of growth plate and chondroepiphysis. J Biomech Eng 120(4):491–496
33. Sergerie K, Lacoursiere MO, Levesque M, Villemure I (2009) Mechanical properties of the porcine growth plate and its three zones from unconfined compression tests. J Biomech 42 (4):510–516
34. Genin GM, Kent A, Birman V, Wopenka B, Pasteris JD, Marquez PJ, Thomopoulos S (2009) Functional grading of mineral and collagen in the attachment of tendon to bone. Biophys J 97 (4):976–985
35. Birch R (2002) Obstetric brachial plexus palsy. J Hand Surg Br 27(1):3–8
36. Mehta SH, Blackwell SC, Bujold E, Sokol RJ (2006) What factors are associated with neonatal injury following shoulder dystocia? J Perinatol 26(2):85–88
37. Moukoko D, Ezaki M, Wilkes D, Carter P (2004) Posterior shoulder dislocation in infants with neonatal brachial plexus palsy. J Bone Joint Surg Am 86-A(4):787–793
38. Smith NC, Rowan P, Benson LJ, Ezaki M, Carter PR (2004) Neonatal brachial plexus palsy. Outcome of absent biceps function at three months of age. J Bone Joint Surg Am 86-A (10):2163–2170
39. Kirkos JM, Kyrkos MJ, Kapetanos GA, Haritidis JH (2005) Brachial plexus palsy secondary to birth injuries. J Bone Joint Surg Br 87(2):231–235
40. Wolff J (1892) Das Gesetz der Transformation der Knochen (Berlin A. Hirchwild). Translated as: The law of bone remodeling. In: Maquet P, Furlong R (eds) Springer-Verlag, Berlin
41. Goldstein SA (1987) The mechanical properties of trabecular bone: dependence on anatomic location and function. J Biomech 20(11–12):1055–1061
42. Mullender MG, Huiskes R (1995) Proposal for the regulatory mechanism of Wolff's law. J Orthop Res 13(4):503–512
43. Lang T, LeBlanc A, Evans H, Lu Y, Genant H, Yu A (2004) Cortical and trabecular bone mineral loss from the spine and hip in long-duration spaceflight. J Bone Miner Res 19 (6):1006–1012
44. Priest JD, Jones HH, Tichenor CJ, Nagel DA (1977) Arm and elbow changes in expert tennis players. Minn Med 60(5):399–404
45. Guilak F, Ratcliffe A, Mow VC (1995) Chondrocyte deformation and local tissue strain in articular cartilage: a confocal microscopy study. J Orthop Res 13(3):410–421

46. Krishnan R, Park S, Eckstein F, Ateshian GA (2003) Inhomogeneous cartilage properties enhance superficial interstitial fluid support and frictional properties, but do not provide a homogeneous state of stress. J Biomech Eng 125(5):569–577
47. Mizuno S, Tateishi T, Ushida T, Glowacki J (2002) Hydrostatic fluid pressure enhances matrix synthesis and accumulation by bovine chondrocytes in three-dimensional culture. J Cell Physiol 193(3):319–327
48. O'Connor KM (1997) Unweighting accelerates tidemark advancement in articular cartilage at the knee joint of rats. J Bone Miner Res 12(4):580–589
49. Carter DR, Beaupre GS, Wong M, Smith RL, Andriacchi TP, Schurman DJ (2004) The mechanobiology of articular cartilage development and degeneration. Clin Orthop Relat Res 427(suppl):S69–S77
50. Magnusson SP, Hansen P, Kjaer M (2003) Tendon properties in relation to muscular activity and physical training. Scand J Med Sci Sports 13(4):211–223
51. Woo SL, Gomez MA, Woo YK, Akeson WH (1982) Mechanical properties of tendons and ligaments. II. The relationships of immobilization and exercise on tissue remodeling. Biorheology 19(3):397–408
52. Amiel D, Woo SL, Harwood FL, Akeson WH (1982) The effect of immobilization on collagen turnover in connective tissue: a biochemical-biomechanical correlation. Acta Orthop Scand 53(3):325–332
53. Walsh S, Frank C, Hart D (1992) Immobilization alters cell metabolism in an immature ligament. Clin Orthop Relat Res 277:277–288
54. Woo SL, Gomez MA, Sites TJ, Newton PO, Orlando CA, Akeson WH (1987) The biomechanical and morphological changes in the medial collateral ligament of the rabbit after immobilization and remobilization. J Bone Joint Surg Am 69(8):1200–1211
55. Vogel KG, Koob TJ (1989) Structural specialization in tendons under compression. Int Rev Cytol 115:267–293
56. Vogel KG, Ordog A, Pogany G, Olah J (1993) Proteoglycans in the compressed region of human tibialis posterior tendon and in ligaments. J Orthop Res 11(1):68–77
57. Vogel KG, Sandy JD, Pogany G, Robbins JR (1994) Aggrecan in bovine tendon. Matrix Biol 14(2):171–179
58. Petersen W, Pufe T, Kurz B, Mentlein R, Tillmann B (2002) Angiogenesis in fetal tendon development: spatial and temporal expression of the angiogenic peptide vascular endothelial cell growth factor. Anat Embryol 205(4):263–270
59. Pufe T, Petersen W, Kurz B, Tsokos M, Tillmann B, Mentlein R (2003) Mechanical factors influence the expression of endostatin—an inhibitor of angiogenesis—in tendons. J Orthop Res 21(4):610–616
60. Thomopoulos S, Das R, Birman V, Smith L, Ku K, Elson E, Pryse KM, Marquez P, Genin GM (2011) Fibrocartilage tissue engineering: the role of the stress environment on cell morphology and matrix expression. Tissue Eng Part A 17(7–8):1039–1053
61. Carter DR, Beaupré GS, Beaupre GS (2007) Skeletal function and form: mechanobiology of skeletal development, aging, and regeneration. Cambridge University Press, Cambridge
62. Nowlan NC, Sharpe J, Roddy KA, Prendergast PJ, Murphy P (2010) Mechanobiology of embryonic skeletal development: insights from animal models. Birth Defects Res C Embryo Today 90(3):203–213
63. Osborne AC, Lamb KJ, Lewthwaite JC, Dowthwaite GP, Pitsillides AA (2002) Short-term rigid and flaccid paralyses diminish growth of embryonic chick limbs and abrogate joint cavity formation but differentially preserve pre-cavitated joints. J Musculoskelet Neuronal Interact 2(5):448–456
64. Nowlan NC, Bourdon C, Dumas G, Tajbakhsh S, Prendergast PJ, Murphy P (2010) Developing bones are differentially affected by compromised skeletal muscle formation. Bone 46 (5):1275–1285

65. Brent AE, Braun T, Tabin CJ (2005) Genetic analysis of interactions between the somitic muscle, cartilage and tendon cell lineages during mouse development. Development 132 (3):515–528
66. Sharir A, Stern T, Rot C, Shahar R, Zelzer E (2011) Muscle force regulates bone shaping for optimal load-bearing capacity during embryogenesis. Development 138(15):3247–3259
67. Mikic B, Johnson TL, Chhabra AB, Schalet BJ, Wong M, Hunziker EB (2000) Differential effects of embryonic immobilization on the development of fibrocartilaginous skeletal elements. J Rehabil Res Dev 37(2):127–133
68. Gomez C, David V, Peet NM, Vico L, Chenu C, Malaval L, Skerry TM (2007) Absence of mechanical loading *in utero* influences bone mass and architecture but not innervation in Myod-Myf5-deficient mice. J Anat 210(3):259–271
69. Kahn J, Shwartz Y, Blitz E, Krief S, Sharir A, Breitel DA, Rattenbach R, Relaix F, Maire P, Rountree RB, Kingsley DM, Zelzer E (2009) Muscle contraction is necessary to maintain joint progenitor cell fate. Dev Cell 16(5):734–743
70. Kardon G (1998) Muscle and tendon morphogenesis in the avian hind limb. Development 125(20):4019–4032
71. Germiller JA, Goldstein SA (1997) Structure and function of embryonic growth plate in the absence of functioning skeletal muscle. J Orthop Res 15(3):362–370
72. Pacifici M, Koyama E, Iwamoto M (2005) Mechanisms of synovial joint and articular cartilage formation: recent advances, but many lingering mysteries. Birth Defects Res C Embryo Today 75(3):237–248
73. Mikic B, Isenstein AL, Chhabra A (2004) Mechanical modulation of cartilage structure and function during embryogenesis in the chick. Ann Biomed Eng 32(1):18–25
74. Reich A, Jaffe N, Tong A, Lavelin I, Genina O, Pines M, Sklan D, Nussinovitch A, Monsonego-Ornan E (2005) Weight loading young chicks inhibits bone elongation and promotes growth plate ossification and vascularization. J Appl Physiol 98(6):2381–2389
75. Reich A, Sharir A, Zelzer E, Hacker L, Monsonego-Ornan E, Shahar R (2008) The effect of weight loading and subsequent release from loading on the postnatal skeleton. Bone 43 (4):766–774
76. Stokes IA, Aronsson DD, Dimock AN, Cortright V, Beck S (2006) Endochondral growth in growth plates of three species at two anatomical locations modulated by mechanical compression and tension. J Orthop Res 24(6):1327–1334
77. Stokes IA, Clark KC, Farnum CE, Aronsson DD (2007) Alterations in the growth plate associated with growth modulation by sustained compression or distraction. Bone 41 (2):197–205
78. Henderson JH, Carter DR (2002) Mechanical induction in limb morphogenesis: the role of growth-generated strains and pressures. Bone 31(6):645–653
79. Ingber DE (2008) Tensegrity and mechanotransduction. J Bodyw Mov Ther 12(3):198–200
80. Wang JH (2006) Mechanobiology of tendon. J Biomech 39(9):1563–1582
81. St-Jacques B, Hammerschmidt M, McMahon AP (1999) Indian hedgehog signaling regulates proliferation and differentiation of chondrocytes and is essential for bone formation. Genes Dev 13(16):2072–2086
82. Vortkamp A, Lee K, Lanske B, Segre GV, Kronenberg HM, Tabin CJ (1996) Regulation of rate of cartilage differentiation by Indian hedgehog and PTH-related protein. Science 273 (5275):613–622
83. Broadus AE, Macica C, Chen X (2007) The PTHrP functional domain is at the gates of endochondral bones. Ann N Y Acad Sci 1116:65–81
84. Huang W, Chung UI, Kronenberg HM, de Crombrugghe B (2001) The chondrogenic transcription factor Sox9 is a target of signaling by the parathyroid hormone-related peptide in the growth plate of endochondral bones. Proc Natl Acad Sci U S A 98(1):160–165
85. Akiyama H, Chaboissier MC, Martin JF, Schedl A, de Crombrugghe B (2002) The transcription factor Sox9 has essential roles in successive steps of the chondrocyte differentiation pathway and is required for expression of Sox5 and Sox6. Genes Dev 16(21):2813–2828

86. Wu Q, Zhang Y, Chen Q (2001) Indian hedgehog is an essential component of mechanotransduction complex to stimulate chondrocyte proliferation. J Biol Chem 276 (38):35290–35296
87. Chen X, Macica C, Nasiri A, Judex S, Broadus AE (2007) Mechanical regulation of PTHrP expression in entheses. Bone 41(5):752–759
88. Shen G (2005) The role of type X collagen in facilitating and regulating endochondral ossification of articular cartilage. Orthod Craniofac Res 8(1):11–17
89. Wu QQ, Chen Q (2000) Mechanoregulation of chondrocyte proliferation, maturation, and hypertrophy: ion-channel dependent transduction of matrix deformation signals. Exp Cell Res 256(2):383–391
90. Villemure I, Chung MA, Seck CS, Kimm MH, Matyas JR, Duncan NA (2005) Static compressive loading reduces the mRNA expression of type II and X collagen in rat growth-plate chondrocytes during postnatal growth. Connect Tissue Res 46(4–5):211–219
91. Cancel M, Grimard G, Thuillard-Crisinel D, Moldovan F, Villemure I (2009) Effects of *in vivo* static compressive loading on aggrecan and type II and X collagens in the rat growth plate extracellular matrix. Bone 44(2):306–315
92. Cserjesi P, Brown D, Ligon KL, Lyons GE, Copeland NG, Gilbert DJ, Jenkins NA, Olson EN (1995) Scleraxis: a basic helix-loop-helix protein that prefigures skeletal formation during mouse embryogenesis. Development 121(4):1099–1110
93. Schweitzer R, Chyung JH, Murtaugh LC, Brent AE, Rosen V, Olson EN, Lassar A, Tabin CJ (2001) Analysis of the tendon cell fate using Scleraxis, a specific marker for tendons and ligaments. Development 128(19):3855–3866
94. Brent AE, Schweitzer R, Tabin CJ (2003) A somitic compartment of tendon progenitors. Cell 113(2):235–248
95. Murchison ND, Price BA, Conner DA, Keene DR, Olson EN, Tabin CJ, Schweitzer R (2007) Regulation of tendon differentiation by scleraxis distinguishes force-transmitting tendons from muscle-anchoring tendons. Development 134(14):2697–2708
96. Scott A, Danielson P, Abraham T, Fong G, Sampaio AV, Underhill TM (2011) Mechanical force modulates scleraxis expression in bioartificial tendons. J Musculoskelet Neuronal Interact 11(2):124–132
97. Maeda T, Sakabe T, Sunaga A, Sakai K, Rivera AL, Keene DR, Sasaki T, Stavnezer E, Iannotti J, Schweitzer R, Ilic D, Baskaran H, Sakai T (2011) Conversion of mechanical force into TGF-beta-mediated biochemical signals. Curr Biol 21(11):933–941
98. Mendias CL, Gumucio JP, Bakhurin KI, Lynch EB, Brooks SV (2012) Physiological loading of tendons induces scleraxis expression in epitenon fibroblasts. J Orthop Res 30(4):606–612
99. Stains JP, Civitelli R (2005) Cell-to-cell interactions in bone. Biochem Biophys Res Commun 328(3):721–727
100. Stains JP, Civitelli R (2005) Cell-cell interactions in regulating osteogenesis and osteoblast function. Birth Defects Res C Embryo Today 75(1):72–80
101. Banes AJ, Horesovsky G, Larson C, Tsuzaki M, Judex S, Archambault J, Zernicke R, Herzog W, Kelley S, Miller L (1999) Mechanical load stimulates expression of novel genes *in vivo* and *in vitro* in avian flexor tendon cells. Osteoarthritis Cartilage 7(1):141–153
102. Waggett AD, Benjamin M, Ralphs JR (2006) Connexin 32 and 43 gap junctions differentially modulate tenocyte response to cyclic mechanical load. Eur J Cell Biol 85(11):1145–1154
103. Grimston SK, Brodt MD, Silva MJ, Civitelli R (2008) Attenuated response to *in vivo* mechanical loading in mice with conditional osteoblast ablation of the connexin43 gene (Gja1). J Bone Miner Res 23(6):879–886
104. Grimston SK, Goldberg DB, Watkins M, Brodt MD, Silva MJ, Civitelli R (2011) Connexin43 deficiency reduces the sensitivity of cortical bone to the effects of muscle paralysis. J Bone Miner Res 26(9):2151–2160
105. Grimston SK, Screen J, Haskell JH, Chung DJ, Brodt MD, Silva MJ, Civitelli R (2006) Role of connexin43 in osteoblast response to physical load. Ann N Y Acad Sci 1068:214–224

106. Grimston SK, Silva MJ, Civitelli R (2007) Bone loss after temporarily induced muscle paralysis by Botox is not fully recovered after 12 weeks. Ann N Y Acad Sci 1116:444–460
107. Fujioka H, Wang GJ, Mizuno K, Balian G, Hurwitz SR (1997) Changes in the expression of type-X collagen in the fibrocartilage of rat Achilles tendon attachment during development. J Orthop Res 15(5):675–681
108. Galatz L, Rothermich S, VanderPloeg K, Petersen B, Sandell L, Thomopoulos S (2007) Development of the supraspinatus tendon-to-bone insertion: localized expression of extracellular matrix and growth factor genes. J Orthop Res 25(12):1621–1628
109. Bland YS, Ashhurst DE (1997) Fetal and postnatal development of the patella, patellar tendon and suprapatella in the rabbit; changes in the distribution of the fibrillar collagens. J Anat 190(Pt 3):327–342
110. Bland YS, Ashhurst DE (2001) The hip joint: the fibrillar collagens associated with development and ageing in the rabbit. J Anat 198(pt 1):17–27
111. Blitz E, Viukov S, Sharir A, Shwartz Y, Galloway JL, Pryce BA, Johnson RL, Tabin CJ, Schweitzer R, Zelzer E (2009) Bone ridge patterning during musculoskeletal assembly is mediated through SCX regulation of Bmp4 at the tendon-skeleton junction. Dev Cell 17(6):861–873
112. Kronenberg HM (2003) Developmental regulation of the growth plate. Nature 423 (6937):332–336
113. Chen X, Macica CM, Dreyer BE, Hammond VE, Hens JR, Philbrick WM, Broadus AE (2006) Initial characterization of PTH-related protein gene-driven lacZ expression in the mouse. J Bone Miner Res 21(1):113–123
114. Asou Y, Nifuji A, Tsuji K, Shinomiya K, Olson EN, Koopman P, Noda M (2002) Coordinated expression of scleraxis and Sox9 genes during embryonic development of tendons and cartilage. J Orthop Res 20(4):827–833
115. Thomopoulos S, Kim HM, Rothermich SY, Biederstadt C, Das R, Galatz LM (2007) Decreased muscle loading delays maturation of the tendon enthesis during postnatal development. J Orthop Res 25(9):1154–1163
116. Kim HM, Galatz LM, Patel N, Das R, Thomopoulos S (2009) Recovery potential after postnatal shoulder paralysis. An animal model of neonatal brachial plexus palsy. J Bone Joint Surg Am 91(4):879–891
117. Das R, Rich J, Kim HM, McAlinden A, Thomopoulos S (2011) Effects of botulinum toxin-induced paralysis on postnatal development of the supraspinatus muscle. J Orthop Res 29(2):281–288
118. Kim HM, Galatz LM, Das R, Patel N, Thomopoulos S (2010) Musculoskeletal deformities secondary to neurotomy of the superior trunk of the brachial plexus in neonatal mice. J Orthop Res 28(10):1391–1398
119. Tatara A, Lipner J, Das R, Kim HM, Patel N, Silva MJ, Thomopoulos S (2010) The effects of muscle load and osteoclast activity on bone formation at the developing tendon enthesis. Trans Orthop Res Soc 57:134
120. Iannotti JP, Naranja RJ, Gartsman GM (1994) Surgical treatment of the intact cuff and repairable cuff defect: arthroscopic and open techniques. In: Norris TR (ed) Orthopaedic knowledge update: shoulder and elbow. American Academy of Orthopaedic Surgeons, Rosemont, IL, pp 151–155
121. Fu FH, Bennett CH, Lattermann C, Ma CB (1999) Current trends in anterior cruciate ligament reconstruction. Part 1: biology and biomechanics of reconstruction. Am J Sports Med 27(6):821–830
122. Kannus P, Jozsa L (1991) Histopathological changes preceding spontaneous rupture of a tendon. A controlled study of 891 patients. J Bone Joint Surg Am 73(10):1507–1525
123. Waggy C, Blaha, JD, Lobosky, DA, Beresford, WA, Clovis E (1994) Healing of tendon to bone insertion site in rabbits: a model of the effect of partial disruption. In: Transaction of the Orthopaedic Research Society, 40:39
124. St Pierre P, Olson EJ, Elliott JJ, O'Hair KC, McKinney LA, Ryan J (1995) Tendon-healing to cortical bone compared with healing to a cancellous trough. A biomechanical and histological evaluation in goats. J Bone Joint Surg Am 77(12):1858–1866

125. Ditsios K, Boyer MI, Kusano N, Gelberman RH, Silva MJ (2003) Bone loss following tendon laceration, repair and passive mobilization. J Orthop Res 21(6):990–996
126. Galatz LM, Rothermich SY, Zaegel M, Silva MJ, Havlioglu N, Thomopoulos S (2005) Delayed repair of tendon to bone injuries leads to decreased biomechanical properties and bone loss. J Orthop Res 23(6):1441–1447
127. Thomopoulos S, Matsuzaki H, Zaegel M, Gelberman RH, Silva MJ (2007) Alendronate prevents bone loss and improves tendon-to-bone repair strength in a canine model. J Orthop Res 25(4):473–479
128. Cadet ER, Vorys GC, Rahman R, Park SH, Gardner TR, Lee FY, Levine WN, Bigliani LU, Ahmad CS (2010) Improving bone density at the rotator cuff footprint increases supraspinatus tendon failure stress in a rat model. J Orthop Res 28(3):308–314
129. Silva MJ, Thomopoulos S, Kusano N, Zaegel MA, Harwood FL, Matsuzaki H, Havlioglu N, Dovan TT, Amiel D, Gelberman RH (2006) Early healing of flexor tendon insertion site injuries: tunnel repair is mechanically and histologically inferior to surface repair in a canine model. J Orthop Res 24(5):990–1000
130. Gimbel JA, Van Kleunen JP, Williams GR, Thomopoulos S, Soslowsky LJ (2007) Long durations of immobilization in the rat result in enhanced mechanical properties of the healing supraspinatus tendon insertion site. J Biomech Eng 129(3):400–404
131. Peltz CD, Dourte LM, Kuntz AF, Sarver JJ, Kim SY, Williams GR, Soslowsky LJ (2009) The effect of postoperative passive motion on rotator cuff healing in a rat model. J Bone Joint Surg Am 91(10):2421–2429
132. Sarver JJ, Peltz CD, Dourte L, Reddy S, Williams GR, Soslowsky LJ (2008) After rotator cuff repair, stiffness—but not the loss in range of motion—increased transiently for immobilized shoulders in a rat model. J Shoulder Elbow Surg 17(1 suppl):108S–113S
133. Dagher E, Hays PL, Kawamura S, Godin J, Deng XH, Rodeo SA (2009) Immobilization modulates macrophage accumulation in tendon-bone healing. Clin Orthop Relat Res 467 (1):281–287
134. Hays PL, Kawamura S, Deng XH, Dagher E, Mithoefer K, Ying L, Rodeo SA (2008) The role of macrophages in early healing of a tendon graft in a bone tunnel. J Bone Joint Surg Am 90 (3):565–579
135. Kawamura S, Ying L, Kim HJ, Dynybil C, Rodeo SA (2005) Macrophages accumulate in the early phase of tendon-bone healing. J Orthop Res 23(6):1425–1432
136. Galatz LM, Charlton N, Das R, Kim HM, Havlioglu N, Thomopoulos S (2009) Complete removal of load is detrimental to rotator cuff healing. J Shoulder Elbow Surg 18(5):669–675
137. Thomopoulos S, Zampiakis E, Das R, Silva MJ, Gelberman RH (2008) The effect of muscle loading on flexor tendon-to-bone healing in a canine model. J Orthop Res 26(12):1611–1617
138. Stasiak M, Imhauser C, Packer J, Bedi A, Brophy R, Kovacevic D, Jackson K, Deng XH, Rodeo S, Torzilli P (2010) A novel *in vivo* joint loading system to investigate the effect of daily mechanical load on a healing anterior cruciate ligament reconstruction. J Med Device 4(1):15003
139. Brophy RH, Kovacevic D, Imhauser CW, Stasiak M, Bedi A, Fox AJ, Deng XH, Rodeo SA (2011) Effect of short-duration low-magnitude cyclic loading versus immobilization on tendon-bone healing after ACL reconstruction in a rat model. J Bone Joint Surg Am 93 (4):381–393
140. Bedi A, Kovacevic D, Fox AJ, Imhauser CW, Stasiak M, Packer J, Brophy RH, Deng XH, Rodeo SA (2010) Effect of early and delayed mechanical loading on tendon-to-bone healing after anterior cruciate ligament reconstruction. J Bone Joint Surg Am 92(14):2387–2401
141. Peltz CD, Sarver JJ, Dourte LM, Wurgler-Hauri CC, Williams GR, Soslowsky LJ (2010) Exercise following a short immobilization period is detrimental to tendon properties and joint mechanics in a rat rotator cuff injury model. J Orthop Res 28(7):841–845
142. Eliasson P, Andersson T, Aspenberg P (2012) Achilles tendon healing in rats is improved by intermittent mechanical loading during the inflammatory phase. J Orthop Res 30(2):274–279

Chapter 12
Soft Tissue to Bone Healing in Rotator Cuff Repair

Leesa M. Galatz

12.1 Introduction

Tears of the rotator cuff tendons from their bony insertions are an extremely important clinical problem. Rotator cuff disease is one of the most common musculoskeletal disorders. In the United States, approximately 200,000 surgeries per year are performed for rotator cuff tears and nearly 400,000 surgeries per year are performed for rotator cuff tendinitis or partial rotator cuff tears [1]. Millions of individuals are at risk for developing pain and disability secondary to rotator cuff-related pathology. A recent analysis of cadaveric studies of rotator cuff tears revealed a 30% prevalence of tears [2]. While the majority of tears are degenerative, resulting from attritional changes in the tendon leading to attenuation, many occur in traumatic settings as well.

Although rotator cuff repair is a common procedure in the orthopaedic setting, healing of the tendons to bone after surgical repair is unpredictable, with failure rates ranging from 20 to 94% [3–5]. Healing in the adult setting is a reparative rather than a regenerative process, occurring via scar formation; the resultant tissue has significantly lower structural and material properties compared to native, uninjured tendon. Recently, innovations have been implemented to improve the strength of the repair and to biologically augment the healing process. The purpose of this chapter is to review the normal anatomy of the rotator cuff and its insertion site, to discuss the factors affecting tendon healing and to highlight recent strategies for improving healing of the injured rotator cuff.

L.M. Galatz (✉)
Department of Orthopaedic Surgery, Washington University, 660 South Euclid, Box 8233, St. Louis, MO 63110, USA
e-mail: galatzl@wudosis.wustl.edu

S. Thomopoulos et al. (eds.), *Structural Interfaces and Attachments in Biology*, DOI 10.1007/978-1-4614-3317-0_12,

12.2 Normal Anatomy of the Rotator Cuff and its Insertion Site

The rotator cuff muscles and tendons of the shoulder are a complex group of muscles that play a critical role in maintaining strength and stability in what is otherwise a biomechanically challenging joint. The shoulder is comprised of a shallow socket (the glenoid), an osseous component of the scapula, and a relatively large humeral head. The osseous structures result in a relatively unstable joint, thus the soft tissue stabilizers of the shoulder are important for normal function of the upper extremity. The static stabilizers of the shoulder include a ring of labral cartilage located circumferentially around the glenoid, which serves to deepen the socket, and the capsuloligamentous structures, which individually tighten at various shoulder positions. The rotator cuff provides dynamic stability and is active in nearly all phases of shoulder motion [6]. The contraction of the rotator cuff effectively centers the humeral head on the glenoid, counteracting the upward vector of the deltoid (Fig. 12.1).

The rotator cuff is comprised of four separate muscles (supraspinatus, infraspinatus, teres minor, and subscapularis), all of which originate from the scapula. The supraspinatus, infraspinatus, and teres minor muscles form the superior and posterior portions of the rotator cuff, and as they course laterally, they merge and join to form a single tendinous structure that inserts on the greater tuberosity (an osseous protuberance on the humeral head). The subscapularis arises from the anterior portion of the scapula and attaches to the lesser tuberosity, forming the anterior musculature of the shoulder.

Mature tendon has a highly organized and aligned structure. It is composed primarily of collagen type I and is relatively acellular [7]. Tendon exhibits high strength in response to tensile force and provides the mode of bony attachment for most muscles in the skeletal system. The rotator cuff has a relatively hypovascular area within what is known as the rotator cuff cable (Fig. 12.2). This hypovascular

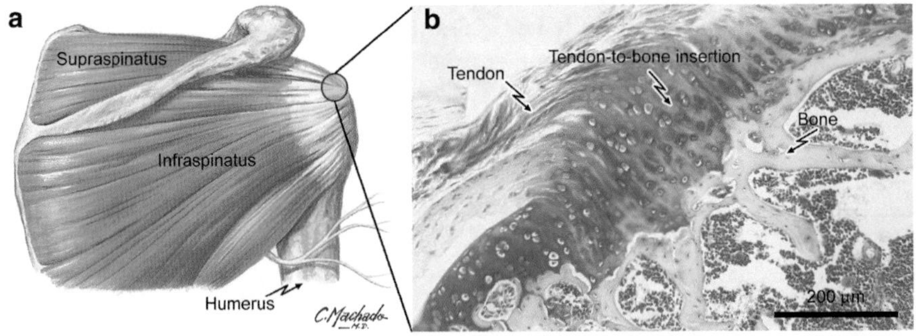

Fig. 12.1 (**a**) The rotator cuff is made up of four muscles that arise from the scapula and insert onto the humeral head. They are active during all phases of shoulder motion, centering the humeral head on the glenoid. (**b**) The rotator cuff insertion site is comprised of tendon, unmineralized fibrocartilage, mineralized fibrocartilage, and bone

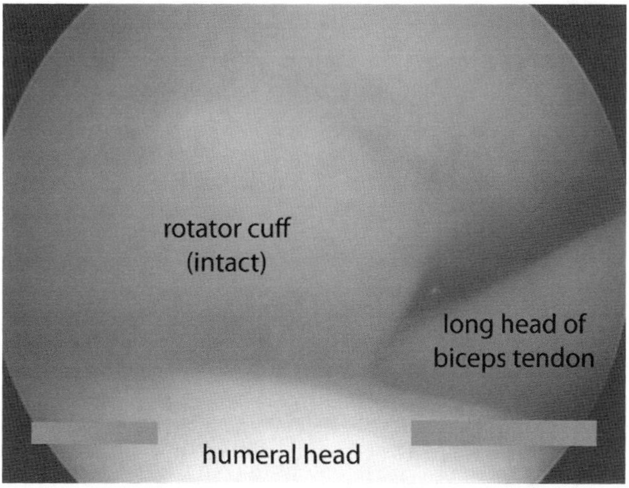

Fig. 12.2 The rotator cuff cable is a relatively hypovascular area near the insertion of the rotator cuff. Most tears arise in this area, which can be best appreciated from the articular side of the tendon

area can be visualized from the articular side of the tendon. There is a thickening of the supraspinatus that forms a cable-like structure, within which is the hypovascular zone. Tears of the rotator cuff often originate in this zone.

The insertion site of the rotator cuff to bone is comprised of four zones; this transition provides a gradual transition from a compliant to a hard material [8, 9]. The zones include tendon, unmineralized fibrocartilage, mineralized fibrocartilage, and bone (Fig. 12.1). There is a distinctive mineral gradient across the zones, transitioning from completely unmineralized tissue in the tendon to highly mineralized tissue in the bone. The purpose of this relatively gradual transition is to reduce the high stresses that would otherwise concentrate at the junction of a compliant material (tendon) to a stiff material (bone) [10]. These high stresses may otherwise result in a tear or attenuation of the tendon. The fibrocartilaginous transition zone may therefore serve a protective role to the tendon as it inserts on the tuberosity, allowing effective load transfer from the muscles to the bone.

12.3 Biology of Rotator Cuff Tendon-to-Bone Healing

Rotator cuff healing is characterized by a reparative rather than a regenerative response [11, 12]. A disorganized fibrous interface develops at the insertion consisting of biomechanically inferior tissue (Fig. 12.3). This tissue is later remodeled, becoming more organized and able to bear higher loads. However, the tissue never remodels to entirely resemble normal uninjured tendon.

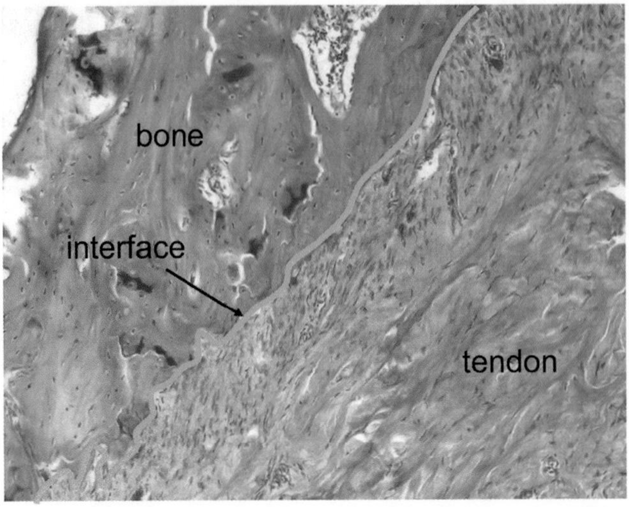

Fig. 12.3 A 4-week specimen after a rotator cuff injury and repair demonstrates relatively disorganized deposition of extracellular matrix components. Repair tissue is hypervascular and hypercellular compared to normal tendon tissue. Toluidine blue stained section, *solid line* indicates interface between healing tendon and bone (reproduced, with permission, from ref. [12])

Histologically, the resultant tissue is hypercellular and hypervascular relative to uninjured tissue. Biomechanical properties likewise never reach those of uninjured tendon.

Tendon healing occurs in phases similar to those seen in typical wound healing scenarios. An initial inflammatory phase is characterized by the presence of multinucleated cells. Most of these cells are replaced by mononuclear cells, which are the predominant cell type present for the next few weeks. In an acute repair rodent rotator cuff model, metabolic activity, growth factor production, and cell proliferation reach a peak at 7–10 days [11], after which there was a gradual decrease to baseline levels. While this timing may differ for repairs of chronic tears, and for healing in humans, there is likely a short time period of cell proliferation and growth factor production; this timing may provide a window for therapeutic manipulation.

The next phase of tendon healing consists of extracellular matrix production. While normal tendon is comprised primarily of collagen type I, the healing response is characterized by an initial production of collagen type III. Collagen type III is typically seen in degenerated and injured tendon, and also in developing tendon. It is a primary component of the early fibrous interface at the healing tendon-to-bone junction. Collagen type I production begins at some point after collagen type III and persists throughout the course of tendon healing.

Many different growth factors have been isolated at the healing rotator cuff tendon-to-bone insertion [12, 13]. These include TGF-β, PDGF-BB, bFGF, and various bone morphogenetic proteins (BMPs). These factors and many others likely play significant roles in the biology of tendon healing. The exact roles they exert remain a subject of continuing investigation.

Experiments in animal models have demonstrated that the healing tendon-to-bone insertion remains biomechanically inferior to the uninjured tissue, even in the long term [14–18]. Structural properties reach approximately one half of normal between 8 and 16 weeks, depending on the model utilized. This gain in strength is due primarily to an increase in the quantity of tissue produced at the healing site. The cross sectional area of the healing tissue at the tendon-to-bone junction largely exceeds that of the native insertion, accounting for the increase in pullout strength. However, when normalizing the structural properties by the amount of tissue present in order to determine tissue material properties, it is clear that the quality of the material produced is vastly inferior to normal tendon. This outcome is characteristic of the scar-like response that typifies early tendon healing.

Importantly, the graded fibrocartilaginous insertion site which characterizes the uninjured rotator cuff attachment to bone is not recreated in the healing scenario. The tendinous tissue that is generated does, with time, form a functional attachment, but the fibrocartilage and mineralized fibrocartilage tissues characteristic of the natural insertion are not reliably recreated. Some fibrocartilage cells may be found at later healing time points, but they are typically few in number and lack the distinct and organized morphology characteristic of the normal insertion site.

12.4 Patient-Specific Factors Affecting Rotator Cuff Tendon Healing

In every published study that has evaluated the anatomic outcome after rotator cuff repair using imaging modalities, a high percentage of unhealed tendons has been reported. Failure rates range from 20 to 94% [3–5, 19]. Multiple factors, including patient-related and technique-related factors, influence tendon healing.

12.4.1 Age

Age is likely the strongest biologic factor influencing rotator cuff healing. Most studies that have stratified patients for age have revealed a significant relationship between increased age and failure of healing [3, 4, 20–24]. The average age of the patients who heal are in their mid-to-late 50s and the average age of the patients who fail to heal is in the mid 60s. This information suggests that somewhere in the early seventh decade of life, changes in biology and/or physiology are such that the likelihood of healing even a small tear decreases dramatically.

This information has significant clinical implications. Surgical decision-making is influenced by patient age. Older patients who are less likely to heal may be better candidates for nonoperative treatment compared to younger patients, who are more likely to heal and also have higher functional demands. These younger individuals will benefit to a greater extent from operative repair.

12.4.2 Tear Size

Tear size has also been shown to influence tendon healing; the larger the tear, the lower the healing rate [25]. The threshold of tear size over which healing rates drop significantly is unknown. Regardless, tears considered large or massive, involving two or more tendons, have much lower healing potential. Care must be taken in interpreting much of this data, however, as older individuals are more likely to have larger tears, making age and tear size covariates. Larger numbers of patients must be studied in order to accurately stratify the effect of these variables separately.

12.4.3 Muscle Degeneration

Muscle tissue is highly sensitive to its loading environment. When tendons detach from their bony insertion sites, their respective muscles are unloaded and shortened, leading to muscle atrophy and the accumulation of fibrous tissue and fat; this is particularly apparent in the setting of a chronic tear [26–30]. Thus far, these changes have been found to be irreversible [31, 32]. Muscle degeneration has clinical implications for the feasibility of the repair. The degenerated muscles are much less compliant than normal muscles, and they often cannot be mobilized from their retracted position to the anatomic insertion on the humeral head. In instances where the tendon can be mobilized and repaired, the construct is under high tension, leading to early failure of the repair. Ideally, rotator cuff tears should be repaired prior to the onset of these chronic degenerative changes in clinically indicated patients.

12.4.4 Smoking

Smoking has been shown to have an effect on tendon healing. In a rodent model, rats were administered nicotine through a subcutaneous, continuous delivery osmotic pump [33]. High nicotine levels resulted in decreased cell proliferation and decreased collagen I production in the healing tissue. Mechanical properties were inferior to saline controls at all time points tested and histological signs of inflammation persisted longer in the nicotine specimens. Mechanical testing revealed increased stiffness at later time points (8 weeks). The clinical implication of the increased stiffness is not yet known. Smoking has also been shown in a human study to increase the likelihood of developing a rotator cuff tear; in patients with shoulder pain, individuals who smoke have a significantly greater chance of having a rotator cuff tear [34]. A more recent history of smoking, a greater quantity of cigarettes smoked, and a higher number of years smoking are all associated with rotator cuff tears. The extent to which these factors influence healing remains a subject of investigation.

12.4.5 Medical Comorbidities

A number of animal studies have been utilized to ascertain the effects of various medical comorbidities commonly seen in humans. Beason et al. performed a study evaluating the healing characteristics of a patellar tendon defect in aged mice with hypercholesterolemia compared to controls [35]. The tendons in the aged mice with hypercholesterolemia had a higher than expected rupture rate as well as a decreased elastic modulus, suggesting a negative cumulative effect of cholesterol. Furthermore, patients with rotator cuff tears had higher total cholesterol, triglycerides, and low density lipoproteins compared to an age matched control group [36]. High-density lipoproteins were lower in the cuff tear group. These results suggest that serum cholesterol may have a significant effect on the development of rotator cuff tears, and this may represent a viable therapeutic target for clinical management.

Non-steroidal anti-inflammatory medications are commonly used for pain relief in the setting of tendon degeneration or injury. Animal studies have suggested that a certain level of inflammation is necessary for normal tendon healing and remodeling. A study investigating the effects of NSAIDs on rotator cuff healing in a rat model found that both indomethacin, a cyclooxygenase 1 and 2 inhibitor, as well as celecoxib, a specific cyclooxygenase 2 inhibitor, had detrimental effects on tendon healing [37]. Histologic findings revealed a less organized tissue at the healing site in comparison to controls, as well as persistent osteoclasts. Biomechanical testing showed lower load to failure in both NSAID-treated groups. Most clinicians recommend that patients not use these medications in the immediate postoperative period, although further studies are necessary to determine the exact period of time and dosing regimen after which it is safe to resume these medications.

Diabetes is another common medical comorbidity that may have an effect on rotator cuff healing. Diabetes is known to affect microvascular environment of tissues. A study utilizing a rodent model of induced diabetes was used to investigate the effect of diabetes on rotator cuff healing [38]. Diabetes was induced preoperatively. Short-term results at 2 weeks showed reduced load-to-failure in the diabetic group compared to the control group. This study may underestimate the effects of diabetes compared to the chronically ill patients; longer term studies are necessary to come to a definitive conclusion. No long-term healing studies exist to answer this question in the human population.

Decreased bone mineral density is also associated with a higher failure rate after rotator cuff repair. In a study of 272 patients evaluated by either computed tomography or ultrasonography for rotator cuff integrity an average of 13 months after repair, decreased BMD and fatty infiltration were associated with unhealed cuffs [39]. These results are substantiated by a rat study in which the failure stress at the supraspinatus insertion was evaluated [40]. The study compared female rats after ovariectomies, half treated with bisphosphonates to improve bone density. Improving bone density improved the failure stress. These studies highlight the role of the bone in the process of degeneration and repair.

12.5 Surgical Factors Affecting Rotator Cuff Tendon Healing

The surgical factor receiving the greatest attention, and having the greatest effect on rotator cuff healing, is repair construct. Historically, the distal end of the rotator cuff tendon has been re-apposed to the bone using a single row of anchors. However, a "double row" repair was popularized several years ago in response to the relatively high failure rate of tendon healing after repair [41–44]. The goals of this repair are to increase the mechanical strength of the repair and to better recreate the anatomic footprint of the native insertion site. Apreleva et al. were the first to evaluate the effect of a double row repair on recreation of a normal footprint after repair in a cadaveric model [45]. They found that a double row construct successfully increased the contact area between the repaired tendon and the bony insertion site.

Several mechanical studies [43, 44, 46–49] evaluated the strength of the double row repair in comparison to a single row repair and found improvement in the overall strength of the repair. However, these results have not necessarily been translated into improvements in structural healing or clinical outcomes. Many studies report excellent results after a single row repair [50], often in spite of a high rate of failure of healing. Furthermore, many studies show no difference or only modest differences in healing between double and single row repair. Duquin et al. [51] performed a systematic review of 23 eligible studies and found re-tear rates significantly lower for double row repairs in tears greater than 1 cm in size. Similarly, several recent high level studies comparing the two methods showed no difference in clinical outcome, except in tears >3 cm, where strength was improved with a double row repair [52, 53]. Further investigation is necessary to ultimately determine the appropriate application of various repair techniques in given patient populations.

12.6 Surgical Repair Techniques and Outcomes

12.6.1 Technique

A rotator cuff repair can be accomplished through either open or arthroscopic techniques. Consistent with the current trend in surgery, there has been a shift toward arthroscopic or minimally invasive techniques. A variety of devices and instruments are commercially available to achieve a tendon-to-bone reattachment in the shoulder.

Access to the joint is achieved via a posterior portal. An anterior portal is established through the rotator interval (Fig. 12.4). A thorough examination of intraarticular structures allows an accurate diagnosis and assessment for concurrent pathology. The long head of the biceps arises from the supraglenoid tubercle and is evaluated for tearing and attenuation. Attritional changes may be seen as the biceps

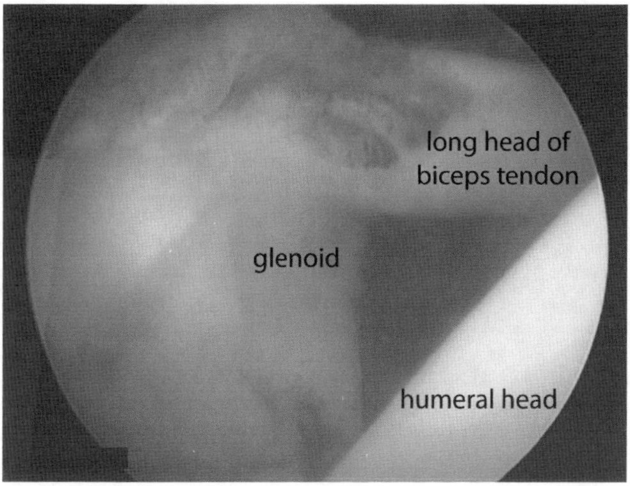

Fig. 12.4 The shoulder joint visualized from the posterior portal with an anterior portal through the rotator interval (the space between the supraspinatus and subscapularis tendons). The humeral head, glenoid, and biceps tendon are seen

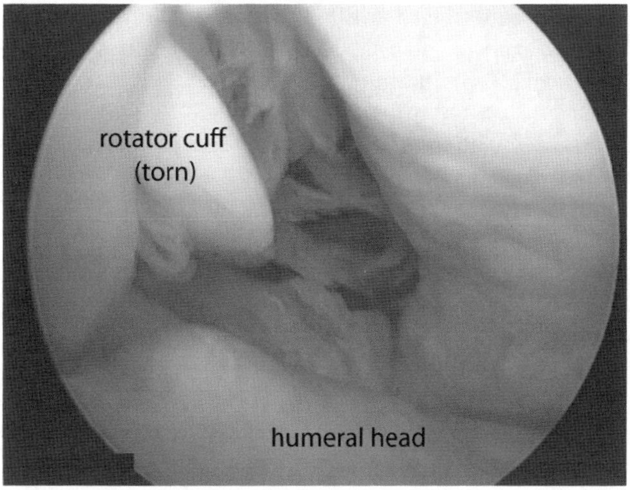

Fig. 12.5 A rotator cuff tear is assessed from the articular side

exit the joint anterior to the supraspinatus through the intertubercular groove. Cartilaginous surfaces are evaluated, as arthritic changes may contribute to pain and mechanical symptoms postoperatively. The rotator cuff is visualized from the articular surface (Fig. 12.5). Tear size and tendon delamination can be appreciated from the intraarticular perspective, guiding surgical strategy during repair.

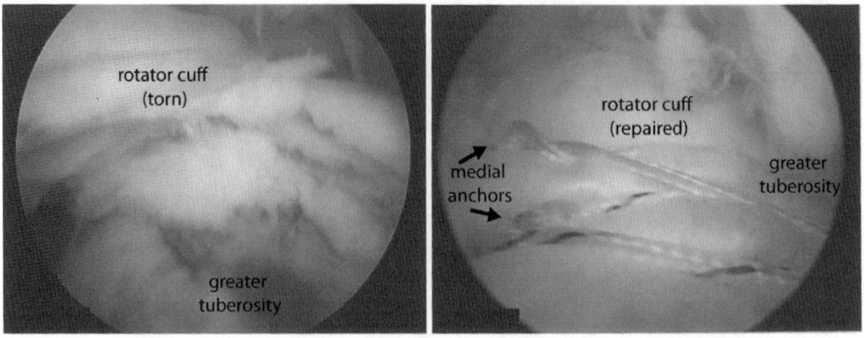

Fig. 12.6 Anchors are placed into the greater tuberosity. The anchor is analogous to a small screw with an eyelet through which sutures pass and is used to repair the tendon to bone. Anchors are made from a variety of materials including metal, bioabsorbable, and nonabsorbable plastics. The final repair of tendon to bone is shown on the *right*

The repair is performed with the arthroscope and working instruments in the subacromial space, between the rotator cuff tendon and the acromial process of the scapula. An anterolateral portal creates access for working instruments. A limited bursectomy allows visualization of the retracted tendon and the greater tuberosity, the insertion site for the supraspinatus tendon. The edge of the tendon is debrided with a shaver. The bone of the tuberosity is likewise debrided, removing remnants of tendon tissue and exposing punctate bleeding bone. The bone is not decorticated, as this will compromise subsequent anchor fixation.

A description of a double row repair follows [54]. As mentioned previously, multiple methods of tendon-to-bone reattachment are possible; however, the basic principles are the same. The tendon is mobilized from surrounding adhesions to reduce tension on the repair. The tendon is then attached to the bone. The attachment should be secure, minimize motion at the tendon bone interface, and maximize contact area at the tendon bone interface, yet not strangulate the tissue [41, 43, 44, 46, 47, 55]. The repair configuration should not be so tight that blood flow is compromised. This may result in a tendon tear subsequent to mechanical attenuation at the suture-tendon interface. Achieving the proper balance in these criteria is challenging.

The suture anchors are then inserted through superior accessory portals; this provides an optimal angle of insertion into the bone. A large cannula through the anterolateral portal facilitates easy passage of instruments in and out of the subacromial space, minimizing trauma to the deltoid muscle. The sutures are retrieved through this cannula, placed in a suture-passing device, and passed through the tendon (Fig. 12.6). Once all sutures have been placed through the tendon, arthroscopic knot tying devices are used to tie the sutures, reducing the tendon to the bone. The long ends of the sutures are brought laterally and anchored to the lateral cortex using another anchor or two (Fig. 12.6). This configuration helps achieve the goals of secure fixation, minimal motion, and maximal contact between the tendon and bone.

12.6.2 Influence of Structural Failure

Rotator cuff repair has a long history of largely good to excellent results, often in spite of structural failure of the repair. However, range of motion and strength are generally compromised to some extent with an unhealed cuff. This clinical scenario often results in a painful shoulder with functional disability. This is particularly important in the younger (ages 40–60 years) patient population, which is generally still of working age. Patients with manual labor jobs, especially those that require shoulder level or overhead activity, and those with high recreational shoulder demands do poorly in the setting of a failed repair.

Gerber et al. reported a series of 27 patients after open rotator cuff repair [56]. At a minimum of 2-year follow-up, 17 patients healed their tear and had an excellent outcome. The patients with re-tears had a poorer outcome based on Constant score, subjective shoulder value, pain, and ability to perform activities of daily living. A series of 20 patients with known structural failure were evaluated at 3-year follow-up [57]. Overall, outcomes were improved over preoperative values. Rotator cuff tendons and muscles were evaluated by MRI and compared to preoperative studies. Fatty degeneration increased over time in the supraspinatus and infraspinatus muscles. Muscle atrophy was also seen in the supraspinatus. Glenohumeral arthritis was also increased over time. Seventeen of the patients were very satisfied or satisfied, and poorer outcomes correlated with larger tear size, severity of fatty degeneration of the muscles, and the presence of arthritis. This same group of patients was reevaluated 9 years after surgery [32]. Overall, the clinical improvement seen initially did not deteriorate, despite increased fatty degeneration in the muscles.

Zumstein et al. reported a series of 27 patients at 3 and 9 years following open rotator cuff repair [58]. Thirty seven percent were re-torn at 3 years and 57% were re-torn at 9 years. The patients with an intact repair had better results, as measured by outcome score and strength. Fatty degeneration progressed in all torn tendons. The size of re-tears progressed over the time interval studied. Healed repairs appeared to protect against progressive fatty degeneration. Interestingly, the same group of investigators reported on clinical and structural results after repair of single tendon tears and found that repair may halt the atrophy of the supraspinatus, but not reverse it [31]. Similarly, fatty degeneration either remained stable or progressed, even in patients with healed tears. Further investigation is necessary to elucidate the pathophysiology of these muscle changes, as well as the potential effect of repair.

Dodson et al. followed a group of patients with known structural repair-site failures an average of 3 years after repair [59]. The initial good clinical results did not decrease over time; however, range of motion and strength measurements decreased. The size of the re-tear increased and none of the tears healed. Muscle architecture was not evaluated in this study. Miller et al. examined rotator cuff repairs with ultrasound for repair-site integrity at regular intervals for 2 years after surgery [60]. All tears were originally greater than 3 cm. Forty-one percent of the tears recurred (9 patients). Seven tears recurred within 3 months. The remaining tear recurred within 6 months. Tears in this study were stable after 6 months. Outcome scores (Western Ontario Rotator Cuff) were worse in the group with recurrent tears compared to the group with healed tears.

Not all patients do poorly after failure of healing after rotator cuff repair. Galatz et al. reported a series of 18 patients 2 years after a single row arthroscopic repair [3]. Seventeen of the cuffs tears had recurred. However, there were significant improvements in function and American Shoulder and Elbow Surgeons outcome scores. This same cohort of patients was reevaluated 10 years after the index procedure (unpublished data). Fifteen of the original 18 were available for review. Only two had subsequent procedures—one had a revision repair and one had a joint replacement. There were no changes in outcome score, range of motion, or level of pain over the time course studies. Many patients, however, had progression of degenerative changes in the glenohumeral joint.

There are many other studies citing no differences between patients with healed and unhealed cuffs [61–64]. Overall, future investigations in both the clinical and basic science realms will help elucidate issues with regard to rotator cuff tendon healing. Measurement tools as well as patient demographics will likely have an important influence on the relationship between healing and outcome. Regardless, it is unusual to have a poor outcome in the setting of a healed repair.

12.7 Future Strategies to Enhance Rotator Cuff Healing

Strong potential exists for improving rotator cuff tendon-to-bone healing using a variety of biological strategies. Platelet rich plasma (PRP) has been safely used for human application; however, use of growth factors, matrix metalloproteinase (MMP) inhibitors, tissue engineered scaffolds, and stem cells have only been studied using animal models.

12.7.1 Growth Factors

In one study, osteoinductive protein extract containing BMPs 2 and 7, transforming growth factor (TGF) β 1 and 3, and fibroblast growth factor (FGF) was delivered via collagen sponge to the rotator cuff healing site in a sheep model [65]. Compared to controls, the treated group had a greater volume of reparative tissue and bone present at the healing interface, a more apparent fibrocartilage interface, and a greater load to failure 6 and 12 weeks after repair. The growth factors BMP 12, 13, and 14 have been identified during tendon fetal development and hold great potential for enhancing tendon repair [13, 66–68]. BMP 12 has been shown to induce the formation of tendon-like tissue in mature animals [69, 70]. BMP 12 application to the rotator cuff healing site using a collagen sponge resulted in increased tensile strength and stiffness of the repair [71]. FGF is active in various phases of tendon healing and promotes connective tissue formation and remodeling. It also activates the release of other growth factors such as TGF βs and BMPs. Used in a rat model, FGF improved biomechanical and histological properties 2 weeks after repair, but the results did not persist at 4 and 6 week time points [72].

TGF β3 is a compelling growth factor for enhancing repair, as it is associated with scarless soft tissue healing of tendon and skin in early stages of development. In one rat study, sustained delivery of the growth factor to the rotator cuff healing site was facilitated using a heparin-binding fibrin matrix [73]. There were improvements in cellularity, vascularity, and cell proliferation in the reparative tissue. Structural properties were improved 4 weeks after repair. In another rat study, a calcium phosphate matrix with TGF β3 was used to augment the repair [74]. The load-to-failure was improved in these repairs compared to untreated controls and compared to the calcium phosphate matrix alone. Bone volume was increased at the attachment site based on computed tomography evaluation. The ratio of collagen I: III was increased, indicating a more regenerative rather than scar-mediated healing response. While no growth factor is currently approved for use in rotator cuff repair, there is great potential for their use in future clinical cuff applications.

12.7.2 Matrix Metalloproteinases

MMPs are a family of proteinases that are involved in the maintenance and remodeling of extracellular matrices on connective tissue. They work in concert with tissue inhibitors of MMPs (TIMPs) to maintain homeostasis of the remodeling process and a balance between reparative and degenerative processes. MMPs have a role in injury response, age related degenerative processes, and repair. Doxycycline is an MMP inhibitor, and its use in a rat model of injury and repair resulted in some biomechanical improvements as well as improved collagen organization at early time points [75]. Alpha 2-macroglobulin is another inhibitor of MMPs. While some qualitative increase in fibrocartilage formation was identified at the healing site using this inhibitor, there were no improvements in biomechanical properties of the repair [76].

12.7.3 Tissue Engineering

Recently, an explosion of interest in tissue engineering strategies for use in rotator cuff repair has occurred, with the goal of not only improving biomechanical strength of the repair, but also utilizing a scaffold for delivery of cells and growth factors. Some early studies have utilized polyurethane mesh patches with some success [77]. Nanofiber scaffolds of PLGA with a novel distribution of mineralized and unmineralized regions have recently been investigated [78]. In one study, human rotator cuff fibroblasts were cultured on the scaffold [79]. The fibroblasts deposited a proteoglycan and collagen matrix onto the scaffold, which contained both collagen types I and II. A fibrocartilage transition zone was also identified.

12.7.4 Stem Cells

There has been recent interest in the field of orthopaedic surgery in utilizing mesenchymal stem cells to assist with regeneration. Studies have evaluated the effect of stem cells specifically in the setting of rotator cuff repair using rodent models. Application of bone marrow derived mesenchymal stem cells alone did not improve rotator cuff healing based on biomechanical and histological evaluation [80]. Similarly, bone marrow derived stem cells transfected with BMP 13 did not effect healing [81]. There was no difference in the amount of new cartilage formation, collagen fiber organization, or biomechanical properties. However, when bone marrow derived stem cells were transduced with scleraxis (a transcription factor necessary for tenogenesis), there was improvement in rotator cuff healing. Its expression in osteoblastic cell lines may also induce chondrocyte-like gene expression, which may be important at the bone-tendon junction. When stem cells transfected with adenoviral-mediated scleraxis were applied to the rotator cuff healing site in a rodent model, there were improvements in biomechanical and histological properties [82]. These studies highlight the potential value of mesenchymal stem cells as a delivery mechanism for factors which may improve healing of the rotator cuff.

12.7.5 Platelet Rich Plasma

PRP is a sample of autologous blood with high concentrations of platelets above baseline values. Its application has been used for tendinopathy, muscle injury, and tendon and ligament healing [83, 84]. PRP use is compelling, as it contains multiple growth factors, cytokines, and other proteins, all of which are active at various phases of muscle or tendon healing. There are several commercially available preparation systems, each one varying slightly from another. Generally, the application of PRP works well *in vitro* [85–87]. Fibroblasts treated with PRP have demonstrated increases in growth factors, MMP production, and collagen production. Increases in cell proliferation and tendon regenerate material have also been noted.

Unfortunately these benefits have not consistently translated to clinical improvements. Randelli et al. demonstrated the safety of application of PRP in the human setting [88]. Multiple other studies have not shown an improvement in tendon healing with the use of PRP. Weber et al. presented a study showing no differences in a randomized controlled study (Weber et al., presented at the

American Shoulder and Elbow Surgeons Open Meeting, 2010). Jo et al. performed a level 2 study which also demonstrated no clinical difference [89]. There was a lower re-tear rate in the treated group, but the difference was not statistically significant. Randelli et al., in a follow-up study of 2 years, showed improvement in pain scores at early timepoints; however, the differences did not persist at longer timepoints and there was no benefit of PRP application in larger tears [90]. Castricini et al. also showed no difference in outcome scores or tendon integrity based on MRI [91]. Bergeson et al. showed no benefit of fibrin matrix in a prospective study [92]. Alternatively, there is one recent human study which showed that the application of PRP fibrin matrix resulted in better healing of rotator cuff tears measuring less than 3 cm [93]. However, there were no differences in clinical outcomes. Taken together, these studies shed concern over the potential applicability of PRP for rotator cuff repair in the clinical setting. Based on currently available scientific information, there is no strong evidence to support its use.

12.8 Conclusions

The repair of the rotator cuff to its humeral head insertion presents a major challenge due to the disparity in the properties of the two tissues. Healing of tendon to bone is characterized by the formation of a fibrovascular scar and bone loss, leading to a repaired attachment that is prone to rupture. Further complicating the repair is the muscle degeneration that is typical in the retracted rotator cuff muscle (s). Current surgical treatment techniques attempt to securely attach the torn tendon to its bony footprint using an arthroscopic approach and a double-row suturing technique. Future treatment approaches may include delivery of growth factors and/ or mesenchymal stem cells to stimulate regeneration of a fibrocartilaginous insertion.

References

1. AAOS by group. The Burden of Musculoskeletal Disease in the U.S. (2011) American Academy of Orthopedic Surgery, Rosemont, IL pp. 129–179
2. Reilly P, Macleod I, Macfarlane R, Windley J, Emery RJH (2006) Dead men and radiologists don't lie: a review of cadaveric and radiological studies of rotator cuff tear prevalence. Ann R Coll Surg Engl 88:116–121
3. Galatz LM, Ball CM, Teefey SA, Middleton WD, Yamaguchi K (2004) The outcome and repair integrity of completely arthroscopically repaired large and massive rotator cuff tears. J Bone Joint Surg Am 86-A:219–224
4. Boileau P, Brassart N, Watkinson DJ, Carles M, Hatzidakis AM, Krishnan SG (2005) Arthroscopic repair of full-thickness tears of the supraspinatus: does the tendon really heal? J Bone Joint Surg Am 87:1229–1240

5. Kamath G, Galatz LM, Keener JD, Teefey S, Middleton W, Yamaguchi K (2009) Tendon integrity and functional outcome after arthroscopic repair of high-grade partial-thickness supraspinatus tears. J Bone Joint Surg Am 91:1055–1062
6. Soslowsky LJ, Carpenter JE, Bucchieri JS, Flatow EL (1997) Biomechanics of the rotator cuff. Orthop Clin North Am 28:17–30
7. Kumagai J, Sarkar K, Uhthoff HK, Okawara Y, Ooshima A (1994) Immunohistochemical distribution of type I II and III collagens in the rabbit supraspinatus tendon insertion. J Anat 185(pt 2):279–284
8. Shaw HM, Benjamin M (2007) Structure-function relationships of entheses in relation to mechanical load and exercise. Scand J Med Sci Sports 17:303–315
9. Benjamin M, Evans EJ, Copp L (1986) The histology of tendon attachments to bone in man. J Anat 149:89–100
10. Thomopoulos S, Williams GR, Gimbel JA, Favata M, Soslowsky LJ (2003) Variation of biomechanical, structural, and compositional properties along the tendon to bone insertion site. J Orthop Res 21:413–419
11. Galatz LM, Sandell LJ, Rothermich SY, Das R, Mastny A, Havlioglu N, Silva MJ, Thomopoulos S (2006) Characteristics of the rat supraspinatus tendon during tendon-to-bone healing after acute injury. J Orthop Res 24:541–550
12. Thomopoulos S, Hattersley G, Rosen V, Mertens M, Galatz L, Williams GR, Soslowsky LJ (2002) The localized expression of extracellular matrix components in healing tendon insertion sites: an in situ hybridization study. J Orthop Res 20:454–463
13. Würgler-Hauri CC, Dourte LM, Baradet TC, Williams GR, Soslowsky LJ (2007) Temporal expression of 8 growth factors in tendon-to-bone healing in a rat supraspinatus model. J Shoulder Elbow Surg 16:S198–S203
14. Carpenter JE, Thomopoulos S, Flanagan CL, DeBano CM, Soslowsky LJ (1998) Rotator cuff defect healing: a biomechanical and histologic analysis in an animal model. J Shoulder Elbow Surg 7:599–605
15. Edelstein L, Thomas SJ, Soslowsky LJ (2011) Rotator cuff tears: what have we learned from animal models? J Musculoskelet Neuronal Interact 11:150–162
16. Coleman SH, Fealy S, Ehteshami JR, Macgillivray JD, Altchek DW, Warren RF, Turner AS (2003) Chronic rotator cuff injury and repair model in sheep. J Bone Joint Surg Am 85-A:2391–2402
17. Derwin KA, Baker AR, Codsi MJ, Iannotti JP (2007) Assessment of the canine model of rotator cuff injury and repair. J Shoulder Elbow Surg 16:S140–S148
18. Gerber C, Schneeberger AG, Perren SM, Nyffeler RW (1999) Experimental rotator cuff repair. A preliminary study. J Bone Joint Surg Am 81:1281–1290
19. Lafosse L, Brozska R, Toussaint B, Gobezie R (2007) The outcome and structural integrity of arthroscopic rotator cuff repair with use of the double-row suture anchor technique. J Bone Joint Surg Am 89:1533–1541
20. Provencher MT, Kercher JS, Galatz LM, Elattrache NS, Frank RM, Cole BJ (2011) Evolution of rotator cuff repair techniques: are our patients really benefiting? Instr Course Lect 60:123–136
21. Tashjian RZ, Hollins AM, Kim H-M, Teefey SA, Middleton WD, Steger-May K, Galatz LM, Yamaguchi K (2010) Factors affecting healing rates after arthroscopic double-row rotator cuff repair. Am J Sports Med 38:2435–2442
22. Keener JD, Wei AS, Kim HM, Paxton ES, Teefey SA, Galatz LM, Yamaguchi K (2010) Revision arthroscopic rotator cuff repair: repair integrity and clinical outcome. J Bone Joint Surg Am 92:590–598
23. Harryman DT, Mack LA, Wang KY, Jackins SE, Richardson ML, Matsen FA (1991) Repairs of the rotator cuff. Correlation of functional results with integrity of the cuff. J Bone Joint Surg Am 73:982–989
24. Lichtenberg S, Liem D, Magosch P, Habermeyer P (2006) Influence of tendon healing after arthroscopic rotator cuff repair on clinical outcome using single-row Mason-Allen suture technique: a prospective, MRI controlled study. Knee Surg Sports Traumatol Arthrosc 14:1200–1206

25. Oh JH, Kim SH, Kang JY, Oh CH, Gong HS (2010) Effect of age on functional and structural outcome after rotator cuff repair. Am J Sports Med 38:672–678
26. Liu X, Manzano G, Kim HT, Feeley BT (2011) A rat model of massive rotator cuff tears. J Orthop Res 29:588–595
27. Cheung S, Dillon E, Tham S-C, Feeley BT, Link TM, Steinbach L, Ma CB (2011) The presence of fatty infiltration in the infraspinatus: its relation with the condition of the supraspinatus tendon. Arthroscopy 27:463–470
28. Zingg PO, Jost B, Sukthankar A, Buhler M, Pfirrmann CWA, Gerber C (2007) Clinical and structural outcomes of nonoperative management of massive rotator cuff tears. J Bone Joint Surg Am 89:1928–1934
29. Kim HM, Dahiya N, Teefey SA, Keener JD, Galatz LM, Yamaguchi K (2010) Relationship of tear size and location to fatty degeneration of the rotator cuff. J Bone Joint Surg Am 92:829–839
30. Kim HM, Galatz LM, Lim C, Havlioglu N, Thomopoulos S (2011) The effect of tear size and nerve injury on rotator cuff muscle fatty degeneration in a rodent animal model. J Shoulder Elbow Surg 61(4):613–621
31. Fuchs B, Gilbart MK, Hodler J, Gerber C (2006) Clinical and structural results of open repair of an isolated one-tendon tear of the rotator cuff. J Bone Joint Surg Am 88:309–316
32. Jost B, Zumstein M, Pfirrmann CWA, Gerber C (2006) Long-term outcome after structural failure of rotator cuff repairs. J Bone Joint Surg Am 88:472–479
33. Galatz LM, Silva MJ, Rothermich SY, Zaegel MA, Havlioglu N, Thomopoulos S (2006) Nicotine delays tendon-to-bone healing in a rat shoulder model. J Bone Joint Surg Am 88:2027–2034
34. Baumgarten KM, Gerlach D, Galatz LM, Teefey SA, Middleton WD, Ditsios K, Yamaguchi K (2010) Cigarette smoking increases the risk for rotator cuff tears. Clin Orthop Relat Res 468:1534–1541
35. Beason DP, Abboud JA, Kuntz AF, Bassora R, Soslowsky LJ (2011) Cumulative effects of hypercholesterolemia on tendon biomechanics in a mouse model. J Orthop Res 29:380–383
36. Abboud JA, Kim JS (2010) The effect of hypercholesterolemia on rotator cuff disease. Clin Orthop Relat Res 468:1493–1497
37. Cohen DB, Kawamura S, Ehteshami JR, Rodeo SA (2006) Indomethacin and celecoxib impair rotator cuff tendon-to-bone healing. Am J Sports Med 34:362–369
38. Bedi A, Fox AJS, Harris PE, Deng X-H, Ying L, Warren RF, Rodeo SA (2010) Diabetes mellitus impairs tendon-bone healing after rotator cuff repair. J Shoulder Elbow Surg 19:978–988
39. Chung SW, Oh JH, Gong HS, Kim JY, Kim SH (2011) Factors affecting rotator cuff healing after arthroscopic repair: osteoporosis as one of the independent risk factors. Am J Sports Med 39:2099–2107
40. Cadet ER, Vorys GC, Rahman R, Park S-H, Gardner TR, Lee FY, Levine WN, Bigliani LU, Ahmad CS (2010) Improving bone density at the rotator cuff footprint increases supraspinatus tendon failure stress in a rat model. J Orthop Res 28:308–314
41. Ahmad CS, Stewart AM, Izquierdo R, Bigliani LU (2005) Tendon-bone interface motion in transosseous suture and suture anchor rotator cuff repair techniques. Am J Sports Med 33:1667–1671
42. Pauly S, Fiebig D, Kieser B, Albrecht B, Schill A, Scheibel M (2011) Biomechanical comparison of four double-row speed-bridging rotator cuff repair techniques with or without medial or lateral row enhancement. Knee Surg Sports Traumatol Arthrosc 19:2090–2097
43. Park MC, Elattrache NS, Tibone JE, Ahmad CS, Jun B-J, Lee TQ (2007) Part I: footprint contact characteristics for a transosseous-equivalent rotator cuff repair technique compared with a double-row repair technique. J Shoulder Elbow Surg 16:461–468
44. Park MC, Tibone JE, Elattrache NS, Ahmad CS, Jun B-J, Lee TQ (2007) Part II: biomechanical assessment for a footprint-restoring transosseous-equivalent rotator cuff repair technique compared with a double-row repair technique. J Shoulder Elbow Surg 16:469–476

45. Apreleva M, Özbaydar M, Fitzgibbons PG, Warner JJP (2002) Rotator cuff tears. Arthroscopy 18:519–526
46. Millett PJ, Mazzocca A, Guanche CA (2004) Mattress double anchor footprint repair: a novel, arthroscopic rotator cuff repair technique. Arthroscopy 20:875–879
47. Burkhart SS, Denard PJ, Obopilwe E, Mazzocca AD (2012) Optimizing pressurized contact area in rotator cuff repair: the Diamondback repair. Arthroscopy 28(2):188–195
48. Tuoheti Y, Itoi E, Yamamoto N, Seki N, Abe H, Minagawa H, Okada K, Shimada Y (2005) Contact area, contact pressure, and pressure patterns of the tendon-bone interface after rotator cuff repair. Am J Sports Med 33:1869–1874
49. Mazzocca AD, Millett PJ, Guanche CA, Santangelo SA, Arciero RA (2005) Arthroscopic single-row versus double-row suture anchor rotator cuff repair. Am J Sports Med 33:1861–1868
50. Galatz LM, Williams GR, Fenlin JM, Ramsey ML, Iannotti JP (2004) Outcome of open reduction and internal fixation of surgical neck nonunions of the humerus. J Orthop Trauma 18:63–67
51. Duquin TR, Buyea C, Bisson LJ (2010) Which method of rotator cuff repair leads to the highest rate of structural healing? A systematic review. Am J Sports Med 38:835–841
52. Franceschi F, Ruzzini L, Longo UG, Martina FM, Zobel BB, Maffulli N, Denaro V (2007) Equivalent clinical results of arthroscopic single-row and double-row suture anchor repair for rotator cuff tears: a randomized controlled trial. Am J Sports Med 35:1254–1260
53. Koh KH, Kang KC, Lim TK, Shon MS, Yoo JC (2011) Prospective randomized clinical trial of single- versus double-row suture anchor repair in 2- to 4-cm rotator cuff tears: clinical and magnetic resonance imaging results. Arthroscopy 27:453–462
54. Park MC, Elattrache NS, Ahmad CS, Tibone JE (2006) "Transosseous-equivalent" rotator cuff repair technique. Arthroscopy 22:1360.e1–1360.e5
55. Park MC, Cadet ER, Levine WN, Bigliani LU, Ahmad CS (2005) Tendon-to-bone pressure distributions at a repaired rotator cuff footprint using transosseous suture and suture anchor fixation techniques. Am J Sports Med 33:1154–1159
56. Gerber C, Fuchs B, Hodler J (2000) The results of repair of massive tears of the rotator cuff. J Bone Joint Surg Am 82:505–515
57. Jost B, Pfirrmann CW, Gerber C, Switzerland Z (2000) Clinical outcome after structural failure of rotator cuff repairs. J Bone Joint Surg Am 82:304–314
58. Zumstein MA, Jost B, Hempel J, Hodler J, Gerber C (2008) The clinical and structural long-term results of open repair of massive tears of the rotator cuff. J Bone Joint Surg Am 90:2423–2431
59. Dodson CC, Kitay A, Verma NN, Adler RS, Nguyen J, Cordasco FA, Altchek DW (2010) The long-term outcome of recurrent defects after rotator cuff repair. Am J Sports Med 38:35–39
60. Miller BS, Downie BK, Kohen RB, Kijek T, Lesniak B, Jacobson JA, Hughes RE, Carpenter JE (2011) When do rotator cuff repairs fail? Serial ultrasound examination after arthroscopic repair of large and massive rotator cuff tears. Am J Sports Med 39:2064–2070
61. Sugaya H, Maeda K, Matsuki K, Moriishi J (2005) Functional and structural outcome after arthroscopic full-thickness rotator cuff repair: single-row versus dual-row fixation. Arthroscopy 21:1307–1316
62. Sugaya H, Maeda K, Matsuki K, Moriishi J (2007) Repair integrity and functional outcome after arthroscopic double-row rotator cuff repair. A prospective outcome study. J Bone Joint Surg Am 89:953–960
63. Charousset C, Grimberg J, Duranthon LD, Bellaiche L, Petrover D (2007) Can a double-row anchorage technique improve tendon healing in arthroscopic rotator cuff repair?: A prospective, nonrandomized, comparative study of double-row and single-row anchorage techniques with computed tomographic arthrography tendon healing assessment. Am J Sports Med 35:1247–1253

64. Charousset C, Bellaïche L, Kalra K, Petrover D (2010) Arthroscopic repair of full-thickness rotator cuff tears: is there tendon healing in patients aged 65 years or older? Arthroscopy 26:302–309
65. Rodeo SA, Potter HG, Kawamura S, Turner AS, Kim HJ, Atkinson BL (2007) Biologic augmentation of rotator cuff tendon-healing with use of a mixture of osteoinductive growth factors. J Bone Joint Surg Am 89:2485–2497
66. Galatz L, Rothermich S, VanderPloeg K, Petersen B, Sandell L, Thomopoulos S (2007) Development of the supraspinatus tendon-to-bone insertion: localized expression of extracellular matrix and growth factor genes. J Orthop Res 25:1621–1628
67. Lee JY, Zhou Z, Taub PJ, Ramcharan M, Li Y, Akinbiyi T, Maharam ER, Leong DJ, Laudier DM, Ruike T, Torina PJ, Zaidi M, Majeska RJ, Schaffler MB, Flatow EL, Sun HB (2011) BMP-12 treatment of adult mesenchymal stem cells *in vitro* augments tendon-like tissue formation and defect repair *in vivo*. PLoS One 6:e17531
68. Wang Q-W, Chen Z-L, Piao Y-J (2005) Mesenchymal stem cells differentiate into tenocytes by bone morphogenetic protein (BMP) 12 gene transfer. J Biosci Bioeng 100:418–422
69. Kovacevic D, Rodeo SA (2008) Biological augmentation of rotator cuff tendon repair. Clin Orthop Relat Res 466:622–633
70. Wolfman NM, Hattersley G, Cox K, Celeste AJ, Nelson R, Yamaji N, Dube JL, DiBlasio-Smith E, Nove J, Song JJ, Wozney JM, Rosen V (1997) Ectopic induction of tendon and ligament in rats by growth and differentiation factors 5, 6, and 7, members of the TGF-beta gene family. J Clin Invest 100:321–330
71. Seeherman HJ, Archambault JM, Rodeo SA, Turner AS, Zekas L, D'Augusta D, Li XJ, Smith E, Wozney JM (2008) rhBMP-12 accelerates healing of rotator cuff repairs in a sheep model. J Bone Joint Surg Am 90:2206–2219
72. Ide J, Kikukawa K, Hirose J, Iyama K-I, Sakamoto H, Fujimoto T, Mizuta H (2009) The effect of a local application of fibroblast growth factor-2 on tendon-to-bone remodeling in rats with acute injury and repair of the supraspinatus tendon. J Shoulder Elbow Surg 18:391–398
73. Manning CN, Kim HM, Sakiyama-Elbert S, Galatz LM, Havlioglu N, Thomopoulos S (2011) Sustained delivery of transforming growth factor beta three enhances tendon-to-bone healing in a rat model. J Orthop Res 29:1099–1105
74. Kovacevic D, Fox AJ, Bedi A, Ying L, Deng X-H, Warren RF, Rodeo SA (2011) Calcium-phosphate matrix with or without TGF-β3 improves tendon-bone healing after rotator cuff repair. Am J Sports Med 39:811–819
75. Bedi A, Fox AJS, Kovacevic D, Deng X-H, Warren RF, Rodeo SA (2010) Doxycycline-mediated inhibition of matrix metalloproteinases improves healing after rotator cuff repair. Am J Sports Med 38:308–317
76. Bedi A, Kovacevic D, Hettrich C, Gulotta LV, Ehteshami JR, Warren RF, Rodeo SA (2010) The effect of matrix metalloproteinase inhibition on tendon-to-bone healing in a rotator cuff repair model. J Shoulder Elbow Surg 19:384–391
77. Encalada-Diaz I, Cole BJ, Macgillivray JD, Ruiz-Suarez M, Kercher JS, Friel NA, Valero-Gonzalez F (2011) Rotator cuff repair augmentation using a novel polycarbonate polyurethane patch: preliminary results at 12 months' follow-up. J Shoulder Elbow Surg 20:788–794
78. Li X, Xie J, Lipner J, Yuan X, Thomopoulos S, Xia Y (2009) Nanofiber scaffolds with gradations in mineral content for mimicking the tendon-to-bone insertion site. Nano Lett 9 (7):2763–2768
79. Moffat KL, Kwei AS-P, Spalazzi JP, Doty SB, Levine WN, Lu HH (2009) Novel nanofiber-based scaffold for rotator cuff repair and augmentation. Tissue Eng Part A 15:115–126
80. Gulotta LV, Kovacevic D, Ehteshami JR, Dagher E, Packer JD, Rodeo SA (2009) Application of bone marrow-derived mesenchymal stem cells in a rotator cuff repair model. Am J Sports Med 37:2126–2133
81. Gulotta LV, Kovacevic D, Packer JD, Ehteshami JR, Rodeo SA (2011) Adenoviral-mediated gene transfer of human bone morphogenetic protein-13 does not improve rotator cuff healing in a rat model. Am J Sports Med 39:180–187

82. Gulotta LV, Kovacevic D, Packer JD, Deng X-H, Rodeo SA (2011) Bone marrow-derived mesenchymal stem cells transduced with scleraxis improve rotator cuff healing in a rat model. Am J Sports Med 39:1282–1289
83. Coombes BK, Bisset L, Vicenzino B (2010) Efficacy and safety of corticosteroid injections and other injections for management of tendinopathy: a systematic review of randomised controlled trials. Lancet 376:1751–1767
84. de Jonge S, de Vos RJ, Weir A, van Schie HTM, Bierma-Zeinstra SMA, Verhaar JAN, Weinans H, Tol JL (2011) One-year follow-up of platelet-rich plasma treatment in chronic Achilles tendinopathy: a double-blind randomized placebo-controlled trial. Am J Sports Med 39:1623–1629
85. de Mos M, van der Windt AE, Jahr H, van Schie HTM, Weinans H, Verhaar JAN, van Osch GJVM (2008) Can platelet-rich plasma enhance tendon repair? A cell culture study. Am J Sports Med 36:1171–1178
86. Tohidnezhad M, Varoga D, Wruck CJ, Brandenburg LO, Seekamp A, Shakibaei M, Sönmez TT, Pufe T, Lippross S (2011) Platelet-released growth factors can accelerate tenocyte proliferation and activate the anti-oxidant response element. Histochem Cell Biol 135:453–460
87. Zhang J, Wang JH-C (2010) Platelet-rich plasma releasate promotes differentiation of tendon stem cells into active tenocytes. Am J Sports Med 38:2477–2486
88. Randelli PS, Arrigoni P, Cabitza P, Volpi P, Maffulli N (2008) Autologous platelet rich plasma for arthroscopic rotator cuff repair. A pilot study. Disabil Rehabil 30:1584–1589
89. Jo CH, Kim JE, Yoon KS, Lee JH, Kang SB, Lee JH, Han HS, Rhee SH, Shin S (2011) Does platelet-rich plasma accelerate recovery after rotator cuff repair? A prospective cohort study. Am J Sports Med 39:2082–2090
90. Randelli P, Arrigoni P, Ragone V, Aliprandi A, Cabitza P (2011) Platelet rich plasma in arthroscopic rotator cuff repair: a prospective RCT study, 2-year follow-up. J Shoulder Elbow Surg 20:518–528
91. Castricini R, Longo UG, De Benedetto M, Panfoli N, Pirani P, Zini R, Maffulli N, Denaro V (2011) Platelet-rich plasma augmentation for arthroscopic rotator cuff repair: a randomized controlled trial. Am J Sports Med 39:258–265
92. Bergeson AG, Tashjian RZ, Greis PE, Crim J, Stoddard GJ, Burks RT (2012) Effects of platelet-rich fibrin matrix on repair integrity of at-risk rotator cuff tears. Am J Sports Med 40 (2):286–293
93. Barber FA, Hrnack SA, Snyder SJ, Hapa O (2011) Rotator cuff repair healing influenced by platelet-rich plasma construct augmentation. Arthroscopy 27:1029–1035

Chapter 13
Soft Tissue-to-Bone Healing in Anterior Cruciate Ligament Reconstruction

John M. Solic and Scott A. Rodeo

13.1 Introduction

The anterior cruciate ligament (ACL) acts as the primary restraint to anterior translation of the tibia and is a secondary restraint to varus and valgus stress [1, 2]. It is estimated that 800,000 ACL tears occur annually in the USA, with the majority occurring in individuals 15–30 years of age; however, this number may rise if activity levels of middle aged patients increase. Nonoperative treatment of ACL ruptures in patients with high activity levels leads to high levels of functional knee instability, as well as meniscal and cartilage injuries [3–5]. The most common treatment for ACL tears in active patients is reconstruction with intra-articular grafts. ACL reconstruction is reliably able to improve knee stability and reduce the incidence of subsequent meniscus tears [6–9]. However graft failure remains a challenge in ACL reconstruction with failure rates ranging from 5 to 27% [7, 10, 11].

The ideal graft choice for ACL reconstruction remains controversial. The ideal graft should have structural properties similar to the native ACL and should allow secure early fixation, rapid biologic incorporation, and minimal donor site morbidity. Graft options include autograft and allograft donor tissue. Autograft options include the patellar, hamstring, and quadriceps tendons. Allograft options include patellar, hamstring, quadriceps, achilles, and anterior and posterior tibialis tendons. Selection of a graft is complex and includes factors such as patient age and activity level, comorbidities, history of previous surgery and graft harvest, and future demand.

J.M. Solic
Sports Medicine and Shoulder Center, Triangle Orthopaedic Associates, Durham, NC, USA
e-mail: SolicJ@hss.edu

S.A. Rodeo (✉)
Department of Orthopaedic Surgery, Sports Medicine and Shoulder Service, The Hospital for Special Surgery/Weill Cornell Medical College, 535 East 70th Street, New York, NY 10021, USA
e-mail: RodeoS@hss.edu

S. Thomopoulos et al. (eds.), *Structural Interfaces and Attachments in Biology*,
DOI 10.1007/978-1-4614-3317-0_13,

Regardless of graft choice, successful ACL reconstruction relies on incorporation of the graft into the bone tunnel. All graft choices except patellar tendon grafts require tendon-to-bone healing within one or both bone tunnels.

13.2 Biology of Normal Tendon-to-Bone Attachments

The attachment of tendon to bone represents a unique biologic and biomechanical challenge. There is a significant difference between the stiffness of the tendon and bone, which creates a high level of stress at their interface. In native tendon-to-bone attachments, this mismatch is dampened by the presence of a unique zone of transitional tissue at the enthesis. This transitional zone acts to transfer stress between tendon and bone by graduated change in the structure, composition, and mechanical properties [12].

Two types of entheses exist: direct and indirect insertions. Direct insertions (fibrocartilagenous entheses) have tendon fibers that pass directly into the cortex over a small surface area. The superficial fibers insert into the periosteum and deep fibers attach to bone at right angles or tangentially [13]. The microscopic structure of direct insertions consists of four zones with gradual transitions between each zone (Fig. 13.1). These zones include: tendon, uncalcified fibrocartilage, calcified

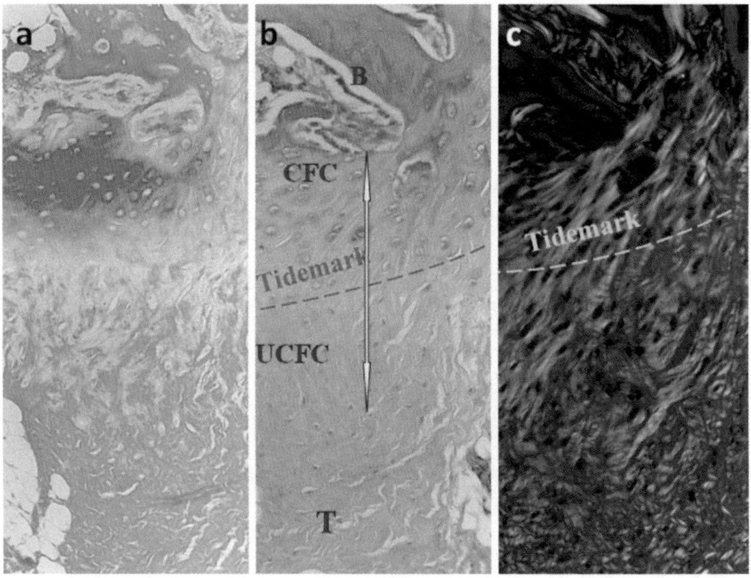

Fig. 13.1 Photomicrographs showing the (**a**) Safranin O staining, (**b**) Hematoxylin & Eosin staining, and (**c**) polarized microscopic image of the direct tendon-to-bone insertion. Note the gradual transition of the four zones at the direct tendon-to-bone insertion. Magnification ×20; *B* bone; *CFC* calcified fibrocartilage; *UCFC* uncalcified fibrocartilage; *T* tendon (reproduced, with permission, from ref. [13])

fibrocartilage, and bone. There is a tidemark representing the mineralization front between the calcified and uncalcified fibrocartilage zones. This gradual change in tissue composition and biomechanical properties is believed to allow more efficient load transfer between tendon and bone. Examples of direct insertions include: the ACL, achilles tendon, patellar tendon, rotator cuff, and femoral insertion of the medial collateral ligament (MCL).

Indirect insertions (fibrous entheses) include the tibial insertion of the MCL and the deltoid insertion on the humerus. There is no fibrocartilage transitional zone and the tendon fibers pass obliquely along the surface and insert over a broader area via Sharpey's fibers [13, 14]. In this way, the tendon collagen fibers become continuous with the underlying bone.

13.3 Tendon Graft-to-Bone Healing in ACL Reconstruction

Healing of a tendon graft in a bone tunnel following ACL reconstruction takes place in four phases: inflammatory phase, proliferative phase, matrix synthesis, and matrix remodeling (Fig. 13.2). The inflammatory phase begins shortly after graft implantation. There is recruitment of inflammatory cells and marrow-derived stem cells to the tendon graft interface as early as 4 days [15]. These inflammatory cells release cytokines and growth factors including transforming growth factor (TGF)-beta and platelet-derived growth factor (PDGF). These cytokines may contribute to the formation of a fibrous scar tissue interface between the bone and tendon graft [15]. There is also an ingrowth of blood vessels and nerves that may be due to growth factor stimulation or hypoxia [16, 17]. The graft is covered by a vascular synovial envelope by 6 weeks and the intrinsic vasculature matures gradually for at least 5–6 months [18].

The acute inflammatory phase is followed by a period of proliferation of the inflammatory and marrow-derived stromal cells. In the matrix synthesis phase, a provisional matrix consisting of type III collagen and some type I collagen is deposited. This is subsequently degraded by matrix metalloproteinases (MMPs) and serine proteases, and new matrix with progressive bony ingrowth is deposited. During matrix remodeling, the graft, interface tissue, and new bone remodel to create a collagen fiber attachment between the graft and host bone [19, 20].

In the normal uninjured ACL, the transition zone is a direct type insertion with a fibrocartilagenous interface. The nature of the healing attachment between the tendon graft and bone tunnel is debatable, with animal models demonstrating both direct and indirect types of insertions. Some animal studies have demonstrated chondrocytes present at the graft bone interface early in the healing process [21–24]. Other studies have demonstrated an indirect attachment with the presence of Sharpey's collagen fibers at the interface (Fig. 13.3) [25–28].

In a dog model, Rodeo et al. evaluated the progression of collagen fiber continuity between the graft and host bone [25]. At 2 weeks, the earliest time point of sectioning, there was evidence of a highly cellular, fibrous interface tissue between

Fig. 13.2 Schematic of basic phases of tendon graft-to-bone healing in animal models

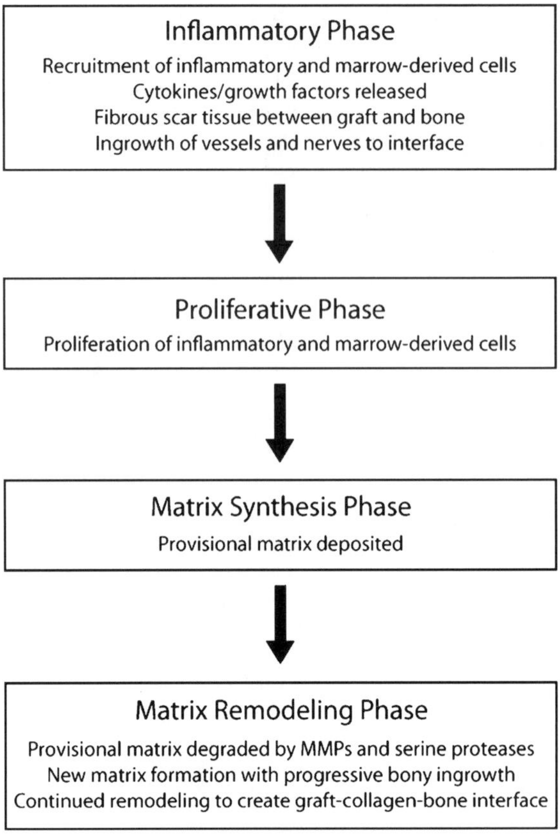
Inflammatory Phase
Recruitment of inflammatory and marrow-derived cells
Cytokines/growth factors released
Fibrous scar tissue between graft and bone
Ingrowth of vessels and nerves to interface
Proliferative Phase
Proliferation of inflammatory and marrow-derived cells
Matrix Synthesis Phase
Provisional matrix deposited
Matrix Remodeling Phase
Provisional matrix degraded by MMPs and serine proteases
New matrix formation with progressive bony ingrowth
Continued remodeling to create graft-collagen-bone interface

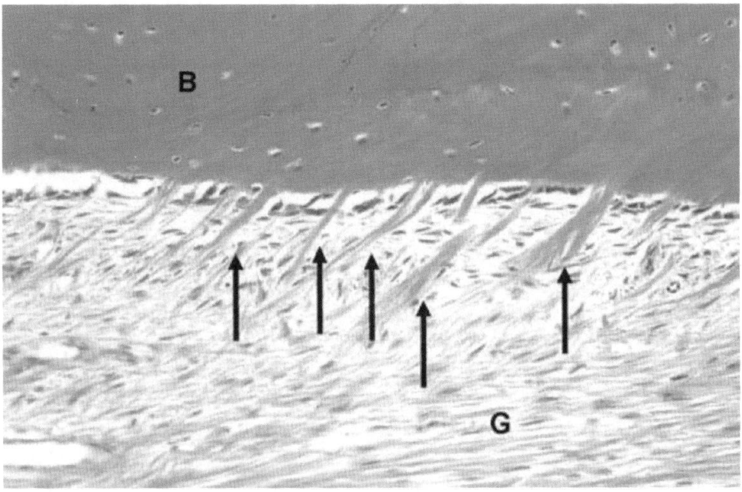

Fig. 13.3 Histological section of bone-graft interface. Present were the Sharpey's-like fibers (*arrows*) anchoring the soft tissue graft (G) to the bone tunnel (B) after 12 weeks of healing in a goat model. The presence of these fibers correlates with the interface strength (Hematoxylin & Eosin stain ×20) (reproduced, with permission, from ref. [31])

the tendon and bone along the length of the bone tunnel. The authors noted progressive maturation of this interface over time. By 12 weeks, Sharpey's fibers were clearly present at the interface. At the 2, 4, and 8-week time points, the specimens failed by pullout of the tendon from the bone tunnel. However, at 12 and 26 weeks, all specimens failed by pullout of the tendon from the loading apparatus or midsubstance rupture. This progressive strength was accompanied by increasing amounts of bone ingrowth and mineralization. Other animal studies have also demonstrated that the mechanical strength of the tendon-to-bone interface can be correlated to the degree of bony ingrowth, mineralization, and maturation of the provisional tissue [29, 30].

The degree of healing and Sharpey's fiber presence between the graft and host bone is not uniform circumferentially along the length of the tunnels [13, 20, 24, 26, 32]. The reasons for this variation are not known, but it may be related to differences in the mechanical and biologic environments at different points along the graft. The graft, along its course, may see different degrees of micromotion as well as different morphologic types of bone with varying capacities to influence ingrowth into the graft. Both rabbit and rat models have demonstrated that healing within the tibial tunnel, as determined by histologic analysis, was inferior compared to the femoral tunnel [19, 33]. It has been suggested that this may be related to the observation that the femoral aspect of the graft is exposed along its length to cancellous bone, but the tibial tunnel has dense cancellous bone only at the segment closest to the articular portion of the graft. This postulation is supported by a study using a rabbit model that showed better healing when the graft was inserted into a cancellous bone tunnel vs. a marrow-filled space [34].

13.4 Factors Affecting Graft Healing in ACL Reconstruction

13.4.1 Graft Source

Allografts have become a viable option for ACL reconstruction and provide some potential advantages compared to autograft, including decreased surgical time and the elimination of donor site morbidity [35]. Shino et al. [36] showed in a dog model that there were no differences in revascularization, mesenchymal cell infiltration, and remodeling between deep frozen patellar tendon allograft and autograft. The mean maximal tensile strength was similar at 30 weeks. Nikolaou et al. also found no differences in the histology and revascularization of patellar tendon autografts and allografts in a dog model [37]. The ultimate load-to-failure and stiffness were similar between both graft types and reached 90% of control ligament strength by 36 weeks.

Several other studies have found significant differences in the biomechanical and histologic properties of allografts vs. autografts. In a goat model, comparing bone-tendon-bone autograft to deep frozen allograft, the autograft group had

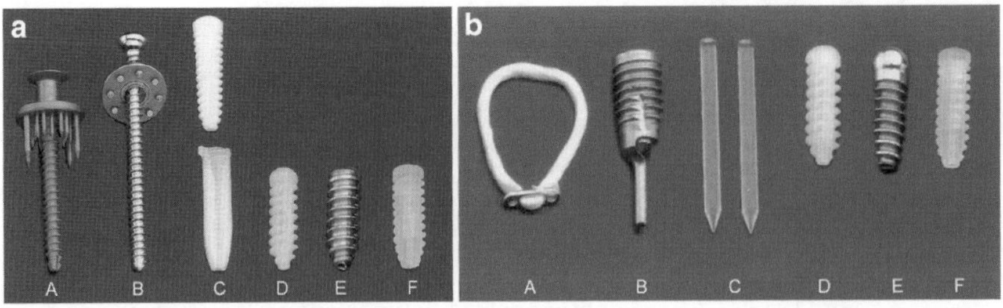

Fig. 13.4 *Left*: Tibial side soft tissue devices. A: WasherLoc, B: spiked washer, C: Intrafix, D: BioScrew, E: SoftSilk, F: SmartScrew. *Right*: Femoral side soft tissue fixation devices. A: EndoButton, B: Bone Mulch Screw, C: RigidFix, D: Bioscrew, E: RCI Screw, F: SmartScrew (*Left panel* reproduced, with permission, from ref. [46]. *Right panel* reproduced, with permission, from ref. [47].)

increased density and number of small diameter collagen fibrils. At 6 months, the autograft group also had higher ultimate load-to-failure and less anterior tibial translation [38]. In a dog model evaluating fresh soft tissue allograft and autograft at 6 months, the autograft group demonstrated a more organized four-layer insertion site compared to a less organized site in the allograft group [39].

Most of the studies using animal models to compare allograft vs. autograft use different processing and sterilization techniques, different graft tissues, and different methods of evaluating histologic and mechanical properties. This makes drawing comparisons between studies difficult.

13.4.2 Graft Fixation Techniques

Graft fixation is a critical aspect of ACL reconstruction. Biomechanical testing has shown that graft materials have higher initial strength than the native ACL [40–42]. However, multiple studies have shown that by 6 weeks after graft transplantation, the strength of the graft material is significantly decreased due to the intrinsic remodeling that takes place within the graft [43, 44]. Therefore, prior to "biologic fixation" by graft incorporation, the initial mechanical fixation must be secure enough to allow for early rehabilitation in the first 3 months, which can produce forces of 450–500 N [45].

There are several different fixation techniques that can be used for initial fixation of soft tissue grafts (Fig. 13.4). These devices can broadly be divided into suspensory (fixation achieved outside the tunnel) and intra-tunnel (fixation achieved within the bone tunnel). Multiple biomechanical studies have evaluated the initial strength of these various devices; however, direct comparisons are difficult due to the wide variation in fixation and testing methods in these studies.

Even less is known about the influence of these various fixation devices on the biologic incorporation of soft tissue grafts. In a sheep model, Weiler et al. evaluated graft-tunnel healing using an Achilles tendon autograft fixed with a biodegradable poly-(D, L-lactide) interference screw [22]. They found that at 6 weeks only a partial interstitial fibrous zone existed between the graft and bone tunnel. At 24 weeks, all specimens had a tunnel entrance site that resembled a normal appearing ligament attachment site with a bony bridge between the intra-tunnel graft and the insertion site. At 52 weeks, the insertion site showed the normal four zones associated with direct tendon-to-bone attachments.

Despite this encouraging result, in their biomechanical analysis the authors found that in the early postoperative period the mechanical properties of the graft were significantly decreased [48]. There was no graft pullout after 24 weeks, suggesting that long-term fixation was not compromised. Other authors have also found similar decreases in early load-to-failure of soft tissue grafts fixed with bio-absorbable interference screws and better early fixation strength with suspensory fixation [49, 50]. The clinical implications of these findings are not clear, as a recent meta-analysis suggested that fixation of hamstring grafts with interference screws on the femoral side may be associated with a lower rate of clinical failures [51]. However, there is a general tendency for many surgeons to recommend a less aggressive rehabilitation protocol and timeline with the use of soft tissue-only grafts.

13.4.3 Bone Tunnel Properties

Although not supported by strong basic science data, it is generally thought that increasing the amount of graft in the tunnel and making the fit as tight as possible increase the security of tunnel healing. In an extra-articular canine model, Greis et al. demonstrated a statistically significant increase in load-to-failure with an intraosseous graft length of 2 cm vs. 1 cm [52]. Additionally, a tighter fit of the graft in a 4.2 mm diameter tunnel also had a significantly higher load-to-failure compared to a 6 mm diameter tunnel.

Other studies have questioned the need for a snug ("line-to-line") graft fit and for maximizing intraosseous length. In an intra-articular canine model, a tunnel diameter difference of 2 mm on the tibial side did not influence ultimate load-to-failure [53]. Using the same model to evaluate the effect of intraosseous graft length, it was shown that with 5 mm of intraosseous graft vs. 15 mm there was no difference in histological and biomechanical parameters of graft healing at 6 weeks [54]. However, in an intra-articular goat model, reconstructions with 15 mm of intraosseous graft resulted in significantly more anterior translation at 6 weeks vs. those with 25 mm of intraosseous graft [55]. At 12 weeks, there were no significant differences with respect to anterior translation, in situ forces, stiffness, ultimate failure load, and ultimate stress.

13.4.4 Tunnel Position

The ideal position of tunnel placement is an important and highly debated topic in current ACL reconstruction. Despite no universal consensus on the optimal tunnel position or method of achieving it, tunnel misplacement is generally accepted to be one of the main causes of failure of ACL reconstruction [56–58]. Several biomechanical lab studies have shown that graft placement in a position closer to the anatomic footprint results in better initial biomechanical stability and knee kinematics [59–61]. There is also data that supports that separately reconstructing the two functional bundles of the ACL (anteromedial and posterolateral) better reproduces native knee kinematics and provides superior clinical results [62–68]. Much less is known about the effect of tunnel position and single vs. double bundle reconstruction on graft healing and incorporation.

In an extra-articular rabbit model, a soft tissue graft was placed perpendicular to the tibia to create an aperture with compressive forces on one side and tensile forces on the other side [69]. The tensile end showed more abundant Sharpey's fibers early and a direct type insertion with four zones after 6 months. On the compressive side, there was chondroid formation and woven bone at the tendon-bone interface. In an intra-articular goat model, Ekdahl et al. [70] evaluated the effects of two nonanatomic reconstructions and one anatomic reconstruction of one of the two bundles of the native ACL. The anatomic tunnel placement group had less tibial tunnel enlargement and fewer osteoclasts within both the tibial and femoral tunnels. There was also more vascularity, which has been previously shown to correlate with graft strength [71] on the femoral side. Biomechanically, the anatomic reconstruction group had less tibial translation and lower in situ forces than the nonanatomic tunnel groups.

13.4.5 Graft-Tunnel Motion and Rehabilitation

The effect of graft motion and subsequent mechanical loading during the healing process is a complex interaction that is not fully understood. In their normal state, ligaments and tendons show sensitivity to variable mechanical demands and tend to demonstrate an increase in tensile modulus in response to increasing loads. Stress deprivation has also been shown to be associated with a decline in mechanical properties [30, 72–75]. It is also well known that bone is sensitive to variable mechanical loads. Stress deprivation leads to decreased bone mineral density and resorption while increasing loads stimulate increased bone formation and improved mechanical properties [76–78].

It is less clearly known how mechanical loads affect tendon-to-bone healing in the setting of tendon repair and ligament reconstruction. In a canine flexor tendon model, Thomopoulos et al. found that muscle loading significantly improved biomechanical properties compared with unloaded repairs [75]. In contrast, the same group found that early exercise after rotator cuff repair in a rat model led to a diminished healing response compared to a group that was immobilized [74].

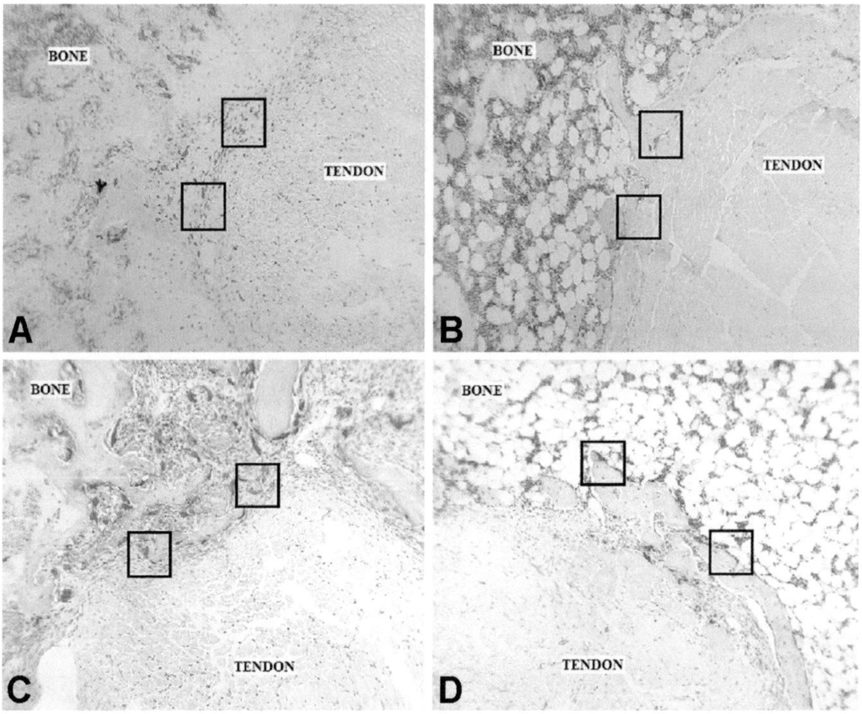

Fig. 13.5 Immunohistochemical staining for ED1+ macrophages on axial section of the tibial tunnel from animals subjected to (**a**) immediate loading and (**b**) delayed loading. The delayed-loading specimen demonstrates significantly reduced quantity of catabolic ED1+ macrophages. A similar finding of decreased number of osteoclasts, identified by tartrate-resistant acid phosphatase (TRAP) staining, is noted in the delayed loading specimen (**d**) vs. the immediate loading specimen (**c**) (adapted, with permission, from ref. [80])

Animal models of ACL reconstruction have also shown variable effects of early loading on graft healing. In a rabbit model, Sakai et al. showed that histologic graft incorporation and graft load-to-failure were improved in animals that were immobilized vs. a group that was allowed normal cage activity postoperatively [79]. Rodeo et al. showed an inverse relationship between graft motion in different locations of the bone tunnel and histologic markers of healing [32]. Using a rat model, Bedi et al. evaluated the effects of cyclical axial loading producing approximately 2% strain performed at various time points [80]. Animals were assigned to immobilization or loading immediately, on postoperative day 4, or on postoperative day 10. The delayed loading groups demonstrated improved mechanical and biologic healing parameters including increased load-to-failure, increased new bone formation inside the bone tunnel, higher levels of anabolic ED2+ macrophages and reduced tendon-bone interface fibrous tissue, catabolic ED1+ macrophages, and osteoclasts (Fig. 13.5). The authors hypothesized that the application of physiologic loads may be most effective if initiated after resolution of the acute inflammatory reaction to surgical trauma.

The significance and translation of these findings to clinical practice is yet to be determined. There is data to support that early aggressive rehabilitation protocols may contribute to tunnel enlargement and theoretically more stress at the tendon-bone interface [81, 82]. There is also good data supporting early motion, early weight bearing, and closed chain kinetic exercises in successful ACL rehabilitation protocols [83–87]. More studies are needed to understand how different postoperative rehabilitation protocols influence biologic healing and clinical outcomes.

13.5 Techniques for Improving Graft Healing

The slower and more variable rates of incorporation of tendon grafts used in ACL reconstruction have generated a strong interest in strategies to augment and improve the healing process. These include growth factors, biomaterial augmentation, biologic modulation, cell therapy, biophysical modalities, and gene therapy [13].

13.5.1 Growth Factors

Bone formation is critical for tendon graft-to-bone healing and the addition of growth factors has been shown to improve the graft healing process. In a sheep model, PDGF increased vascular density and collagen fibril number at 6 and 12 weeks and increased load-to-failure at 6 weeks [88]. In an intra-articular canine model, transforming growth factor-β1 (TGF-β1) improved the density of perpendicular collagen fibrils and load-to-failure vs. controls [89].

In a rabbit model, Anderson et al. used a type I collagen sponge carrier that contained a mixture of bovine bone-derived bone morphogenetic protein (BMP)-2, BMP-7, TGF-β1, TGF-β2, TGF-β1, and fibroblastic growth factor [90]. Compared to controls, the treatment group had significantly higher load-to-failure values and more extensive new bone and cartilage formation at the graft bone interface. Other growth factors including vascular endothelial growth factor (VEGF) [91] and granulocyte colony stimulating factor [92] have shown improved histological and biomechanical properties when introduced at the tendon-bone interface.

13.5.2 Biomaterials

Calcium phosphate has a chemical composition similar to bone and has been used as a bone void filler and osteoconductive material in the setting of fractures with bone loss. These properties make it an attractive option as an augment to the tendon-bone interface to encourage bone formation and inhibit fibrous tissue deposition. Various forms have been investigated in lab studies and show encouraging early results. These include integrating the calcium into the tendon graft [24], injectable tricalcium phosphate [93], hydroxyapatite (HA) cement [94], HA powder in collagen gel [95], and magnesium-based bone adhesive [96].

Another scaffold that has been studied extensively is the periosteum. Periosteum contains multipotent mesodermal cells, chondroprogenitor, and osteoprogenitor cells [97–100]. Periosteum-enveloped grafts have been shown to have improved histologic and biomechanical parameters [101]. There has been some clinical experience with periosteum graft augmentation. Robert and Es-Sayeh used a periosteal flap harvested from the superior and medial metaphysis of the tibia and wrapped it around the proximal aspect of the four-strand graft near the outlet of the femoral tunnel [102]. The augmented group demonstrated a significant reduction in enlargement of the articular side of the tunnel. In a prospective case series, Chen et al. reported good clinical results as measured by instrumented laxity, Lysholm, and International Knee Documentation Committee scores in 62 patients who were evaluated at 2 years after reconstruction with hamstring graft augmented with periosteum [103]. The same group published a larger series of 312 patients with a similar graft technique and good clinical objective and subjective outcomes at mean follow-up of 4.6 years [104]. It is important to note that none of these series had a control group of standard hamstring ACL reconstruction for comparison.

13.5.3 Cell and Gene Therapy

The concept of using periosteum as a natural source of delivering progenitor cells to the tendon-bone interface has been expanded to include the delivery of various cell types through many different mechanisms. Chen et al. used a hydrogel with photoencapsulated periosteal progenitor cells and BMP-2 to improve histologic healing, pullout strength, and stiffness in a rabbit ACL reconstruction model [105]. Others have used autologous mesenchymal stem cells [23, 106, 107], synovial mesenchymal stem cells [108], and bone marrow aspirates [109] to demonstrate improved graft-tunnel healing.

One of the limitations of direct delivery of growth factors and biomaterials is the inability to provide a sustained and prolonged exposure. This challenge may be able to be met with advancements in gene therapy. Martinek et al. used a tendon graft infected with adenovirus-BMP-2 gene to significantly improve histologic healing parameters as well as stiffness and ultimate load-to-failure [110]. Wang et al. demonstrated similar results using a plasmid cytomegalovirus BMP-2 delivery system in a rabbit model [111]. While promising, gene therapy techniques have additional safety and regulatory issues that add complexity to their transition into clinical practice.

13.5.4 Biologic Modulation

Opportunities exist for modulating several biologically active agents that have been shown to play a role in the healing process after ACL reconstruction. Following ACL injury [112] and reconstruction [113], the level of MMPs increases in the intra-articular environment. In a rabbit model, the use of an intra-articular injection of alpha-2-macroglobulin (a known MMP inhibitor) after ACL reconstruction was evaluated [27]. The control group demonstrated an increased concentration of intra-articular MMPs and less organized and vascular connective tissue at the bone-tendon interface. The treatment group had more mature interface tissue, more Sharpey's fibers between the graft and bone, and a significantly higher load-to-failure at both 2 and 5 weeks.

Given that healing of the graft within the tunnel is dependent on bone ingrowth, it is believed that excessive osteoclast activity within the tunnel may contribute to bone resorption, tunnel widening, and poor healing. Rodeo et al. evaluated the effects of osteoprotegerin (OPG), an inhibitor of osteoclast activity, and receptor activator of nuclear factor-kappa B ligand [114], an osteoclast activator in a rabbit ACL reconstruction model [115]. In the OPG-treated limbs, there were significantly fewer osteoclasts and significantly more bone at the tendon-bone interface when compared to controls and the receptor activator of nuclear factor-kappa B ligand (RANKL)-treated limbs. The OPG group also had a smaller average tunnel area and significantly increased stiffness compared to the RANKL group. Other techniques of biomodulation, including macrophage inhibition [116] and enhanced angiogenesis using hyperbaric oxygen [117], have shown promise in improving histologic and biomechanical parameters of graft healing.

13.5.5 Biophysical Modalities

Mechanical stimulation, electrical stimulation, pulsed electric magnetic fields, and ultrasound therapy have been applied in various clinical settings to augment soft tissue and fracture healing. Ultrasound therapy is a noninvasive mechanism of delivering mechanical energy transcutaneously. It has been shown to promote osteoblast proliferation and angiogenesis in the lab setting [118–120]. Clinically it has been shown to accelerate delayed fracture healing and soft tissue repair [121, 122]. In an ovine ACL model, Walsh et al. demonstrated that low-intensity pulsed ultrasound (LIPUS) could improve tendon osteointegration, vascularity, stiffness, and peak load [71]. Furthermore, other studies have shown similar promise in applying LIPUS to tendon-bone healing in animal models [123].

13.5.6 Effect of Mechanical Load

Further information about the effect of mechanical load on healing between soft tissue and bone may help identify methods to improve healing by modulating the postoperative mechanical environment. It is likely that specific types and magnitudes of mechanical loading, as well as specific timing, will affect healing. Moreover, it is possible that "biologic augmentation" modalities, such as cytokines and stem cells, will be affected by the concurrent mechanical environment. It is clear that there is a complex interaction between biology and biomechanics. For example, it may be found that exogenous agents to improve healing may be more effective if applied after early tendon-to-bone healing has occurred. Further investigations are required to expand our understanding of the complex interplay between biomechanical factors and the cellular and molecular events in soft tissue healing.

13.6 Conclusions

ACL reconstruction is a commonly performed procedure; given the demand of an increasingly active middle-age population, its prevalence is likely to increase. Essential to successful ACL reconstruction is biologic incorporation of the graft, regardless of the type of graft or source. Basic science and clinical data suggests that graft healing depends on many factors including but not limited to graft source, graft fixation technique, tunnel position and bone quality, and timing and magnitude of load applied during the rehabilitation period. The effects of changes in these variables, as well as their interactions, are the subjects of ongoing investigation. Recent data also suggest that modifying the graft healing process with growth factors and biologic augmentation will have a role in improving ACL reconstruction outcomes in the future.

References

1. Paulos L, Noyes FR, Grood E, Butler DL (1991) Knee rehabilitation after anterior cruciate ligament reconstruction and repair. J Orthop Sports Phys Ther 13(2):60–70
2. Markolf KL, Amstutz HC (1976) *In vitro* measurement of bone-acrylic interface pressure during femoral component insertion. Clin Orthop Relat Res 121:60–66
3. Schachter AK, Rokito AS (2007) ACL injuries in the skeletally immature patient. Orthopedics 30(5):365–370; quiz 362–371
4. Henry J, Chotel F, Chouteau J, Fessy MH, Berard J, Moyen B (2009) Rupture of the anterior cruciate ligament in children: early reconstruction with open physes or delayed reconstruction to skeletal maturity? Knee Surg Sports Traumatol Arthrosc 17(7):748–755
5. Jones HP, Appleyard RC, Mahajan S, Murrell GA (2003) Meniscal and chondral loss in the anterior cruciate ligament injured knee. Sports Med 33(14):1075–1089

6. Aglietti P, Giron F, Buzzi R, Biddau F, Sasso F (2004) Anterior cruciate ligament reconstruction: bone-patellar tendon-bone compared with double semitendinosus and gracilis tendon grafts. A prospective, randomized clinical trial. J Bone Joint Surg Am 86-A (10):2143–2155
7. Fithian DC, Paxton EW, Stone ML, Luetzow WF, Csintalan RP, Phelan D, Daniel DM (2005) Prospective trial of a treatment algorithm for the management of the anterior cruciate ligament-injured knee. Am J Sports Med 33(3):335–346
8. Spindler KP, Warren TA, Callison JC Jr, Secic M, Fleisch SB, Wright RW (2005) Clinical outcome at a minimum of five years after reconstruction of the anterior cruciate ligament. J Bone Joint Surg Am 87(8):1673–1679
9. Roe J, Pinczewski LA, Russell VJ, Salmon LJ, Kawamata T, Chew M (2005) A 7-year follow-up of patellar tendon and hamstring tendon grafts for arthroscopic anterior cruciate ligament reconstruction: differences and similarities. Am J Sports Med 33(9):1337–1345
10. Freedman KB, D'Amato MJ, Nedeff DD, Kaz A, Bach BR Jr (2003) Arthroscopic anterior cruciate ligament reconstruction: a metaanalysis comparing patellar tendon and hamstring tendon autografts. Am J Sports Med 31(1):2–11
11. Yunes M, Richmond JC, Engels EA, Pinczewski LA (2001) Patellar versus hamstring tendons in anterior cruciate ligament reconstruction: a meta-analysis. Arthroscopy 17(3):248–257
12. Benjamin M, Ralphs JR (1998) Fibrocartilage in tendons and ligaments—an adaptation to compressive load. J Anat 193(pt 4):481–494
13. Lui P, Zhang P, Chan K, Qin L (2010) Biology and augmentation of tendon-bone insertion repair. J Orthop Surg Res 5:59
14. Petersen W, Laprell H (2000) Insertion of autologous tendon grafts to the bone: a histological and immunohistochemical study of hamstring and patellar tendon grafts. Knee Surg Sports Traumatol Arthrosc 8(1):26–31
15. Kawamura S, Ying L, Kim HJ, Dynybil C, Rodeo SA (2005) Macrophages accumulate in the early phase of tendon-bone healing. J Orthop Res 23(6):1425–1432
16. Haus J, Refior HJ (1987) A study of the synovial and ligamentous structure of the anterior cruciate ligament. Int Orthop 11(2):117–124
17. Aune AK, Hukkanen M, Madsen JE, Polak JM, Nordsletten L (1996) Nerve regeneration during patellar tendon autograft remodelling after anterior cruciate ligament reconstruction: an experimental and clinical study. J Orthop Res 14(2):193–199
18. Arnoczky SP, Tarvin GB, Marshall JL (1982) Anterior cruciate ligament replacement using patellar tendon. An evaluation of graft revascularization in the dog. J Bone Joint Surg Am 64 (2):217–224
19. Wen CY, Qin L, Lee KM, Wong MW, Chan KM (2010) Grafted tendon healing in tibial tunnel is inferior to healing in femoral tunnel after anterior cruciate ligament reconstruction: a histomorphometric study in rabbits. Arthroscopy 26(1):58–66
20. Deehan DJ, Cawston TE (2005) The biology of integration of the anterior cruciate ligament. J Bone Joint Surg Br 87(7):889–895
21. Panni AS, Milano G, Lucania L, Fabbriciani C (1997) Graft healing after anterior cruciate ligament reconstruction in rabbits. Clin Orthop Relat Res 343:203–212
22. Weiler A, Hoffmann RF, Bail HJ, Rehm O, Sudkamp NP (2002) Tendon healing in a bone tunnel. Part II: histologic analysis after biodegradable interference fit fixation in a model of anterior cruciate ligament reconstruction in sheep. Arthroscopy 18(2):124–135
23. Lim JK, Hui J, Li L, Thambyah A, Goh J, Lee EH (2004) Enhancement of tendon graft osteointegration using mesenchymal stem cells in a rabbit model of anterior cruciate ligament reconstruction. Arthroscopy 20(9):899–910
24. Mutsuzaki H, Sakane M, Nakajima H, Ito A, Hattori S, Miyanaga Y, Ochiai N, Tanaka J (2004) Calcium-phosphate-hybridized tendon directly promotes regeneration of tendon-bone insertion. J Biomed Mater Res A 70(2):319–327

25. Rodeo SA, Arnoczky SP, Torzilli PA, Hidaka C, Warren RF (1993) Tendon-healing in a bone tunnel. A biomechanical and histological study in the dog. J Bone Joint Surg Am 75(12):1795–1803
26. Grana WA, Egle DM, Mahnken R, Goodhart CW (1994) An analysis of autograft fixation after anterior cruciate ligament reconstruction in a rabbit model. Am J Sports Med 22(3):344–351
27. Demirag B, Sarisozen B, Ozer O, Kaplan T, Ozturk C (2005) Enhancement of tendon-bone healing of anterior cruciate ligament grafts by blockage of matrix metalloproteinases. J Bone Joint Surg Am 87(11):2401–2410
28. Blickenstaff KR, Grana WA, Egle D (1997) Analysis of a semitendinosus autograft in a rabbit model. Am J Sports Med 25(4):554–559
29. Wen CY, Qin L, Lee KM, Chan KM (2009) Peri-graft bone mass and connectivity as predictors for the strength of tendon-to-bone attachment after anterior cruciate ligament reconstruction. Bone 45(3):545–552
30. Hannafin JA, Arnoczky SP, Hoonjan A, Torzilli PA (1995) Effect of stress deprivation and cyclic tensile loading on the material and morphologic properties of canine flexor digitorum profundus tendon: an *in vitro* study. J Orthop Res 13(6):907–914
31. Ekdahl M, Wang JH, Ronga M, Fu FH (2008) Graft healing in anterior cruciate ligament reconstruction. Knee Surg Sports Traumatol Arthrosc 16(10):935–947
32. Rodeo SA, Kawamura S, Kim HJ, Dynybil C, Ying L (2006) Tendon healing in a bone tunnel differs at the tunnel entrance versus the tunnel exit: an effect of graft-tunnel motion? Am J Sports Med 34(11):1790–1800
33. Lui PP, Ho G, Shum WT, Lee YW, Ho PY, Lo WN, Lo CK (2010) Inferior tendon graft to bone tunnel healing at the tibia compared to that at the femur after anterior cruciate ligament reconstruction. J Orthop Sci 15(3):389–401
34. Grassman SR, McDonald DB, Thornton GM, Shrive NG, Frank CB (2002) Early healing processes of free tendon grafts within bone tunnels is bone-specific: a morphological study in a rabbit model. Knee 9(1):21–26
35. West RV, Harner CD (2005) Graft selection in anterior cruciate ligament reconstruction. J Am Acad Orthop Surg 13(3):197–207
36. Shino K, Kawasaki T, Hirose H, Gotoh I, Inoue M, Ono K (1984) Replacement of the anterior cruciate ligament by an allogeneic tendon graft. An experimental study in the dog. J Bone Joint Surg Br 66(5):672–681
37. Nikolaou PK, Seaber AV, Glisson RR, Ribbeck BM, Bassett FH III (1986) Anterior cruciate ligament allograft transplantation. Long-term function, histology, revascularization, and operative technique. Am J Sports Med 14(5):348–360
38. Jackson DW, Grood ES, Goldstein JD, Rosen MA, Kurzweil PR, Cummings JF, Simon TM (1993) A comparison of patellar tendon autograft and allograft used for anterior cruciate ligament reconstruction in the goat model. Am J Sports Med 21(2):176–185
39. Zhang CL, Fan HB, Xu H, Li QH, Guo L (2006) Histological comparison of fate of ligamentous insertion after reconstruction of anterior cruciate ligament: autograft vs allograft. Chin J Traumatol 9(2):72–76
40. Cooper DE, Small J, Urrea L (1998) Factors affecting graft excursion patterns in endoscopic anterior cruciate ligament reconstruction. Knee Surg Sports Traumatol Arthrosc 6(suppl 1): S20–S24
41. Noyes FR, Butler DL, Grood ES, Zernicke RF, Hefzy MS (1984) Biomechanical analysis of human ligament grafts used in knee-ligament repairs and reconstructions. J Bone Joint Surg Am 66(3):344–352
42. Woo SL, Hollis JM, Adams DJ, Lyon RM, Takai S (1991) Tensile properties of the human femur-anterior cruciate ligament-tibia complex. The effects of specimen age and orientation. Am J Sports Med 19(3):217–225
43. Butler DL (1989) Kappa Delta Award paper. Anterior cruciate ligament: its normal response and replacement. J Orthop Res 7(6):910–921

44. Papageorgiou CD, Ma CB, Abramowitch SD, Clineff TD, Woo SL (2001) A multidisciplinary study of the healing of an intraarticular anterior cruciate ligament graft in a goat model. Am J Sports Med 29(5):620–626
45. Frank CB, Jackson DW (1997) The science of reconstruction of the anterior cruciate ligament. J Bone Joint Surg Am 79(10):1556–1576
46. Kousa P, Jarvinen TL, Vihavainen M, Kannus P, Jarvinen M (2003) The fixation strength of six hamstring tendon graft fixation devices in anterior cruciate ligament reconstruction. Part II: tibial site. Am J Sports Med 31(2):182–188
47. Kousa P, Jarvinen TL, Vihavainen M, Kannus P, Jarvinen M (2003) The fixation strength of six hamstring tendon graft fixation devices in anterior cruciate ligament reconstruction. Part I: femoral site. Am J Sports Med 31(2):174–181
48. Weiler A, Peine R, Pashmineh-Azar A, Abel C, Sudkamp NP, Hoffmann RF (2002) Tendon healing in a bone tunnel. Part I: biomechanical results after biodegradable interference fit fixation in a model of anterior cruciate ligament reconstruction in sheep. Arthroscopy 18 (2):113–123
49. Singhatat W, Lawhorn KW, Howell SM, Hull ML (2002) How four weeks of implantation affect the strength and stiffness of a tendon graft in a bone tunnel: a study of two fixation devices in an extraarticular model in ovine. Am J Sports Med 30(4):506–513
50. Zantop T, Weimann A, Wolle K, Musahl V, Langer M, Petersen W (2007) Initial and 6 weeks postoperative structural properties of soft tissue anterior cruciate ligament reconstructions with cross-pin or interference screw fixation: an *in vivo* study in sheep. Arthroscopy 23 (1):14–20
51. Colvin A, Sharma C, Parides M, Glashow J (2011) What is the best femoral fixation of hamstring autografts in anterior cruciate ligament reconstruction?: A meta-analysis. Clin Orthop Relat Res 469(4):1075–1081
52. Greis PE, Burks RT, Bachus K, Luker MG (2001) The influence of tendon length and fit on the strength of a tendon-bone tunnel complex. A biomechanical and histologic study in the dog. Am J Sports Med 29(4):493–497
53. Yamazaki S, Yasuda K, Tomita F, Minami A, Tohyama H (2002) The effect of graft-tunnel diameter disparity on intraosseous healing of the flexor tendon graft in anterior cruciate ligament reconstruction. Am J Sports Med 30(4):498–505
54. Yamazaki S, Yasuda K, Tomita F, Minami A, Tohyama H (2006) The effect of intraosseous graft length on tendon-bone healing in anterior cruciate ligament reconstruction using flexor tendon. Knee Surg Sports Traumatol Arthrosc 14(11):1086–1093
55. Zantop T, Ferretti M, Bell KM, Brucker PU, Gilbertson L, Fu FH (2008) Effect of tunnel-graft length on the biomechanics of anterior cruciate ligament-reconstructed knees: intra-articular study in a goat model. Am J Sports Med 36(11):2158–2166
56. Johnson DL, Swenson TM, Irrgang JJ, Fu FH, Harner CD (1996) Revision anterior cruciate ligament surgery: experience from Pittsburgh. Clin Orthop Relat Res 325:100–109
57. Corsetti JR, Jackson DW (1996) Failure of anterior cruciate ligament reconstruction: the biologic basis. Clin Orthop Relat Res 325:42–49
58. Goradia VK, Rochat MC, Kida M, Grana WA (2000) Natural history of a hamstring tendon autograft used for anterior cruciate ligament reconstruction in a sheep model. Am J Sports Med 28(1):40–46
59. Loh JC, Fukuda Y, Tsuda E, Steadman RJ, Fu FH, Woo SL (2003) Knee stability and graft function following anterior cruciate ligament reconstruction: comparison between 11 o'clock and 10 o'clock femoral tunnel placement. 2002 Richard O'Connor Award paper. Arthroscopy 19(3):297–304
60. Musahl V, Plakseychuk A, VanScyoc A, Sasaki T, Debski RE, McMahon PJ, Fu FH (2005) Varying femoral tunnels between the anatomical footprint and isometric positions: effect on kinematics of the anterior cruciate ligament-reconstructed knee. Am J Sports Med 33 (5):712–718

61. Zavras TD, Race A, Amis AA (2005) The effect of femoral attachment location on anterior cruciate ligament reconstruction: graft tension patterns and restoration of normal anterior-posterior laxity patterns. Knee Surg Sports Traumatol Arthrosc 13(2):92–100
62. Adachi N, Ochi M, Uchio Y, Iwasa J, Kuriwaka M, Ito Y (2004) Reconstruction of the anterior cruciate ligament. Single- versus double-bundle multistranded hamstring tendons. J Bone Joint Surg Br 86(4):515–520
63. Buoncristiani AM, Tjoumakaris FP, Starman JS, Ferretti M, Fu FH (2006) Anatomic double-bundle anterior cruciate ligament reconstruction. Arthroscopy 22(9):1000–1006
64. Colombet P, Robinson J, Jambou S, Allard M, Bousquet V, de Lavigne C (2006) Two-bundle, four-tunnel anterior cruciate ligament reconstruction. Knee Surg Sports Traumatol Arthrosc 14(7):629–636
65. Cha PS, Brucker PU, West RV, Zelle BA, Yagi M, Kurosaka M, Fu FH (2005) Arthroscopic double-bundle anterior cruciate ligament reconstruction: an anatomic approach. Arthroscopy 21(10):1275
66. Muneta T, Sekiya I, Yagishita K, Ogiuchi T, Yamamoto H, Shinomiya K (1999) Two-bundle reconstruction of the anterior cruciate ligament using semitendinosus tendon with endobuttons: operative technique and preliminary results. Arthroscopy 15(6):618–624
67. Muneta T, Koga H, Mochizuki T, Ju YJ, Hara K, Nimura A, Yagishita K, Sekiya I (2007) A prospective randomized study of 4-strand semitendinosus tendon anterior cruciate ligament reconstruction comparing single-bundle and double-bundle techniques. Arthroscopy 23 (6):618–628
68. Yasuda K, Kondo E, Ichiyama H, Kitamura N, Tanabe Y, Tohyama H, Minami A (2004) Anatomic reconstruction of the anteromedial and posterolateral bundles of the anterior cruciate ligament using hamstring tendon grafts. Arthroscopy 20(10):1015–1025
69. Yamakado K, Kitaoka K, Yamada H, Hashiba K, Nakamura R, Tomita K (2002) The influence of mechanical stress on graft healing in a bone tunnel. Arthroscopy 18(1):82–90
70. Ekdahl M, Nozaki M, Ferretti M, Tsai A, Smolinski P, Fu FH (2009) The effect of tunnel placement on bone-tendon healing in anterior cruciate ligament reconstruction in a goat model. Am J Sports Med 37(8):1522–1530
71. Walsh WR, Stephens P, Vizesi F, Bruce W, Huckle J, Yu Y (2007) Effects of low-intensity pulsed ultrasound on tendon-bone healing in an intra-articular sheep knee model. Arthroscopy 23(2):197–204
72. Woo SL, Gomez MA, Sites TJ, Newton PO, Orlando CA, Akeson WH (1987) The biomechanical and morphological changes in the medial collateral ligament of the rabbit after immobilization and remobilization. J Bone Joint Surg Am 69(8):1200–1211
73. Gelberman RH, Woo SL, Lothringer K, Akeson WH, Amiel D (1982) Effects of early intermittent passive mobilization on healing canine flexor tendons. J Hand Surg Am 7 (2):170–175
74. Thomopoulos S, Williams GR, Soslowsky LJ (2003) Tendon to bone healing: differences in biomechanical, structural, and compositional properties due to a range of activity levels. J Biomech Eng 125(1):106–113
75. Thomopoulos S, Zampiakis E, Das R, Silva MJ, Gelberman RH (2008) The effect of muscle loading on flexor tendon-to-bone healing in a canine model. J Orthop Res 26(12):1611–1617
76. Woo SL, Kuei SC, Amiel D, Gomez MA, Hayes WC, White FC, Akeson WH (1981) The effect of prolonged physical training on the properties of long bone: a study of Wolff's Law. J Bone Joint Surg Am 63(5):780–787
77. Jones HH, Priest JD, Hayes WC, Tichenor CC, Nagel DA (1977) Humeral hypertrophy in response to exercise. J Bone Joint Surg Am 59(2):204–208
78. Burstein AH, Currey JD, Frankel VH, Reilly DT (1972) The ultimate properties of bone tissue: the effects of yielding. J Biomech 5(1):35–44
79. Sakai H, Fukui N, Kawakami A, Kurosawa H (2000) Biological fixation of the graft within bone after anterior cruciate ligament reconstruction in rabbits: effects of the duration of postoperative immobilization. J Orthop Sci 5(1):43–51

80. Bedi A, Kovacevic D, Fox AJ, Imhauser CW, Stasiak M, Packer J, Brophy RH, Deng XH, Rodeo SA (2010) Effect of early and delayed mechanical loading on tendon-to-bone healing after anterior cruciate ligament reconstruction. J Bone Joint Surg Am 92(14):2387–2401
81. Wilson TC, Kantaras A, Atay A, Johnson DL (2004) Tunnel enlargement after anterior cruciate ligament surgery. Am J Sports Med 32(2):543–549
82. Hoher J, Moller HD, Fu FH (1998) Bone tunnel enlargement after anterior cruciate ligament reconstruction: fact or fiction? Knee Surg Sports Traumatol Arthrosc 6(4):231–240
83. Beynnon BD, Fleming BC, Johnson RJ, Nichols CE, Renstrom PA, Pope MH (1995) Anterior cruciate ligament strain behavior during rehabilitation exercises *in vivo*. Am J Sports Med 23 (1):24–34
84. Beynnon BD, Johnson RJ, Fleming BC (2002) The science of anterior cruciate ligament rehabilitation. Clin Orthop Relat Res 402:9–20
85. Beynnon BD, Johnson RJ, Fleming BC, Stankewich CJ, Renstrom PA, Nichols CE (1997) The strain behavior of the anterior cruciate ligament during squatting and active flexion-extension. A comparison of an open and a closed kinetic chain exercise. Am J Sports Med 25 (6):823–829
86. Noyes FR, Mangine RE, Barber S (1987) Early knee motion after open and arthroscopic anterior cruciate ligament reconstruction. Am J Sports Med 15(2):149–160
87. Tyler TF, McHugh MP, Gleim GW, Nicholas SJ (1998) The effect of immediate weightbearing after anterior cruciate ligament reconstruction. Clin Orthop Relat Res 357:141–148
88. Weiler A, Forster C, Hunt P, Falk R, Jung T, Unterhauser FN, Bergmann V, Schmidmaier G, Haas NP (2004) The influence of locally applied platelet-derived growth factor-BB on free tendon graft remodeling after anterior cruciate ligament reconstruction. Am J Sports Med 32 (4):881–891
89. Yamazaki S, Yasuda K, Tomita F, Tohyama H, Minami A (2005) The effect of transforming growth factor-beta1 on intraosseous healing of flexor tendon autograft replacement of anterior cruciate ligament in dogs. Arthroscopy 21(9):1034–1041
90. Anderson K, Seneviratne AM, Izawa K, Atkinson BL, Potter HG, Rodeo SA (2001) Augmentation of tendon healing in an intraarticular bone tunnel with use of a bone growth factor. Am J Sports Med 29(6):689–698
91. Yoshikawa T, Tohyama H, Katsura T, Kondo E, Kotani Y, Matsumoto H, Toyama Y, Yasuda K (2006) Effects of local administration of vascular endothelial growth factor on mechanical characteristics of the semitendinosus tendon graft after anterior cruciate ligament reconstruction in sheep. Am J Sports Med 34(12):1918–1925
92. Sasaki K, Kuroda R, Ishida K, Kubo S, Matsumoto T, Mifune Y, Kinoshita K, Tei K, Akisue T, Tabata Y, Kurosaka M (2008) Enhancement of tendon-bone osteointegration of anterior cruciate ligament graft using granulocyte colony-stimulating factor. Am J Sports Med 36 (8):1519–1527
93. Huangfu X, Zhao J (2007) Tendon-bone healing enhancement using injectable tricalcium phosphate in a dog anterior cruciate ligament reconstruction model. Arthroscopy 23 (5):455–462
94. Tien YC, Chih TT, Lin JH, Ju CP, Lin SD (2004) Augmentation of tendon-bone healing by the use of calcium-phosphate cement. J Bone Joint Surg Br 86(7):1072–1076
95. Ishikawa H, Koshino T, Takeuchi R, Saito T (2001) Effects of collagen gel mixed with hydroxyapatite powder on interface between newly formed bone and grafted achilles tendon in rabbit femoral bone tunnel. Biomaterials 22(12):1689–1694
96. Gulotta LV, Kovacevic D, Ying L, Ehteshami JR, Montgomery S, Rodeo SA (2008) Augmentation of tendon-to-bone healing with a magnesium-based bone adhesive. Am J Sports Med 36 (7):1290–1297
97. Breitbart AS, Grande DA, Kessler R, Ryaby JT, Fitzsimmons RJ, Grant RT (1998) Tissue engineered bone repair of calvarial defects using cultured periosteal cells. Plast Reconstr Surg 101(3):567–574; discussion 566–575

98. Ritsila V, Alhopuro S, Gylling U, Rintala A (1972) The use of free periosteum for bone formation in congenital clefts of the maxilla. A preliminary report. Scand J Plast Reconstr Surg 6(1):57–60
99. Rubak JM (1983) Osteochondrogenesis of free periosteal grafts in the rabbit iliac crest. Acta Orthop Scand 54(6):826–831
100. Liu SH, Wei FC, Zhang D, Sun SZ, Zhao HQ, Li GJ (2006) [Experimental study of mandibular periosteal distraction in rabbits]. Hua Xi Kou Qiang Yi Xue Za Zhi 24 (3):273–275
101. Chen CH, Chen WJ, Shih CH, Yang CY, Liu SJ, Lin PY (2003) Enveloping the tendon graft with periosteum to enhance tendon-bone healing in a bone tunnel: a biomechanical and histologic study in rabbits. Arthroscopy 19(3):290–296
102. Robert H, Es-Sayeh J (2004) The role of periosteal flap in the prevention of femoral widening in anterior cruciate ligament reconstruction using hamstring tendons. Knee Surg Sports Traumatol Arthrosc 12(1):30–35
103. Chen CH, Chen WJ, Shih CH, Chou SW (2004) Arthroscopic anterior cruciate ligament reconstruction with periosteum-enveloping hamstring tendon graft. Knee Surg Sports Traumatol Arthrosc 12(5):398–405
104. Chen CH, Chang CH, Su CI, Wang KC, Liu HT, Yu CM, Wong CB, Wang IC (2010) Arthroscopic single-bundle anterior cruciate ligament reconstruction with periosteum-enveloping hamstring tendon graft: clinical outcome at 2 to 7 years. Arthroscopy 26 (7):907–917
105. Chen CH, Liu HW, Tsai CL, Yu CM, Lin IH, Hsiue GH (2008) Photoencapsulation of bone morphogenetic protein-2 and periosteal progenitor cells improve tendon graft healing in a bone tunnel. Am J Sports Med 36(3):461–473
106. Ge Z, Goh JC, Lee EH (2005) The effects of bone marrow-derived mesenchymal stem cells and fascia wrap application to anterior cruciate ligament tissue engineering. Cell Transplant 14(10):763–773
107. Soon MY, Hassan A, Hui JH, Goh JC, Lee EH (2007) An analysis of soft tissue allograft anterior cruciate ligament reconstruction in a rabbit model: a short-term study of the use of mesenchymal stem cells to enhance tendon osteointegration. Am J Sports Med 35 (6):962–971
108. Ju YJ, Muneta T, Yoshimura H, Koga H, Sekiya I (2008) Synovial mesenchymal stem cells accelerate early remodeling of tendon-bone healing. Cell Tissue Res 332(3):469–478
109. Karaoglu S, Celik C, Korkusuz P (2009) The effects of bone marrow or periosteum on tendon-to-bone tunnel healing in a rabbit model. Knee Surg Sports Traumatol Arthrosc 17 (2):170–178
110. Martinek V, Latterman C, Usas A, Abramowitch S, Woo SL, Fu FH, Huard J (2002) Enhancement of tendon-bone integration of anterior cruciate ligament grafts with bone morphogenetic protein-2 gene transfer: a histological and biomechanical study. J Bone Joint Surg Am 84-A(7):1123–1131
111. Wang CJ, Weng LH, Hsu SL, Sun YC, Yang YJ, Chan YS, Yang YL (2010) pCMV-BMP-2-transfected cell-mediated gene therapy in anterior cruciate ligament reconstruction in rabbits. Arthroscopy 26(7):968–976
112. Amiel D, Ishizue KK, Harwood FL, Kitabayashi L, Akeson WH (1989) Injury of the anterior cruciate ligament: the role of collagenase in ligament degeneration. J Orthop Res 7 (4):486–493
113. Roseti L, Buda R, Cavallo C, Desando G, Facchini A, Grigolo B (2008) Ligament repair: a molecular and immunohistological characterization. J Biomed Mater Res A 84(1):117–127
114. Rosenberg TD, Franklin JL, Baldwin GN, Nelson KA (1992) Extensor mechanism function after patellar tendon graft harvest for anterior cruciate ligament reconstruction. Am J Sports Med 20(5):519–525; discussion 516–525

115. Rodeo SA, Kawamura S, Ma CB, Deng XH, Sussman PS, Hays P, Ying L (2007) The effect of osteoclastic activity on tendon-to-bone healing: an experimental study in rabbits. J Bone Joint Surg Am 89(10):2250–2259
116. Hays PL, Kawamura S, Deng XH, Dagher E, Mithoefer K, Ying L, Rodeo SA (2008) The role of macrophages in early healing of a tendon graft in a bone tunnel. J Bone Joint Surg Am 90 (3):565–579
117. Yeh WL, Lin SS, Yuan LJ, Lee KF, Lee MY, Ueng SW (2007) Effects of hyperbaric oxygen treatment on tendon graft and tendon-bone integration in bone tunnel: biochemical and histological analysis in rabbits. J Orthop Res 25(5):636–645
118. Einhorn TA, Lane JM (1998) Significant advances have been made in the way surgeons treat fractures. Clin Orthop Relat Res 355(suppl):S2–S3
119. Klassen JF, Trousdale RT (1997) Treatment of delayed and nonunion of the patella. J Orthop Trauma 11(3):188–194
120. Qin L, Wang L, Wong MW, Wen C, Wang G, Zhang G, Chan KM, Cheung WH, Leung KS (2010) Osteogenesis induced by extracorporeal shockwave in treatment of delayed osteotendinous junction healing. J Orthop Res 28(1):70–76
121. Qin L, Lu H, Fok P, Cheung W, Zheng Y, Lee K, Leung K (2006) Low-intensity pulsed ultrasound accelerates osteogenesis at bone-tendon healing junction. Ultrasound Med Biol 32 (12):1905–1911
122. Malizos KN, Papachristos AA, Protopappas VC, Fotiadis DI (2006) Transosseous application of low-intensity ultrasound for the enhancement and monitoring of fracture healing process in a sheep osteotomy model. Bone 38(4):530–539
123. Lu H, Qin L, Cheung W, Lee K, Wong W, Leung K (2008) Low-intensity pulsed ultrasound accelerated bone-tendon junction healing through regulation of vascular endothelial growth factor expression and cartilage formation. Ultrasound Med Biol 34(8):1248–1260

Chapter 14
Engineering Graded Tissue Interfaces

Neethu Mohan and Michael Detamore

14.1 Complexity at the Interface

Tissues in biological systems are arranged in discrete layers with gradient interfaces, in which each layer has a definite role. Together they form a functional organ. The interface has a complex structure with tissue-specific cell types, extracellular matrix, biological signals, and mechanical properties. At the interface, there is a well-defined pattern of chemical and physical gradients to enable a smooth transition from one tissue to another with different functions. The importance of protein and chemical gradients during development, chemotaxis [1, 2], capillary sprouting, wound healing [3–5], and axonal growth in nervous tissue [6] is well documented. Developmental biologists have for many years known the importance of cell organization, boundaries, and interfaces between tissues in regulating tissue development. The three-dimensional form of organisms is achieved through a process called pattern formation. The general features of animal body plans are initially laid out during embryogenesis in broad strokes. The differential fates are specified along the rostral–caudal axis. During subsequent development, the cells that make up the field itself are defined; further specific signaling centers are established within the field, which serve to provide positional information; and finally, cells differentiate in response to additional cues according to their already-encoded positional information [7].

A similar patterning is present at tissue interfaces. The most widely studied interfaces include cartilage–bone, ligament–bone, tendon–bone, tendon–ligament, and dentin–enamel junctions. Transitions are observed in composition, architecture, mechanical properties, and biological functions. The chemical gradients constitute the gradient in extracellular matrix (ECM) proteins, growth factors, and other biochemical components. The spatial localization and gradient length of

N. Mohan • M. Detamore (✉)
Department of Chemical and Petroleum Engineering, University of Kansas, Lawrence, KS, USA
e-mail: n788m511@ku.edu; detamore@ku.edu

S. Thomopoulos et al. (eds.), *Structural Interfaces and Attachments in Biology*,
DOI 10.1007/978-1-4614-3317-0_14, © Springer Science+Business Media New York 2013

these signals are integral to their function. A gradient is also observed in physical properties such as stiffness, porosity, and topology. A gradual transition in physico-chemical and biological properties is required to connect these mechanically mismatched tissues for smooth coordination of their functions. The cues present in the ECM guide major cellular processes such as cell–cell interaction, proliferation, migration, and differentiation. Cells in turn interact and remodel the surrounding ECM to maintain the respective tissue phenotype at the interface.

Studies have also shown that tissue interfaces undergo gradual changes in their properties with age and play important roles in diseases [8]. For example, the zone of calcified cartilage forms the interface between cartilage and bone for transmitting force, attaching cartilage to bone, and limiting diffusion of nutrients from bone to the deep layers of cartilage [9]. The structure and the height of this interface is a relatively constant percent of articular cartilage. The permeability of the bone–cartilage interface to water and solutes varies with age [10]. Advancement of the calcified region toward the articular surface is observed with age and has been associated with traumatic osteochondral defects [11] and in diseases like osteochondritis dissecans (OCD) and osteoarthritis [12] that affect both the articular cartilage and bone. Damage to interfaces affects the function of two integrated tissues and efforts to restore the interface using artificial implants have not been successful to a great extent. Tissue engineering offers a promising approach to recreate the interface using a combination of tissue-specific cells, three-dimensional scaffolds, and biological signals. *In vitro* engineering of these gradient interfaces requires creation of biomimetic materials with controlled spatial and temporal features to direct cell response, tissue formation, and tissue function.

14.2 Major Tissue Interfaces

14.2.1 Cartilage–Bone Interface

Cartilage is a smooth, white, glistening tissue that lines diarthroidal joints and helps in the very low friction movement of joints and in resisting compression. It is a highly hydrated, avascular, aneural tissue, consisting of chondrocytes dispersed in an interpenetrating network of type II collagen and proteoglycans. Bone, on the other hand, is a highly organized rigid connective tissue composed of osteoclasts, osteocytes, and osteoblasts with abundant intercellular matrix in the form of type I collagen fibers and stiffening inorganic substances. The articular cartilage–bone transitional junction possesses a complex, zonal architecture that varies in composition, structure, and biomechanical properties to allow for smooth transition from articulation at the joint surface to rigid attachment at the subchondral bone. This strong and stable interface, termed the "tidemark", is characterized by an undulating basophilic band. A major contributing factor to the stability of this interface is the smooth compositional transition from un-mineralized cartilage to mineralized bone. This continuous interface has a gradual increase in calcium phosphate mineral content from 0 to 75% across the zone from articular cartilage to subchondral bone. The collagen fibrils extend across this tidemark, ensuring a continuous organic phase [13, 14]. The arrangement of hypertrophic chondrocyte cells, type X collagen, and the orientation of collagen fibrils form a definite pattern at the interface. The height of the interface is maintained by a balance between the progression of the tidemark into the un-mineralized cartilage and changing into bone by vascular invasion and bony remodeling. The permeability of this interface to nutrients varies with age.

The interface plays an important role in diseases affecting both bone and cartilage. Osteochondral defects due to trauma may lead to necrosis of chondrocytes, loss of proteoglycans, and empty lacunae in the subchondral bone with multiple extensive fracture lines through the zone of calcified cartilage. An osteochondral defect is a lesion that initiates in the subchondral bone that leads to separation and instability of the overlying articular cartilage [15]. The zone of calcified cartilage that is quiescent in adults gets reactivated in osteoarthritis and progressively calcifies the un-mineralized cartilage. This might contribute to cartilage thinning, which would increase the intensity of forces across the uncalcified cartilage, leading to more damage. Moreover, parallel cracks at the tidemark would result from the shear forces at the interface [16]. The horizontal splitting was found at increasing frequency with increased age and degree of osteoarthritic involvement [12].

14.2.2 Ligament–Bone/Tendon–Bone Interface

This tissue interface exhibits a multi-tissue transition consisting of four distinct, continuous regions of ligament, un-mineralized fibrocartilage, mineralized fibrocartilage, and lamellar bone [17]. The insertion of ligaments or tendons into bone is mainly achieved through a fibrocartilage interface. The non-mineralized fibrocartilage matrix consists of ovoid chondrocytes and collagen types I and II within the proteoglycan-rich matrix. The mineralized fibrocartilage zone contains hypertrophic chondrocytes surrounded by a mineralized matrix and type X collagen [17–19]. The fibrocartilage transformation from an un-mineralized to a mineralized state adds significant insertional strength to the interface and makes it highly resistant to avulsion. The gradient structure eliminates high levels of stress at the interface, providing effective transfer of mechanical load from tendon to bone [20]. An injured anterior cruciate ligament (ACL) fails to regenerate the intervening fibrocartilage at the enthesis. Failure rates for rotator cuff repair (which requires tendon to bone healing) have been reported to be as high as 94% [21].

14.3 Regenerative Medicine Strategies to Engineer Tissue Interfaces

Regeneration is defined as restoration of a tissue/organ to normal function following an injury. Tissue engineering aims to create a biological substitute to replace or repair tissue function by combining cells, scaffolds, and signaling molecules. *In vivo* tissue engineering offers a tremendous advantage over traditional *in vitro* approaches in that a functional tissue is fully integrated within the host physiology by allowing cells to grow in an environment that physically and chemically represents the microenvironment of the damage and repair process. Engineering connective tissue interfaces is rather complex, as this requires combination of cells of different phenotypes, scaffolds of different material types and physico-chemical properties, and signals for different biological functions. The scaffolds aid in the presentation of this information that includes a 3D template to form the tissue structure, biological cues for cell adhesion, differentiation, and maturation. Different approaches employed to regenerate tissue interfaces and fabricate biomimetic scaffolds are briefly discussed in the following section.

14.3.1 Cells in Engineering Interfaces

The importance of cell–cell interactions for the formation of tissue interfaces have been examined by coculturing cells relevant to the tissue types like fibroblasts, osteoblasts and chondrocytes [22, 23] in specific 3D microenvironments. A study by Jiang et al. [24] looked into the effect of coculture of chondrocytes and osteoblasts for osteochondral regeneration. Their results indicated that chondrocytes and osteoblasts supported the formation of a mineralized tissue within the proteoglycan-collagen-rich matrix. A promising approach is to promote tissue synthesis, derived from single source progenitor cells that will be differentiated in the construct to chondrocytes and osteoblasts. A recent study by Cheng et al. [25] created a stem cell-derived osteochondral interface using an interface-specific microenvironment in 3D configuration, via multilayered cocultures. Mesenchymal stem cells (MSCs) were encapsulated in collagen microspheres and differentiated to chondrogenic and osteogenic functional units. These pre-differentiated functional microspheres were aggregated to form a trilayer scaffold with chondrogenic microspheres on top, osteogenic microspheres at the bottom, and an intermediate undifferentiated layer of MSCs in collagen microspheres. The study identified chondrogenic medium as the optimal medium for the culture of the trilayered constructs that generated a continuous calcified interface with hypertrophic chondrocytes and type X collagen. Coculture of cell types relevant to the interface might enhance the integration of different tissues at the interface, but the use of progenitor cells from a single source and differentiating them to respective phenotypes in response to biological cues is a more promising approach.

14.3.2 Engineering Graded Scaffolds: Why Are Graded Structures Required?

Gradients in porosity, pore size, and mineral composition have functional consequences with regard to stiffness, permeability, and biological activity in tissues. These parameters are highly interrelated; a gradient in mineral content and porosity results in a gradient in stiffness. Porosity and pore size have an effect on permeability, while pore size and surface morphology are likely to influence phenotypic expression. Studies have indicated that graded patterns of biologic molecules were the driving force for migrating cells [26]. Gradients of secreted signaling proteins were found to guide the growth of blood vessels during normal and pathological angiogenesis [27]. Earlier attempts to engineer the osteochondral interface used methods to fabricate independent layers and further integrated the two components together by suturing or gluing [28, 29]. Fabrication of bi/tri/multilayered scaffolds with distinct phases resulted in an abrupt or discrete interface created by the joining of two materials [30]. There was a severe lack of integration at the interface, limiting the biological performance of the regenerated tissue. Consequently, investigators explored methods to construct scaffolds with graded structures and better integration for a smooth transition of properties at the interface. Malafaya and Reis [31] fabricated a chitosan-based bilayered scaffold by a particle aggregation method where cross-linked chitosan served as the chondrogenic layer and hydroxyapatite (HA) incorporated collagen formed the osteogenic phase. HA was incorporated into collagen by random assembly of particles. The cross-linking of collagen and the contact points of adjacent HA particles formed the bonding sites, thereby creating a highly interconnected network to overcome any risk of delamination. Ahn et al. [32] designed a biphasic scaffold combining hyaluronic acid and atellocollagen for the chondral (i.e., cartilage) phase and HA and beta-tricalcium phosphate for the osseous (i.e., bone) phase. The two phases were freeze-dried together to create the intermediate zone in which both the chondral phase and the osseous phase coexisted. Thus scaffolds that can guide the chondrogenic and osteogenic differentiation of cells in different regions of the same matrix were developed. Furthermore the challenge was in maintaining the appropriate chondrogenic and osteogenic phenotypes under a single set of cell culture conditions [28, 33]. Spalazzi et al. [34] designed a triphasic scaffold system mimicking the multi-tissue organization of the native ACL-to-bone interface. Polyglactin knitted mesh sheets formed the ligament phase, PLGA microspheres were used for the unmineralized fibrocartilage interface, and PLGA microspheres with bioactive glass formed the osteogenic phase. The three phases were further sintered to form the trilayer scaffold. Osteoblasts seeded on the osteogenic phase and fibroblasts seeded on the ligament phase migrated to PLGA microspheres to form a fibrocartilage interface. The study pointed out that tissue-specific gene expression was observed in each of these phases and cocultured scaffolds maintained a higher degree of structural integrity than the acellular scaffolds.

A continuously graded osteochondral construct that simultaneously regenerates both cartilage and bone and promotes proper integration at the interface may be the most promising way to firmly anchor a cartilage substitute to natural surrounding tissues. Graded variations in extracellular matrix architecture and properties at the tissue interface are nature's solution for connecting mechanically mismatched tissues. Creating chemical and material gradients to mimic the heterogeneity of cellular environments may be beneficial for engineering of interfaces.

14.3.3 Gradients in Growth Factor Concentrations

Cells in developing organs and tissues have the ability to detect and respond to various types of signaling gradients by chemotaxis [35] for viability, migration, proliferation and differentiation. A variety of growth factors, like the members of transforming growth factor (TGF)-β family and bone morphogenetic proteins (BMPs) [36, 37], insulin-like growth factors (e.g., IGF-1) [38], and fibroblast growth factors (FGFs) [39], have shown promising roles in the regeneration of cartilage, bone, and ligament. Independent deliveries and cocktails of these growth factors have been delivered through scaffolds at various dose and release regimes in an attempt to optimize the engineered tissue growth [40–42]. Oh et al. fabricated fibril-based scaffolds with increasing gradients of three different growth factors as a tool to investigate the cell response to chemotaxis (Fig. 14.1). Cylindrical scaffolds with a surface area gradient were fabricated by centrifugation of PCL/F127 fibers. Growth factors were immobilized onto heparin that was further linked to these fibers via hydrogen bonding [43].

The presence or absence of these signaling molecules, their relative amounts, spatial arrangements, and the temporal sequence in which they are presented need to be carefully examined while engineering interfaces. Wang et al. [44] reported the use of a single concentration gradient or reverse gradient of (BMP-2) and (IGF-1), encapsulated in microspheres for osteochondral tissue engineering. They found that calcium deposition and osteogenic markers, Collagen I, and bone-sialoprotein (BSP) showed a corresponding increase of transcription level along the (BMP-2) gradient. The presence of the hypertrophic chondrogenic marker Col X also showed an increasing trend along the gradient. The presence of (IGF-1) enhanced the effect of (BMP-2) in inducing osteogenesis and chondrogenesis. However not much has been discussed in detail about the structure of the interfaces. Engineering dual tissues and their interfaces require coordinated activity of multiple growth factors. This can involve cooperative or opposing activities between the signals and cross-talk and reciprocal interactions between signaling pathways. The ability of graded signals to control patterning of cell phenotype and tissue-specific extracellular matrix at the interface was also investigated by Dormer et al. [45]. Phillips et al. [46] looked at zonal organization of osteoblastic and fibroblastic cellular phenotypes for bone–soft tissue interface by a one-step seeding of fibroblasts onto scaffolds containing a spatial distribution

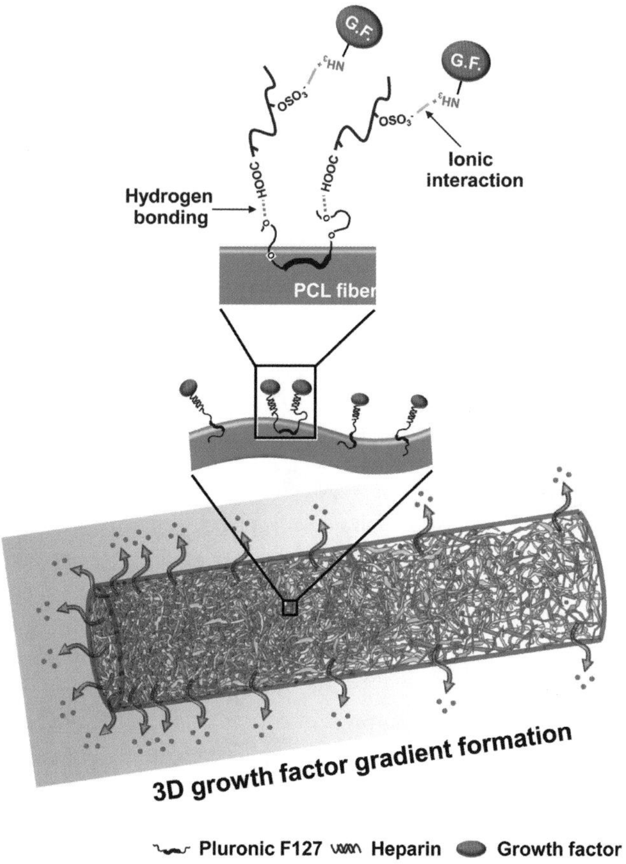

Fig. 14.1 Schematic diagrams for the successive binding of heparin and growth factor onto the fibril surface of a PCL/F127 cylindrical scaffold and the formation of 3D growth factor gradient on the scaffold (reproduced, with permission, from [43])

of retrovirus encoding the osteogenic transcription factor Runx2/Cbfa1. Gradients of immobilized retrovirus, achieved via deposition of controlled poly(L-lysine) densities, resulted in spatial patterns of transcription factor expression, osteoblastic differentiation, and mineralized matrix deposition. They found that the graded distribution of mineral deposition and mechanical properties were maintained when implanted *in vivo* in an ectopic site.

Even though many growth factor cocktails have been investigated, due to the complexity of the biological environment at the interface, an appropriate composition and pattern have yet to be determined. Great care must be given in the design of appropriate carriers and to tailor the retention time, biological activity, and release kinetics of growth factors at specific sites within two engineered tissues and their interface.

14.3.4 Graded Structure in Hydrogels and Stiff Polymers

Gradient scaffolds made from both hydrogels and stiffer materials have been explored in an effort to match the soft tissue–bone interfaces. Hydrogels may mimic the ECM in terms of their high water content, viscoelasticity, and/or diffusive transport characteristics [47, 48]. They can further be tailored to mimic a 3D microenvironment within a tissue. Due to advances in material chemistry, a wide range of hydrogels have been synthesized with tunable physical, chemical, and functional properties. Commonly employed polymers for 3D hydrogel fabrication include blends or copolymers of alginate, agarose, gelatin, hyaluronic acid, chitosan, poly (ethylene glycol) (PEG), and collagen. Various methods have been developed to create chemical and physical gradients on hydrogel scaffolds. Holland et al. [42] used a multi-step cross-linking procedure to fabricate multilayered oligo(poly(ethylene glycol) fumarate) (OPF) osteochondral scaffolds with good integration between layers. Hydrogels with concentration gradients in the cell-adhesion ligand Arg-Gly-Asp-Ser (RGDS) [49], gradients in elastic modulus or pore size [50, 51], and fibril density have been widely explored. Physical gradients that were several hundreds of microns in length were fabricated by making different concentrations of pre-polymer solutions that were allowed to diffuse into each other and further stabilized by appropriate cross-linking methods. Multiple growth factors and proteins have been immobilized in different directions in hydrogels and their concentration-dependent response in rate and orientation of cell migration has been studied. Chemical gradients of encapsulated signals were also made by microfluidic channels embedded in hydrogels [52], or by pumping different polymer solutions at controllable flow rates [53] that were further stabilized by photo or thermal cross-linking methods [54, 55]. Stepwise stiffness gradients and patterned interlocking blocks of different stiffnesses have been produced in hydrogels [56]. These techniques have been used to create gradients of soluble factors, proteins, beads, and even cells within hydrogel networks [44, 57, 58]. Du et al. [58] demonstrated a technique to rapidly produce centimeter scale concentration gradients of cells and microbeads by flow convection and high fluidic shear in a microfluidic channel. They were able to generate cross-gradients in particles and hydrogels by using alternating flows, superposing gradients of two species resulting in anisotropic material gradients. Chatterjee et al. showed that scaffolds with increasing gradients of compressive modulus can direct osteoblast differentiation and mineralization [59]. Hydrogels with mineral gradients were generated when osteoblasts were encapsulated in PEG hydrogels with an increasing gradient of modulus from 10 to 300 KPa (Fig. 14.2). This is a promising approach for engineering seamless tissue interfaces for hard and soft tissues without the use of expensive growth factors [59].

Chemical and physical gradient structures to mimic tissue interfaces can be developed by combining these gradient protocols with appropriate cross-linking methods. A recent review on "Biomimetic gradient hydrogels for tissue engineering" [60, 61] elaborately discussed all of these aspects that have been investigated

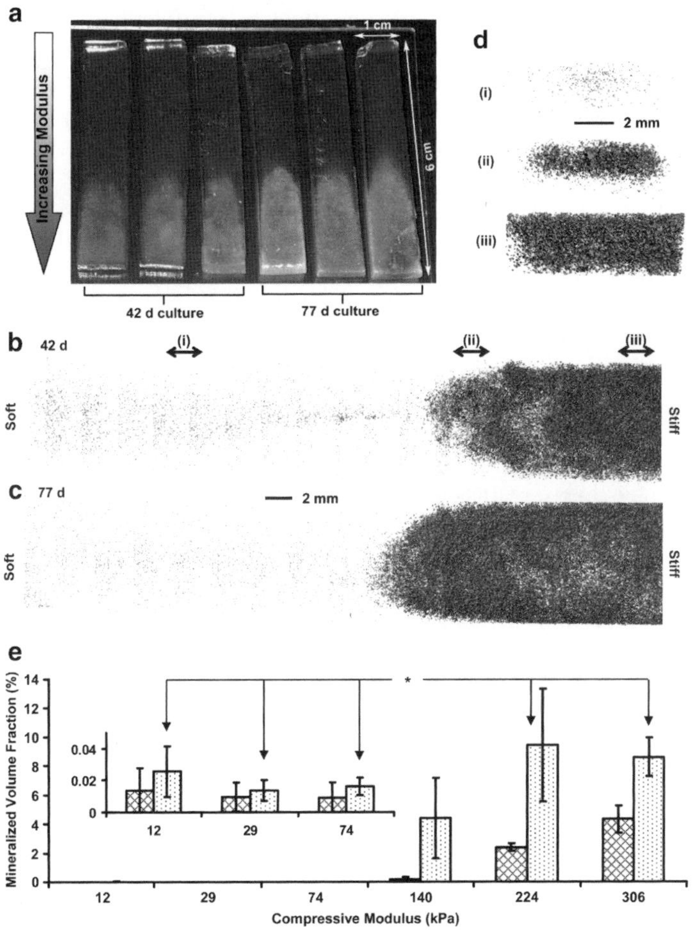

Fig. 14.2 Deposited mineral gradients induced by hydrogel stiffness gradients after 42 days and 77 days culture of encapsulated osteoblasts. Deposition of mineral at the stiffer ends of the gradients caused a change in appearance from transparent to *white* (reproduced, with permission, from [59])

for *in vitro* engineering tissues. However, these strategies have not been widely explored to recreate all the complexities at the interfacial junction of tissues.

Bone substitute materials, calcium phosphates, hydroxyapatite (HA), and bioglasses are biocompatible and have the capacity to bond directly to bone. When combined with polymeric materials, these components impart high stiffness and compressive strength. Li et al. [62] made a continuous linear gradient in calcium phosphate content across the surface of a nanofiber mat that could be used for repairing the tendon-to-bone insertion. This gradient was obtained by varying the incubation time of the nanofiber mat in simulated body fluid. The graded material design produced a change in the mechanical properties of material that reduced the stress concentrations at the interface. Pre-osteoblasts preferentially adhered and proliferated in regions with higher calcium phosphate content along the gradated scaffold. Liu et al. [63] prepared a gradient collagen/nano-HA composite scaffold, by a biomimetic diffusion-precipitate method. Nano-HA was crystallized in the interior of a collagen scaffold to form a compositional and structural gradient. Kon et al. [64] looked into fabrication of multilayered gradient artificial ECMs composed of type I collagen and HA. The cartilaginous layer, consisting of Type I collagen, had a smooth surface. The mineral phase, represented by magnesium-hydroxyapatite, was directly nucleated onto collagen fibers during their self-assembling. The intermediate (tidemark-like) layer consisted of a combination of collagen and HA. The compositions of type I collagen and HA varied in each region (cartilage region: 100% type I collagen; transition region: 40% HA and 60% type I collagen; and bone region: 70% HA and 30% type I collagen). The intermediate and the lower layers were obtained by nucleating nanostructured nonstoichiometric hydroxyapatite into self-assembling collagen fibers, similar to the natural biological neo-ossification process. Chondrocytes were seeded only in the cartilage region and the scaffolds were transplanted into the osteochondral defect. The regeneration of bone and cartilage was found to significantly enhance with these graded artificial ECMs compared to that of the control group in sheep model as well as in early clinical trials in human beings [65].

Hydrogel scaffolds are good candidates for engineering the soft tissues at the interface. They can be chemically modified to couple peptides to enhance cell adhesion, and are good delivery vehicles for bioactive signals and cells. Gradients in these encapsulated components can be obtained by simple diffusion, flow convection or by creating microfluidic channels within the hydrogels. Hydrogels with gradients in material composition, porosity, and mechanical properties can be fabricated by interdiffusion of two different polymers and by effective cross-linking. A gradient in osteoconductive hydroxyapatite is a promising approach to enhance mineralization as well as stiffness to match the mechanical properties of the soft–hard tissue interface. Osteoconductive inorganic materials can be efficiently nucleated within the hydrogels and integration at the interface can be achieved by diffusion of hydrogels into the bony phase along with appropriate cross-linking methods.

14.3.5 Gradients in Pore Architecture

The scaffold design should incorporate anisotropic pore architecture to accommodate the different types of cells and ECM distribution at the interface. Studies have suggested that the pore size and substrate surface influence the cell morphology and phenotypic expression, while porosity influences the cell proliferation. Research has revealed that 70–120 μm pores were suitable for chondrocyte ingrowth [66],

40–150 μm for fibroblast binding [67], and 100–400 μm for bone regeneration [30], depending on the porosity and the scaffold materials used [68, 69]. Thus, the dimensions of scaffold pores can depend on the cell type. A well-engineered scaffold should be tailored with the appropriate pore sizes and porosities to meet the needs of the specific cells and tissues.

One method reported for generating a porosity gradient was to stack porogen mixture layers containing different volume fractions and/or particle sizes. O'Brien et al. [68] fabricated collagen-based, porous tubular scaffolds with a graded structure to facilitate the study of myofibroblast migration during peripheral nerve regeneration. Oh et al. [70] fabricated scaffolds with a porosity and pore size gradient along the cylindrical axis by a centrifugation method. They reported that the porosity and the pore size ranges of the scaffold could easily be varied by adjusting the angular velocity. The *in vitro* and the *in vivo* studies on this gradient scaffold indicated that 380–405 μm pore sizes showed better cell proliferation for chondrocytes and osteoblasts, while the scaffold section with 186–200 μm pore sizes was better for fibroblast growth. Fu et al. [71] looked into the influence of pore architecture on bone regeneration. Hydroxyapatite scaffolds with approximately the same porosity (65–70%) but two differently oriented microstructures, described as "columnar" (pore diameter 90–110 μm) and "lamellar" (pore width 20–30 μm), were prepared by unidirectional freezing of suspensions. The columnar scaffolds with the larger pore width provided the most favorable substrate for cell proliferation and function. They concluded that HA scaffolds with the columnar microstructure and unidirectional pores favored bone repair applications *in vivo*. Hsu et al. [72] fabricated porous ceramic implants with graded pore structures to mimic the bimodal structure of cortical and cancellous bone. Functionally graded scaffolds were made by vacuum impregnating an HA and tricalcium phosphate (TCP) ceramic slurry into a polyurethane foam that was stitched or press fitted to form gradient templates. No interfacial weakness was observed by the three point bending testing in these scaffolds. Sun et al. [73] reported that minute pores that determine the surface topography had an influence on the osteoconductivity. Osteoblasts cultured on porous silicon with pores on the order of 1 μm enhanced osteoblast viability and mineralization, and maintained the expression of the biomarkers of bone formation when compared to nanoscale pores (50 nm or less). The pores and the surface topography influenced cell spreading, mechanical signal transduction, and osteoconductivity.

Previous studies have suggested that different pore sizes favor the growth of chondrocytes, fibroblasts, and osteocytes. Porosity and pore size play a role in directing cell migration and altering permeability of the scaffolds. Scaffolds with gradients in porosity have been obtained by stacking porogens of different sizes, by centrifugation, varying the freeze drying conditions, or by using 3D plotters. Even though gradients in pore architecture are not a critical element in the design of scaffold for interface engineering, they were found to have significant influence on the cell infiltration and behavior, vasculature, and mechanical properties at the interface.

14.3.6 Gradients in Mechanical Properties

Mechanics-based differentiation may be critically interdependent with extracellular matrix composition, and this may regulate cell behavior. Matrix stiffness affects cytoskeletal signaling elements that regulate differentiation, cell spreading [74], cell motility [75], and matrix assembly [76]. Specific ligands together with substrate compliance regulate differentiation [77]. To better suit the functions at the interface, the scaffold needs to be designed for varying mechanical properties which can be achieved by changing the porosity across the scaffold, as porosity is more dominant in determining the scaffold mechanical properties than pore size. It has been hypothesized that this stepwise transition in stiffness is important for the proper functioning of cartilage and distribution of forces. Sharma et al. [78] identified that a mechanical gradient in substrate and ligand loading could direct tenogenic and osteogenic differentiation of stem cells, so these could be considered as potential design variables for engineering a functional interface between tendon and bone. More recently, biphasic but monolithic materials were fabricated by joint freeze-drying and chemical cross-linking of collagen-based materials (mineralized or coupled with hyaluronic acid), as well as by ionotropic gelation of alginate-based materials (with or without hydroxyapatite ceramic particles), which achieved specific mechanical properties (e.g., elasticity or compression strength) [79].

To engineer a functional muscle-tendon tissue, Ladd et al. [80] developed a scaffold with regional variations in mechanical properties and strain profiles to mimic native muscle-tendon junction (MTJ). Muscle tissue is highly compliant, with reported moduli values ranging from 0.012 to 2.8 MPa [81, 82]. Tendon tissue is stiffer in terms of tensile loading with reported moduli of 500–1850 MPa [83–86]. The junction serves as an interface to reduce stress-concentrations and failure at this interface [87]. The scaffold possessed both a compliant/high strain region, a stiff/low strain region, and an intermediate region fabricated by a co-electrospinning method. PLLA fibers with high stiffness, strength, and low ductility were used to engineer tendon, and PCL fibers that were less stiff and more ductile were used as the muscle scaffolding system. Co-electrospinning resulted in a scaffold that had high stiffness and low compliance on one end yet low stiffness and high compliance on the other. The middle region possessed an intermediate stiffness and strain, which are analogous to the tendon, muscle, and junction. The dual scaffolding system promoted the attachment of myoblasts and allowed them to differentiate into myotubes and also supported fibroblasts.

The application of medical imaging systems together with computer-aided design (CAD) has largely dealt with the problem of matching anatomical requirements of the tissue engineered scaffolds [88]. A bio-plotter system can control design factors, including pore size and shape, porosity, strand orientation, strand distance, and interconnectivity. In stereolithography, a gradient in size and volume fraction of the pores can be introduced by adding a linear term to the equation used to describe the pore architecture [89]. Park et al. [90] reported that PCL scaffolds fabricated with controlled pore architecture using rapid prototyping methods have a higher mechanical strength and promote better cell infiltration than scaffolds fabricated by salt leaching methods.

Liu et al. [91] used a multi-nozzle low-temperature deposition and manufacturing (M-LDM) system to make mechanically graded scaffolds using heterogeneous materials, hierarchical porous structures, and different hydrophilicity. This system could be effectively used for designing interfaces. Using CAD, the structure, pore sizes, and porosity of two phases and interface could be designed initially. Further graded structures could be fabricated using multi-nozzle and appropriate polymer combinations. A Computer Aided System for Tissue Scaffolds (CASTS) aims to bring automated production of graded scaffolds by providing a scaffold library database that correlates scaffold porosity values and the corresponding compressive stiffness and integrates this into the design process [92].

The soft tissue–bone interface has varying mechanical properties. Cell spreading, motility, and phenotypic expression are found to be influenced by substrate stiffness. A gradient in mechanical properties may be considered a key element for engineering two tissues for smooth transfer of stress at the interface as well as for regulating cell behavior. Scaffolds with gradients in mechanical properties can be fabricated by blending polymers of different stress/strain behavior or by nucleation of osteoconductive inorganic materials to mimic the tissue properties at the interface. A gradient in porosity is also found to affect the mechanical properties of the scaffolds. Advanced medical imaging systems like MRI and microCT help to capture the micro-architecture of the interface, which together with the bio-plotters/CAM can be used to recreate the complex tissue-interface structures with specific mechanical requirements.

14.3.7 Graded Structures Using Nanofibers

Attempts have been made to fabricate graded scaffolds using nanofibers that mimic the native ECM structure. Nanofibers have the advantage that they can be conveniently functionalized by encapsulation or attachment of bioactive species to control the differentiation and proliferation of seeded cells. Additionally, the nanofibers can be readily assembled into a range of arrays or hierarchically structured by manipulating their alignment, stacking, or folding [93]. Nie and Wang [94] reported the use of PLGA/hydroxyapatite composite nanofibers to deliver BMP-2 plasmid DNA. Coaxial electrospinning was designed to produce a core-shell structure of the nanofiber, which can encapsulate and release drugs more efficiently [95]. Nanofibers were fabricated combining biodegradable polymers with inorganic bioactive materials for osteogenic differentiation and calcification of bone matrix. This design was to mimic the collagen fibers with hydroxyapatite nanocrystallites in the native bone [96]. Organic–inorganic composite nanofibers made of gelatin-HA, collagen-HA, and chitosan-HA have been designed to mimic the ECM of bone [97–99]. Furthermore, instead of adding particulate inorganic materials, degradable and bioactive hybrid nanofibers were produced through the hybridization of inorganic and organic phases in solution, by the sol-gel process. This process increased the chemical stability by forming a hybridized network [100]. The approach of using bioactive inorganic phases in concert with degradable polymers is continuing to attract attention

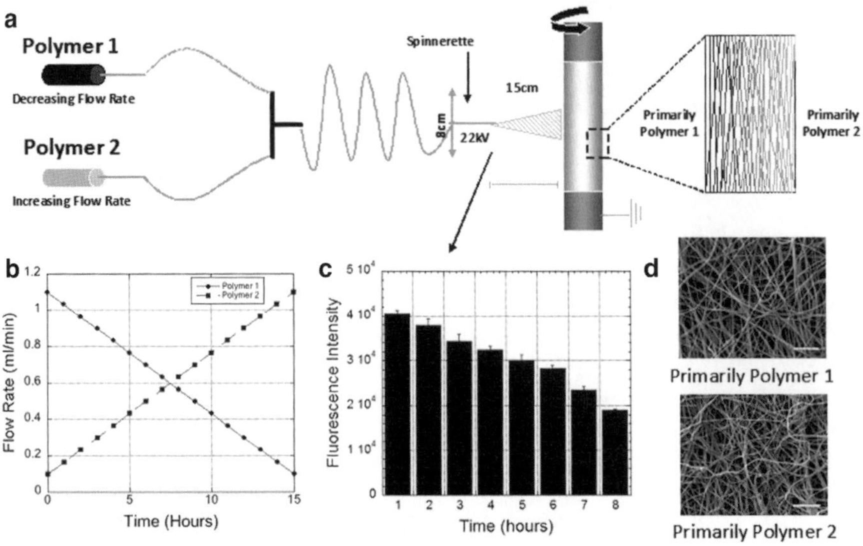

Fig. 14.3 (**a**) Schematic of electrospinning apparatus. Gradients were created in the z direction (scaffold depth) by modulating flow rates of Polymer 1 and Polymer 2, which were mixed prior to the spinnerette and electrospinning. (**b**) Change in pump flow rate with time for Polymer 1 and Polymer 2. (**c**) Electrospinning solution (Polymer 1 solution contained a fluorescent dye, whereas Polymer 2 solution did not) was collected from the spinnerette every hour for 8h, prior to electrospinning, and the fluorescence was measured as shown. A decrease in fluorescence intensity with time verifies the potential gradient formation at the spinnerette and therefore potential gradient formation in the electrospun mat. (**d**) SEM micrographs show similar fiber morphology on the top and bottom of an electrospun gradient scaffold (scale bar = 10 μ) (reproduced, with permission, from [103])

in finding suitable matrices for the regeneration of bone and its interfaced zone. Patterned electrospun mats were developed using electro-conducting templates [101].

A functionally graded nonwoven mesh of polycaprolactone incorporated with TCP nanoparticles was fabricated using a hybrid twin-screw extrusion/electrospinning (TSEE) process to engineer the fibrocartilage–bone interface [102]. This technology utilized a time-dependent feeding of various solid and liquid ingredients. Their melting, dispersion, de-aeration, and pressurization together with electrospinning were confined within a single process. Three distinct yet continuous phases were fabricated for the ligament, interface, and bone regions. The interface-relevant cell types fibroblasts, chondrocytes, and osteoblasts were tri-cultured on this scaffold and implanted subcutaneously in athymic rats. The results indicated that the multiphase scaffold design and tissue-specific distribution of cells resulted in the formation of a fibrocartilage-interface like tissue. A phase-specific distribution of mineralized matrix was observed corresponding to the bone region. In a recent study, haptotactic and durotactic gradients were introduced in hyaluronic acid-based electrospun scaffolds by varying the extent of methacrylation units and the amount of RGD peptide. These gradients were made by modifying electrospinning protocols as shown in Fig. 14.3. Gradients were found to enhance cell infiltration and direct cell migration [103].

It should be emphasized that while multiphase scaffolds consist of different phases, a key criterion for interface engineering is that these phases must be interconnected and pre-integrated with each other, thereby supporting the formation of distinct yet continuous multi-tissue regions. Furthermore, interactions between cells relevant to the interface will help in the formation, maintenance, and repair of interfacial tissue.

Electrospinning is an efficient technique to recreate the hierarchical structures present in the ECM. Nanofibers made from collagen, their blends with other polymers and hydroxyapatite have been found to favor tissue-specific cell response. However, depth of cell infiltration and diffusion constraints are some of the major concerns with this technique. Thus, refinements need to be introduced into the existing electrospinning parameters to make scaffolds of larger size, with graded structures and mechanical properties, and for co-spinning of cells and bioactive molecules.

14.4 Limitations of Discrete Layers and Approaches for Strengthening the Interface Using Continuous Gradients

Discrete layers can severely affect the interconnection between pores of two layers at the interface. This can severely hinder cellular infiltration and migration into the scaffold. The discontinuities at the scaffold interface could also negatively influence the fluid flow between the two regions, which would in turn affect nutrient and waste transport. Moreover, abrupt stress transfer can occur at the interface and can result in stress concentrations which may weaken the scaffold and cause delamination at the interface between two regions. The evolution to continuous gradient scaffolds from biphasic scaffolds is schematically represented in Fig. 14.4. As such, there is a need for a strategy to design and build scaffolds with appropriate continuous functional gradients to support interface regeneration.

Harley et al. [104] described a method called liquid phase co-synthesis to fabricate a multilayered scaffold with a continuous gradual interface. The scaffolds were made by interdiffusion of a type II collagen-glycosaminoglycan copolymer to mineralized, type I collagen-glycosaminoglycan suspensions followed by freezing at a constant rate and lyophilization. Liquid-phase co-synthesis produced an interface across a zone of interdiffusion, inside which intermixing of the two suspensions was obtained to form a soft continuous interface.

Bretcanu et al. [86] made a continuous gradient scaffold by casting a bioglass slurry on preformed polyurethane sponge templates that were compressed at different rates in an aluminum mold to obtain a continuous gradient in porosity. The organic polyurethane foam was then burned out by sintering at high temperatures. This simple method could be used for scaffolds with different shapes and porosity profiles.

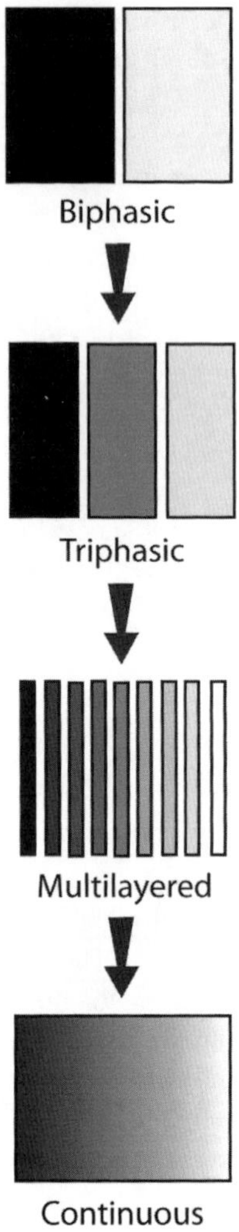

Fig. 14.4 Continuously graded designs attempt to make higher resolution in physical and chemical properties (adapted, with permission, from [108])

Continuous gradient-based bioactive signal delivery systems have recently been applied in the area of interfacial tissue regeneration. Various strategies have been developed to create gradients of bioactive signals. Studies have shown that within a tissue and at the interface the biological activity is maintained by the coordinated activity of multiple signals. At the interface, the presence of biological signals in the adjacent neighboring tissue enhances the stability of the other.

Wang et al. [44] looked into the influence of a continuous linear or reverse gradient of IGF-1 and BMP-2 for osteochondral regeneration. The growth factors were encapsulated in PLGA or silk microspheres and suspended in alginate/silk solution. A continuous gradient of growth factors in alginate/silk scaffolds was fabricated. Representative sections of the scaffold along the linear gradient were analyzed for osteogenic and chondrogenic markers. The results of the study indicated that hMSCs

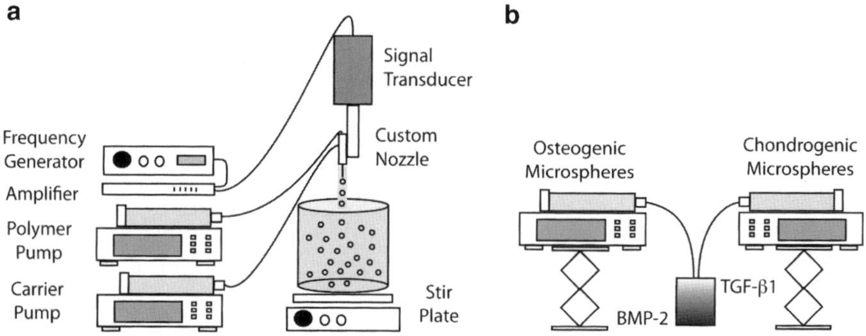

Fig. 14.5 Microparticle and scaffold fabrication process. (**a**) Microspheres were made from a polymer stream (20%w/v PLGA containing growth factors) and annular carrier stream (0.5%w/v PVA in ddH_2O) with an ultrasonic transducer; (**b**) Programmable syringe pumps created a gradient in microsphere types (adapted, with permission, from [108])

exhibited osteogenic and chondrogenic differentiation along the concentration gradients in the single gradient of BMP-2 and reverse gradient of BMP-2/IGF-1, but not the IGF-1 gradient system. They also pointed out that the carrier systems also have a significant role in the delivery and release kinetics of growth factors that might influence gene expression.

Our group followed the approach of making continuous gradients of bioactive signals using a microsphere-based technology [105]. Microspheres allowed encapsulation of bioactive signals and the gradient technology enabled localization of signals at specific sites within the scaffold. A precision particle fabrication process was used to make monodisperse microparticles and programmable syringe pumps were used to create the gradient profiles. Continuous gradient osteochondral scaffolds were fabricated using PLGA microspheres encapsulated with a chondrogenic signal TGF-β1 or osteogenic signal BMP-2. A schematic representation of fabrication process is shown in Fig. 14.5. These microspheres were collected in a mold and sintered to form a 3D osteochondral scaffold with continuous opposing gradients of chondrogenic and osteogenic signals. Microspheres enabled control over growth factor concentrations and release kinetics and the sintering conditions and the microsphere size enabled control over the pore sizes of the scaffold. The microspheres together with our gradient technology enabled spatial localization of bioactive signals, and this approach was useful for fabricating an integrated scaffold that favored simultaneous triggering of osteochondral induction. The continuous gradient scaffolds outperformed the biphasic constructs in GAG and calcium content when seeded with human umbilical cord mesenchymal stromal cells over a 6-week period [45]. We also explored the possibility of making continuous stiffness gradient scaffolds by orienting the PLGA microspheres and $CaCO_3$ incorporated PLGA microspheres using this technology [106].

Scaffolds with a continuous gradient in bioactive signals and material composition might guide tissue-specific differentiation of progenitor cells at the interface.

A continuous gradient in porosity and mechanical properties also enables smooth stress transfer at the interface. Thus, scaffolds with a continuous gradient in their properties can be a promising candidate for interface tissue engineering.

14.5 Conclusions

From a surgical and commercial standpoint, an ideal graft for regeneration of a tissue interface would be an off-the-shelf product. The option of creating a cell-free implant capable of inducing orderly and durable tissue regeneration is still under investigation. An ideal scaffold is expected to have innate ability to stimulate organogenesis rather than serving as a structural template for three-dimensional deposition of ECM. Engineering of functional interfaces with structural hierarchy, bioactive signal patterning, and appropriate mechanical properties is emerging as a major challenge for the current generation of tissue engineers.

Cells play the most important role in co-engineering of two tissues and their interface. Even though co-culture of relevant cells is straightforward, the use of a single progenitor cell source and differentiating them into cells of an appropriate phenotype at the interface in response to biological cues will be a more efficient method. Patterning of biological signals is nature's approach for tissue development. During the development and wound healing process, growth factor patterns enable the homing of progenitor cells that result in appropriate cell density; this is followed by condensation and tissue-specific differentiation of cells. This homing and condensation process could be effectively activated during *in vivo* tissue repair by patterning of biological signals on 3D scaffolds [107]. Bioactive growth factors have a significant influence on maintaining cell phenotype at the interface. Use of single or multiple signaling molecules, their relative amounts, spatial arrangements, and the temporal sequence in which they are presented need to be carefully examined while engineering interfaces. The growth factor carriers need to be tailored for proper encapsulation to retain the bioactivity and release kinetics. Hydrogels have been widely explored as a matrix for engineering soft tissue–bone interfaces. They are flexible for signal encapsulation, bio-functionalization, and are suitable for engineering soft tissues. Multiphase scaffolds using hydrogels and stiff polymers with a continuous interface are good candidates for interfacial tissue engineering. Integration at the interface can be obtained by interdiffusion of the two polymers and appropriate cross-linking methods to attain a smooth gradient in properties. Studies have shown that gradients of pore size influence cell behavior by regulating cell morphology, proliferation, ECM deposition, and vascularization. The porosity and mechanical properties of the scaffolds must be tailored to improve the stress transfer at the interfacial junction. Gradient distribution of osteoconductive materials like hydroxyapatite, $CaCO_3$, and TCP in a monolithic scaffold may be a promising approach to enhance stiffness and osteoconduction. The cell types at the interface respond to the different micromechanical environments experienced locally and remodel their surroundings. Continuous gradients can overcome the limitations of abrupt distinct layers and enable a smooth transition of properties, and may be better suited for addressing the regeneration of interfaces between tissues with drastically different mechanical behaviors. Electrospinning is a good technique to engineer graded structures that mimic the native ECM, but the ability to recreate the mechanical properties of the tissue with electrospinning may be questionable. Recent approaches to incorporate bioactive molecules and osteoconductive materials and methods to make layer by layer scaffolds show a promising trend. Advanced fabrication designs using CAD enable the fabrication of gradient structures similar to tissue interfaces. Therefore, use of biomimetic scaffolds with transitions in physico-chemical and biological signals similar to native tissue interfaces may significantly improve our efforts for *in vitro* and *in vivo* engineering of interfaces.

Native (uninjured) tissue interfaces show transitions in cell type, structure, composition, organization of ECM, chemical signals, mineralization, mechanical properties, and biological function. An ideal scaffold should be able to accommodate all of these transitions to transmit the properties of one tissue to another. However, it is rather complex to incorporate all of these transitions in the engineering of graded scaffolds for interfaces. It should be remembered that the scaffolds are only temporary structures that signal the host cells to infiltrate and synthesize the native tissue. Therefore, the importance is not in the complexity of the architecture or the physico-chemical properties of the 3D scaffolds, but rather in the ability of this temporary matrix to direct cells to form an interface similar to native tissue.

References

1. Li Jeon N, Baskaran H, Dertinger SK, Whitesides GM, Van de Water L, Toner M (2002) Neutrophil chemotaxis in linear and complex gradients of interleukin-8 formed in a microfabricated device. Nat Biotechnol 20(8):826–830
2. Shamloo A, Ma N, Poo MM, Sohn LL, Heilshorn SC (2008) Endothelial cell polarization and chemotaxis in a microfluidic device. Lab Chip 8(8):1292–1299
3. Gillitzer R, Goebeler M (2001) Chemokines in cutaneous wound healing. J Leukoc Biol 69 (4):513–521
4. Middleton J, Patterson AM, Gardner L, Schmutz C, Ashton BA (2002) Leukocyte extravasation: chemokine transport and presentation by the endothelium. Blood 100(12):3853–3860
5. Metz CN (2003) Fibrocytes: a unique cell population implicated in wound healing. Cell Mol Life Sci 60(7):1342–1350
6. Mennicken F, Maki R, de Souza EB, Quirion R (1999) Chemokines and chemokine receptors in the CNS: a possible role in neuroinflammation and patterning. Trends Pharmacol Sci 20 (2):73–78
7. Johnson RL, Tabin CJ (1997) Molecular models for vertebrate limb development. Cell 90 (6):979–990
8. Pan J, Zhou X, Li W, Novotny JE, Doty SB, Wang L (2009) In situ measurement of transport between subchondral bone and articular cartilage. J Orthop Res 27(10):1347–1352
9. Arkill KP, Winlove CP (2008) Solute transport in the deep and calcified zones of articular cartilage. Osteoarthritis Cartilage 16(6):708–714
10. Lane LB, Villacin A, Bullough PG (1977) The vascularity and remodelling of subchondrial bone and calcified cartilage in adult human femoral and humeral heads. An age- and stress-related phenomenon. J Bone Joint Surg Br 59(3):272–278

11. Mori S, Harruff R, Burr DB (1993) Microcracks in articular calcified cartilage of human femoral heads. Arch Pathol Lab Med 117(2):196–198
12. Oegema TR Jr, Carpenter RJ, Hofmeister F, Thompson RC Jr (1997) The interaction of the zone of calcified cartilage and subchondral bone in osteoarthritis. Microsc Res Tech 37 (4):324–332
13. Poole AR, Kojima T, Yasuda T, Mwale F, Kobayashi M, Laverty S (2001) Composition and structure of articular cartilage: a template for tissue repair. Clin Orthop Relat Res (391 Suppl):S26-33.
14. Cohen NP, Foster RJ, Mow VC (1998) Composition and dynamics of articular cartilage: structure, function, and maintaining healthy state. J Orthop Sports Phys Ther 28(4):203–215
15. Pape D, Filardo G, Kon E, van Dijk CN, Madry H (2010) Disease-specific clinical problems associated with the subchondral bone. Knee Surg Sports Traumatol Arthrosc 18(4):448–462
16. Burr DB, Radin EL (2003) Microfractures and microcracks in subchondral bone: are they relevant to osteoarthrosis? Rheum Dis Clin North Am 29(4):675–685
17. Cooper RR, Misol S (1970) Tendon and ligament insertion. A light and electron microscopic study. J Bone Joint Surg Am 52(1):1–20
18. Benjamin M, Evans EJ, Copp L (1986) The histology of tendon attachments to bone in man. J Anat 149:89–100
19. Thomopoulos S, Williams GR, Gimbel JA, Favata M, Soslowsky LJ (2003) Variation of biomechanical, structural, and compositional properties along the tendon to bone insertion site. J Orthop Res 21(3):413–419
20. Sagarriga Visconti C, Kavalkovich K, Wu J, Niyibizi C (1996) Biochemical analysis of collagens at the ligament-bone interface reveals presence of cartilage-specific collagens. Arch Biochem Biophys 328(1):135–142
21. Galatz LM, Ball CM, Teefey SA, Middleton WD, Yamaguchi K (2004) The outcome and repair integrity of completely arthroscopically repaired large and massive rotator cuff tears. J Bone Joint Surg Am 86-A(2):219–224
22. Jiang J, Nicoll SB, Lu HH (2005) Co-culture of osteoblasts and chondrocytes modulates cellular differentiation *in vitro*. Biochem Biophys Res Commun 338(2):762–770
23. Wang IE, Shan J, Choi R, Oh S, Kepler CK, Chen FH, Lu HH (2007) Role of osteoblast-fibroblast interactions in the formation of the ligament-to-bone interface. J Orthop Res 25 (12):1609–1620
24. Jiang J, Tang A, Ateshian GA, Guo XE, Hung CT, Lu HH (2010) Bioactive stratified polymer ceramic-hydrogel scaffold for integrative osteochondral repair. Ann Biomed Eng 38 (6):2183–2196
25. Cheng HW, Luk KD, Cheung KM, Chan BP (2011) *In vitro* generation of an osteochondral interface from mesenchymal stem cell-collagen microspheres. Biomaterials 32 (6):1526–1535
26. DeLong SA, Moon JJ, West JL (2005) Covalently immobilized gradients of bFGF on hydrogel scaffolds for directed cell migration. Biomaterials 26(16):3227–3234
27. Barkefors I, Le Jan S, Jakobsson L, Hejll E, Carlson G, Johansson H, Jarvius J, Park JW, Li Jeon N, Kreuger J (2008) Endothelial cell migration in stable gradients of vascular endothelial growth factor A and fibroblast growth factor 2: effects on chemotaxis and chemokinesis. J Biol Chem 283(20):13905–13912
28. Mano JF, Reis RL (2007) Osteochondral defects: present situation and tissue engineering approaches. J Tissue Eng Regen Med 1(4):261–273
29. Schaefer D, Martin I, Shastri P, Padera RF, Langer R, Freed LE, Vunjak-Novakovic G (2000) *In vitro* generation of osteochondral composites. Biomaterials 21(24):2599–2606
30. Place ES, Evans ND, Stevens MM (2009) Complexity in biomaterials for tissue engineering. Nat Mater 8(6):457–470
31. Malafaya PB, Reis RL (2009) Bilayered chitosan-based scaffolds for osteochondral tissue engineering: influence of hydroxyapatite on *in vitro* cytotoxicity and dynamic bioactivity studies in a specific double-chamber bioreactor. Acta Biomater 5(2):644–660

32. Ahn JH, Lee TH, Oh JS, Kim SY, Kim HJ, Park IK, Choi BS, Im GI (2009) Novel hyaluronate-atelocollagen/beta-TCP-hydroxyapatite biphasic scaffold for the repair of osteochondral defects in rabbits. Tissue Eng Part A 15(9):2595–2604
33. Sharma B, Elisseeff JH (2004) Engineering structurally organized cartilage and bone tissues. Ann Biomed Eng 32(1):148–159
34. Spalazzi JP, Doty SB, Moffat KL, Levine WN, Lu HH (2006) Development of controlled matrix heterogeneity on a triphasic scaffold for orthopedic interface tissue engineering. Tissue Eng 12(12):3497–3508
35. Iijima M, Huang YE, Devreotes P (2002) Temporal and spatial regulation of chemotaxis. Dev Cell 3(4):469–478
36. Fan H, Hu Y, Qin L, Li X, Wu H, Lv R (2006) Porous gelatin-chondroitin-hyaluronate tri-copolymer scaffold containing microspheres loaded with TGF-beta1 induces differentiation of mesenchymal stem cells *in vivo* for enhancing cartilage repair. J Biomed Mater Res A 77(4):785–794
37. Tamai N, Myoui A, Hirao M, Kaito T, Ochi T, Tanaka J, Takaoka K, Yoshikawa H (2005) A new biotechnology for articular cartilage repair: subchondral implantation of a composite of interconnected porous hydroxyapatite, synthetic polymer (PLA-PEG), and bone morphogenetic protein-2 (rhBMP-2). Osteoarthritis Cartilage 13(5):405–417
38. Hunziker EB, Kapfinger E, Martin J, Buckwalter J, Morales TI (2008) Insulin-like growth factor (IGF)-binding protein-3 (IGFBP-3) is closely associated with the chondrocyte nucleus in human articular cartilage. Osteoarthritis Cartilage 16(2):185–194
39. Huang X, Yang D, Yan W, Shi Z, Feng J, Gao Y, Weng W, Yan S (2007) Osteochondral repair using the combination of fibroblast growth factor and amorphous calcium phosphate/poly(L-lactic acid) hybrid materials. Biomaterials 28(20):3091–3100
40. Guo X, Park H, Liu G, Liu W, Cao Y, Tabata Y, Kasper FK, Mikos AG (2009) *In vitro* generation of an osteochondral construct using injectable hydrogel composites encapsulating rabbit marrow mesenchymal stem cells. Biomaterials 30(14):2741–2752
41. Holland TA, Bodde EW, Baggett LS, Tabata Y, Mikos AG, Jansen JA (2005) Osteochondral repair in the rabbit model utilizing bilayered, degradable oligo(poly(ethylene glycol) fumarate) hydrogel scaffolds. J Biomed Mater Res A 75(1):156–167
42. Holland TA, Bodde EW, Cuijpers VM, Baggett LS, Tabata Y, Mikos AG, Jansen JA (2007) Degradable hydrogel scaffolds for *in vivo* delivery of single and dual growth factors in cartilage repair. Osteoarthritis Cartilage 15(2):187–197
43. Oh SH, Kim TH, Lee JH (2011) Creating growth factor gradients in three dimensional porous matrix by centrifugation and surface immobilization. Biomaterials 32(32):8254–8260
44. Wang X, Wenk E, Zhang X, Meinel L, Vunjak-Novakovic G, Kaplan DL (2009) Growth factor gradients via microsphere delivery in biopolymer scaffolds for osteochondral tissue engineering. J Control Release 134(2):81–90
45. Dormer NH, Singh M, Wang L, Berkland CJ, Detamore MS (2010) Osteochondral interface tissue engineering using macroscopic gradients of bioactive signals. Ann Biomed Eng 38 (6):2167–2182
46. Phillips JE, Burns KL, Le Doux JM, Guldberg RE, Garcia AJ (2008) Engineering graded tissue interfaces. Proc Natl Acad Sci U S A 105(34):12170–12175
47. Lutolf MP (2009) Integration column: artificial ECM: expanding the cell biology toolbox in 3D. Integr Biol (Camb) 1(3):235–241
48. Slaughter BV, Khurshid SS, Fisher OZ, Khademhosseini A, Peppas NA (2009) Hydrogels in regenerative medicine. Adv Mater 21(32–33):3307–3329
49. He J, Du Y, Villa-Uribe JL, Hwang C, Li D, Khademhosseini A (2010) Rapid generation of biologically relevant hydrogels containing long-range chemical gradients. Adv Funct Mater 20(1):131–137
50. Tripathi A, Kathuria N, Kumar A (2009) Elastic and macroporous agarose-gelatin cryogels with isotropic and anisotropic porosity for tissue engineering. J Biomed Mater Res A 90 (3):680–694

51. Annabi N, Nichol JW, Zhong X, Ji C, Koshy S, Khademhosseini A, Dehghani F (2010) Controlling the porosity and microarchitecture of hydrogels for tissue engineering. Tissue Eng Part B Rev 16(4):371–383
52. Choi NW, Cabodi M, Held B, Gleghorn JP, Bonassar LJ, Stroock AD (2007) Microfluidic scaffolds for tissue engineering. Nat Mater 6(11):908–915
53. Cooksey GA, Sip CG, Folch A (2009) A multi-purpose microfluidic perfusion system with combinatorial choice of inputs, mixtures, gradient patterns, and flow rates. Lab Chip 9 (3):417–426
54. Kloxin AM, Benton JA, Anseth KS (2010) In situ elasticity modulation with dynamic substrates to direct cell phenotype. Biomaterials 31(1):1–8
55. Marklein RA, Burdick JA (2010) Controlling stem cell fate with material design. Adv Mater 22(2):175–189
56. Cheung YK, Azeloglu EU, Shiovitz DA, Costa KD, Seliktar D, Sia SK (2009) Microscale control of stiffness in a cell-adhesive substrate using microfluidics-based lithography. Angew Chem Int Ed Engl 48(39):7188–7192
57. He J, Du Y, Guo Y, Hancock MJ, Wang B, Shin H, Wu J, Li D, Khademhosseini A (2011) Microfluidic synthesis of composite cross-gradient materials for investigating cell-biomaterial interactions. Biotechnol Bioeng 108(1):175–185
58. Du Y, Hancock MJ, He J, Villa-Uribe JL, Wang B, Cropek DM, Khademhosseini A (2010) Convection-driven generation of long-range material gradients. Biomaterials 31 (9):2686–2694
59. Chatterjee K, Lin-Gibson S, Wallace WE, Parekh SH, Lee YJ, Cicerone MT, Young MF, Simon CG Jr (2010) The effect of 3D hydrogel scaffold modulus on osteoblast differentiation and mineralization revealed by combinatorial screening. Biomaterials 31(19):5051–5062
60. Nakajima S, Ohshima K, Kyogoku M, Miyachi Y, Kabashima K (2010) A case of intravascular large B-cell lymphoma with atypical clinical manifestations and analysis of CXCL12 and CXCR4 expression. Arch Dermatol 146(6):686–687
61. Sant S, Hancock M, Donnelly J, Iyer D, Khademhosseini A (2010) Biomimetic gradient hydrogels for tissue engineering. Can J Chem Eng 88(6):899–911
62. Li X, Xie J, Lipner J, Yuan X, Thomopoulos S, Xia Y (2009) Nanofiber scaffolds with gradations in mineral content for mimicking the tendon-to-bone insertion site. Nano Lett 9 (7):2763–2768
63. Liu C, Han Z, Czernuszka JT (2009) Gradient collagen/nanohydroxyapatite composite scaffold: development and characterization. Acta Biomater 5(2):661–669
64. Kon E, Delcogliano M, Filardo G, Fini M, Giavaresi G, Francioli S, Martin I, Pressato D, Arcangeli E, Quarto R, Sandri M, Marcacci M (2010) Orderly osteochondral regeneration in a sheep model using a novel nano-composite multilayered biomaterial. J Orthop Res 28 (1):116–124
65. Kon E, Delcogliano M, Filardo G, Pressato D, Busacca M, Grigolo B, Desando G, Marcacci M (2010) A novel nano-composite multi-layered biomaterial for treatment of osteochondral lesions: technique note and an early stability pilot clinical trial. Injury 41(7):693–701
66. Griffon DJ, Sedighi MR, Schaeffer DV, Eurell JA, Johnson AL (2006) Chitosan scaffolds: interconnective pore size and cartilage engineering. Acta Biomater 2(3):313–320
67. Salem AK, Stevens R, Pearson RG, Davies MC, Tendler SJ, Roberts CJ, Williams PM, Shakesheff KM (2002) Interactions of 3T3 fibroblasts and endothelial cells with defined pore features. J Biomed Mater Res 61(2):212–217
68. O'Brien FJ, Harley BA, Yannas IV, Gibson LJ (2005) The effect of pore size on cell adhesion in collagen-GAG scaffolds. Biomaterials 26(4):433–441
69. Karageorgiou V, Kaplan D (2005) Porosity of 3D biomaterial scaffolds and osteogenesis. Biomaterials 26(27):5474–5491
70. Oh SH, Park IK, Kim JM, Lee JH (2007) *In vitro* and *in vivo* characteristics of PCL scaffolds with pore size gradient fabricated by a centrifugation method. Biomaterials 28(9):1664–1671

71. Fu Q, Rahaman MN, Bal BS, Brown RF (2009) Proliferation and function of MC3T3-E1 cells on freeze-cast hydroxyapatite scaffolds with oriented pore architectures. J Mater Sci Mater Med 20(5):1159–1165
72. Hsu YH, Turner IG, Miles AW (2007) Fabrication of porous bioceramics with porosity gradients similar to the bimodal structure of cortical and cancellous bone. J Mater Sci Mater Med 18(12):2251–2256
73. Sun W, Puzas JE, Sheu TJ, Lieu X, Fauchet PM (2007) Nano- to microscale porous silicon as a cell interface for bone-tissue engineering. Adv Mater 19:921–924
74. McBeath R, Pirone DM, Nelson CM, Bhadriraju K, Chen CS (2004) Cell shape, cytoskeletal tension, and RhoA regulate stem cell lineage commitment. Dev Cell 6(4):483–495
75. Lo CM, Wang HB, Dembo M, Wang YL (2000) Cell movement is guided by the rigidity of the substrate. Biophys J 79(1):144–152
76. Halliday NL, Tomasek JJ (1995) Mechanical properties of the extracellular matrix influence fibronectin fibril assembly *in vitro*. Exp Cell Res 217(1):109–117
77. Rowlands AS, George PA, Cooper-White JJ (2008) Directing osteogenic and myogenic differentiation of MSCs: interplay of stiffness and adhesive ligand presentation. Am J Physiol Cell Physiol 295(4):C1037–C1044
78. Sharma RI, Snedeker JG (2010) Biochemical and biomechanical gradients for directed bone marrow stromal cell differentiation toward tendon and bone. Biomaterials 31(30):7695–7704
79. Gelinsky M, Welzel PB, Simon P, Bernhardt A, König U (2008) Porous three-dimensional scaffolds made of mineralised collagen: preparation and properties of a biomimetic nanocomposite material for tissue engineering of bone. Chem Eng J 137(1):84–96
80. Ladd MR, Lee SJ, Stitzel JD, Atala A, Yoo JJ (2011) Co-electrospun dual scaffolding system with potential for muscle-tendon junction tissue engineering. Biomaterials 32(6):1549–1559
81. Engler AJ, Griffin MA, Sen S, Bonnemann CG, Sweeney HL, Discher DE (2004) Myotubes differentiate optimally on substrates with tissue-like stiffness: pathological implications for soft or stiff microenvironments. J Cell Biol 166(6):877–887
82. Myers BS, Woolley CT, Slotter TL, Garrett WE, Best TM (1998) The influence of strain rate on the passive and stimulated engineering stress–large strain behavior of the rabbit tibialis anterior muscle. J Biomech Eng 120(1):126–132
83. Pollock CM, Shadwick RE (1994) Relationship between body mass and biomechanical properties of limb tendons in adult mammals. Am J Physiol 266(3 Pt 2):R1016–R1021
84. Mohan N, Nair PD (2010) A synthetic scaffold favoring chondrogenic phenotype over a natural scaffold. Tissue Eng Part A 16(2):373–384
85. Wren TA, Yerby SA, Beaupre GS, Carter DR (2001) Mechanical properties of the human achilles tendon. Clin Biomech (Bristol, Avon) 16(3):245–251
86. Bretcanu O, Samaille C, Boccaccini A (2008) Simple methods to fabricate bioglass-derived glass-ceramic scaffolds exhibiting porosity gradient. J Mater Sci 43:4127–4134
87. Trotter JA (2002) Structure-function considerations of muscle-tendon junctions. Comp Biochem Physiol A Mol Integr Physiol 133(4):1127–1133
88. Leong KF, Chua CK, Sudarmadji N, Yeong WY (2008) Engineering functionally graded tissue engineering scaffolds. J Mech Behav Biomed Mater 1(2):140–152
89. Melchels FP, Bertoldi K, Gabbrielli R, Velders AH, Feijen J, Grijpma DW (2010) Mathematically defined tissue engineering scaffold architectures prepared by stereolithography. Biomaterials 31(27):6909–6916
90. Park S, Kim G, Jeon YC, Koh Y, Kim W (2009) 3D polycaprolactone scaffolds with controlled pore structure using a rapid prototyping system. J Mater Sci Mater Med 20 (1):229–234
91. Liu L, Xiong Z, Yan Y, Zhang R, Wang X, Jin L (2009) Multinozzle low-temperature deposition system for construction of gradient tissue engineering scaffolds. J Biomed Mater Res B Appl Biomater 88(1):254–263

92. Sudarmadji N, Tan JY, Leong KF, Chua CK, Loh YT (2011) Investigation of the mechanical properties and porosity relationships in selective laser-sintered polyhedral for functionally graded scaffolds. Acta Biomater 7(2):530–537
93. Erisken C, Kalyon DM, Wang H (2008) Functionally graded electrospun polycaprolactone and beta-tricalcium phosphate nanocomposites for tissue engineering applications. Biomaterials 29(30):4065–4073
94. Nie H, Wang CH (2007) Fabrication and characterization of PLGA/HAp composite scaffolds for delivery of BMP-2 plasmid DNA. J Control Release 120(1–2):111–121
95. Jiang H, Hu Y, Zhao P, Li Y, Zhu K (2006) Modulation of protein release from biodegradable core-shell structured fibers prepared by coaxial electrospinning. J Biomed Mater Res B Appl Biomater 79(1):50–57
96. Olszta M, Cheng X, Jee S, Kumar R, Kim Y, Kaufman M, Douglas E, Gower L (2007) Bone structure and formation: a new perspective. Mater Sci Eng 58(2):77–116
97. Song JH, Kim HE, Kim HW (2008) Electrospun fibrous web of collagen-apatite precipitated nanocomposite for bone regeneration. J Mater Sci Mater Med 19(8):2925–2932
98. Zhang Y, Venugopal JR, El-Turki A, Ramakrishna S, Su B, Lim CT (2008) Electrospun biomimetic nanocomposite nanofibers of hydroxyapatite/chitosan for bone tissue engineering. Biomaterials 29(32):4314–4322
99. Chen F, Tang QL, Zhu YJ, Wang KW, Zhang ML, Zhai WY, Chang J (2010) Hydroxyapatite nanorods/poly(vinyl pyrolidone) composite nanofibers, arrays and three-dimensional fabrics: electrospun preparation and transformation to hydroxyapatite nanostructures. Acta Biomater 6(8):3013–3020
100. Song JH, Yoon BH, Kim HE, Kim HW (2008) Bioactive and degradable hybridized nanofibers of gelatin-siloxane for bone regeneration. J Biomed Mater Res A 84(4):875–884
101. Zhang D, Chang J (2007) Patterning of electrospun fibers using electroconductive templates. Adv Mater 19:3664–4667
102. Spalazzi JP, Dagher E, Doty SB, Guo XE, Rodeo SA, Lu HH (2008) *In vivo* evaluation of a multiphased scaffold designed for orthopaedic interface tissue engineering and soft tissue-to-bone integration. J Biomed Mater Res A 86(1):1–12
103. Sundararaghavan HG, Burdick JA (2011) Gradients with depth in electrospun fibrous scaffolds for directed cell behavior. Biomacromolecules 12(6):2344–2350
104. Harley BA, Lynn AK, Wissner-Gross Z, Bonfield W, Yannas IV, Gibson LJ (2010) Design of a multiphase osteochondral scaffold III: fabrication of layered scaffolds with continuous interfaces. J Biomed Mater Res A 92(3):1078–1093
105. Singh M, Morris CP, Ellis RJ, Detamore MS, Berkland C (2008) Microsphere-based seamless scaffolds containing macroscopic gradients of encapsulated factors for tissue engineering. Tissue Eng Part C Methods 14(4):299–309
106. Singh M, Dormer N, Salash JR, Christian JM, Moore DS, Berkland C, Detamore MS (2010) Three-dimensional macroscopic scaffolds with a gradient in stiffness for functional regeneration of interfacial tissues. J Biomed Mater Res A 94(3):870–876
107. Ingber DE, Mow VC, Butler D, Niklason L, Huard J, Mao J, Yannas I, Kaplan D, Vunjak-Novakovic G (2006) Tissue engineering and developmental biology: going biomimetic. Tissue Eng 12(12):3265–3283
108. Dormer NH, Berkland CJ, Detamore MS (2010) Emerging techniques in stratified designs and continuous gradients for tissue engineering of interfaces. Ann Biomed Eng 38 (6):2121–2141

Chapter 15
Engineering Fibrous Tissues and Their Interfaces with Bone

Jennifer Lei and Johnna S. Temenoff

15.1 Introduction

Each year, musculoskeletal injuries in the United States (of which 45% result in damage to tendons and ligaments) result in costs of approximately $30 billion [1]. Surgical treatment is necessary in fibrous tissue injuries because tendons and ligaments are relatively non-vascular and acellular, making natural healing slow and ineffective [2, 3]. Unfortunately, surgical repair using autografts, or graft tissue from the injured patient, can create problems of donor site morbidity. Additionally, surgical repair using allografts, or frozen tissues taken from cadavers, can potentially induce an immune response [4–6]. For these reasons, significant research on tissue engineering of fibrous tissues and their interface to bone is underway with the goal of generating new methods for injured tendon and ligament regeneration. Tissue engineering combines the use of cells, scaffolds, and exogenous factors. However, before these techniques are implemented in the clinic, it is important to optimize the cell types, materials, and external factors to best recreate and regenerate the tissue.

To successfully design a tissue-engineered replacement, the normal function, structure, and mechanical properties of the tendon or ligament must be understood and mimicked. The process of tendon and ligament healing is also an important factor in developing tissue engineering approaches because diverse injuries and subsequent secondary pathologies require different methods of regeneration. Furthermore, next-generation tissue-engineered graft alternatives must consider

J. Lei
George W. Woodruff School of Mechanical Engineering, Georgia Institute of Technology and Emory University, Atlanta, GA, USA

J.S. Temenoff (✉)
Wallace H. Coulter Department of Biomedical Engineering, Georgia Institute of Technology and Emory University, Atlanta, GA, USA
e-mail: johnna.temenoff@bme.gatech.edu

S. Thomopoulos et al. (eds.), *Structural Interfaces and Attachments in Biology*,
DOI 10.1007/978-1-4614-3317-0_15,

the best means, biologically and mechanically, to anchor these fibrous tissues to the surrounding joint to restore full function to the patient.

In this chapter, background information about the structure, composition, and function of tendons and ligaments is reviewed. Different types of injuries and the events of native tissue healing are summarized, as well as current reconstruction techniques for injured tissues. This basis will facilitate the understanding of current tissue engineering approaches for fibrous tissues and their interfaces, reviewed in the second half of this chapter. In particular, a discussion of the advantages and disadvantages of the cell sources, scaffolds, and exogenous factors currently used for creating tissue-engineered tendon/ligaments, as well as their interfaces with surrounding bone, is presented, followed by an examination of the remaining challenges that must be overcome before clinical adaptation of these strategies can be realized.

15.2 Physiology and Function

Successful tissue engineering and regenerative medicine methods are based on the structure–function relationship of tendons and ligaments. Tendons and ligaments are bands of connective tissue that transmit forces and facilitate joint movement [7, 8]. The tensile and compressive strength of these tissues is derived from the hierarchical organization of the fiber structure and is a key aspect in tissue replacement. Therefore, this section summarizes the structure-function relationship in tendon/ligament tissue.

Tendons and ligaments are similar in biochemical structure, but differ in function. The tendon is a fibrous band of connective tissue that connects muscle to bone. Tendons transmit forces, in the form of muscle contractions, to bones, thereby facilitating locomotion and joint stability [9, 10]. Ligaments connect bones to adjacent bones. They restrict and guide joint motion and provide joint stability. In contrast to tendons, ligaments are pliable but not elastic [11]. The structure of these fibrous tissues enables them to withstand large tensile loads generated by musculoskeletal components during active motion along the longitudinal direction of the tissue [12].

15.2.1 Structure and Biochemical Composition

Tendons and ligaments have a hierarchical structure. Tropocollagen, a triple helix molecule with two alpha-1 collagen chains and one alpha-2 collagen chain, is the basic structural unit of fibrous tissues. These molecules self-assemble and crosslink to form collagen microfibrils, the smallest unit in the fibrillar structure [12]. Microfibrils arrange end-to-end in bundles to form fibril structures. Crosslinking of fibrils increases Young's modulus, increases tensile strength, and reduces strain at failure [10, 13]. Fibrils are arranged into units of fibers surrounded by the endotenon or endoligament, a layer of loose connective tissue that interfaces with blood vessels, lymphatics, and nerves [14].

Fiber bundles gather into fascicles or secondary fiber bundles that form the characteristic crimp pattern seen in many tendons and ligaments. Secondary fiber bundles are surrounded by epitenon or epiligament, which serve as a loose connective layer for blood vessels, lymphatics, and nerves. Surrounding the connective tissue layer is the paratenon that reduces friction and enables smooth movement between neighboring tissues [15]. Long tendons and ligaments are sometimes enclosed in a synovial sheath to further decrease friction [11, 16]. The size of the fiber bundles is related to the macroscopic size and function of the tendon and affects the mechanical strength of the tissue [17]. Larger fascicles are found in big, weight-bearing tendons such as the Achilles tendon, and smaller fibrils are generally found in the digital tendons.

Biochemically, the composition of tendon and ligaments is similar. In addition to collagen that comprises the fiber bundles, these tissues contain water (55–70% by weight), cells, and other extracellular matrix (ECM) components such as elastin, proteoglycans, and glycoproteins [11]. Each component is discussed in more detail in the following sections.

15.2.2 Cells

Cells compose only 20% of total tendon volume [18]. Fibroblasts, elongated and spindle-shaped, are the main cell type found in fibrous tissues and lie parallel with the collagen fibers [11]. Communication among neighboring cells occurs through the formation of gap junctions [16, 19]. The main action of fibroblasts is to secrete molecules that form the ECM to provide structural support during mechanical loading of the tissue. Thus, these cells have the ability to adapt to an environment of increased mechanical loading through changes in gene expression and ECM protein synthesis [3, 10, 20].

15.2.3 Extracellular Matrix

The ECM of tendon and ligament tissues consists of collagen, elastin, proteoglycans, and glycoproteins. The ECM components comprise 80% by dry weight of the total tissue volume [3, 21–23]. The interactions of the ECM molecules provide the mechanical strength and properties of the fibrous tissue. Each component is discussed in detail in the following sections.

15.2.3.1 Collagen

Besides water, the largest component of the ECM of tendons and ligaments is collagen. In tendons, 75–85% of the dry weight of the tissue consists of collagen, compared to the 70–80% in ligaments [18, 21]. Collagen type I is the predominant fiber in tendon and ligaments, constituting 95 and 90% of the total collagen content in each tissue, respectively [10, 18, 21]. In this molecule, three left-handed helices with a base peptide unit of glycine-proline-hydroxyproline assemble to form fibers with a right-handed superhelix in a coiled structure [13]. The superhelical strands then pack next to each other to form collagen microfibrils [14], as previously described. This structure accounts for the tissue's high tensile strength and relative inelasticity [21].

Other major collagens found in tendon and ligament include types III and V. Collagen type III forms smaller and less organized fibrils than collagen type I, which can decrease mechanical strength. It is present in the endotenon/endoligament and the epitenon/epiligament and is synthesized during early phases of remodeling and repair [24]. Collagen V is cross-linked to other collagen types and regulates fibril growth [25, 26]. Additionally, collagens II, VI, IX, X, XI, and XII are all found in trace amounts [27, 28].

15.2.3.2 Elastin

In tendons and ligaments, elastin accounts for 2–3% and up to 10–15% of the dry weight of the tissue, respectively [10, 21]. Elastin is an insoluble globular protein that contains large hydrophobic domains and adopts a coiled arrangement in a relaxed state [10]. Stretching causes the coils to unravel and exposes the hydrophobic domains to water, creating a thermodynamic driving force for the coils to return to their original configuration. Elastin and microfibrillar proteins contribute to the recovery of a crimped structure after an applied strain [10].

15.2.3.3 Proteoglycans

Proteoglycans contain protein cores with covalently attached glycosaminoglycans. Glycosaminoglycans are complex carbohydrate molecules that provide proteoglycans with unique properties [25]. Two groups of proteoglycans exist in fibrous tissues: small leucine-rich proteoglycans and large modular proteoglycans. In fibrous tissues, proteoglycans are found in relatively small amounts (1–5% dry weight) trapped between collagen fibers and fibrils [14]. Their negative charge plays a large role in attracting water in the tendon and ligament tissue and creates repulsion forces in proteoglycans that provide the tissue with the ability to resist high tensile and compressive loads [25]. Proteoglycans also can create space between collagen fibers, thus enabling diffusion of water-soluble molecules, the migration of cells, as well as allowing fibers to slide past each other in response to compressive or tensile load [16, 25].

Decorin is the most abundant proteoglycan found in tendons. Its main function is to maintain and regulate collagen fibril structure. Decorin is considered a key regulator in matrix organization and is associated with remodeling in a tendon under tensile forces as evidenced by the observation that the skin of decorin-deficient mice was not able to withstand tensile strain [29, 30]. Fibromodulin, similar to decorin, binds to collagen fibers and acts as a modulator of collagen fibrogenesis [25]. It is expressed in high levels in tendons and contributes to tendon strength [31]. Biglycan is another proteoglycan found in tensile regions of tendons and ligaments. It can bind to collagen fibrils as well as transforming growth factor-β (TGF-β) in the tissue, thus participating in collagen fiber maturation and contributing to the regulation of cell proliferation [32, 33]. Aggrecan, a large aggregating proteoglycan found particularly in areas subject to compression, possesses more than 100 chondroitin sulfate and keratin sulfate glycosaminoglycan chains attached to the core. This negatively charged proteoglycan increases osmotic pressure, resulting in better hydration and higher compressive stiffness of the tissue [25].

15.2.3.4 Glycoproteins

Tendons and ligaments contain scarce amounts of several types of glycoproteins in the ECM. Glycoproteins are made up of proteins with attached carbohydrates. Tenascin-C and fibronectin are the main glucoproteins present in fibrous tissues. Tenascin-C interacts with collagen fibrils to provide mechanical stability in the ECM [34]. It is upregulated in response to mechanical loading or growth factors like TGF-β and can inhibit cell adhesion by blocking β1-integrin receptor interactions [35–37]. Tenascin-C can also bind to fibronectin, which is located on collagen surfaces and can facilitate wound healing [38–40]. Fibronectin may be involved in the organization of collagen type III into bundles and has been shown to act as a template in collagen fiber formation during remodeling [41].

15.2.4 Tendon- and Ligament-Bone Interface

The structure of the tendon-/ligament-bone interface is distinct from the structure of the rest of the tissue. Insertion structure and composition of the fibrous tissue into the bone varies depending on the specific attachment [7]. However, the insertion site can be generally characterized as a fibrous enthesis (indirect) or a fibrocartilaginous enthesis (direct) [42]. In indirect interfaces, the tendon or ligament attaches to the bone through collagen fibers (known as Sharpy's fibers) that directly extend into the bone at an acute angle. In direct interfaces, four transition zones of tissue exist (Fig. 15.1). The first zone is characterized as fibrous connective tissue and contains a similar structure and composition to that of normal tendon and ligament. Collagen fibrils lay parallel to each other and fibroblasts surround the fiber matrix. The next zone, uncalcified fibrocartilage, contains larger fibril bundles that are not aligned in a parallel manner. Collagen type II and aggrecan are the predominant proteins found in this region. Their presence enables resistance to compression and dissipation of stress at the interface. This ensures that the deformation and loading of the fibrous tissue is not concentrated at the bone surface [43]. Other collagen types, including collagen type VI, IX, X, XI, and XII, are found in trace amounts in this area and

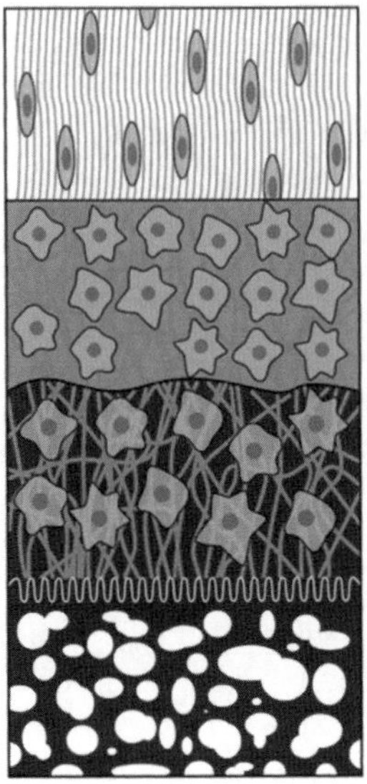

Fig. 15.1 Tendon-/ligament-bone interface. The fibrocartilaginous enthesis (direct insertion) is composed of four transitional zones: fibrous tissue region, uncalcified fibrocartilage region, calcified fibrocartilage region, calcified bone region. (Reproduced, with permission, from Yang and Temenoff [7])

can strengthen the bone insertion connection by reducing stress concentrations at the bone interface [10]. The following zone, calcified fibrocartilage, contains hypertrophic chondrocytes and collagen X. This region is characterized as similar to mineralized tissue. The fourth zone is characterized as calcified bone and provides a secure attachment of the tissue to the bone interface. This region contains osteoblasts, osteoclasts, osteocytes, and mineralized collagen I fibers [43]. Fibrous interfaces are typically found on the shafts of long bones and fibrocartilaginous interfaces are typically found at joint surfaces, such as the knee joint, or at short bones, such as the wrist or ankle [16, 44].

Because the two components of this interface have opposing mechanical properties (tendons and ligaments are strong in tension and bone is optimized for compression) [10, 21], there is a need to gradually transition the mechanical properties from one tissue to another. The uncalcified and calcified regions in a fibrocartilaginous enthesis (direct insertion) are able to effectively transmit loads and have been shown to increase Young's modulus across the different zones [45, 46]. When using tissue engineering methods to reconstruct the interface, results must ensure that this mechanical transition is recreated to reduce stress concentrations and prevent failure at the insertion site.

15.2.5 Mechanical Properties

Tendon and ligaments are viscoelastic tissues that exhibit time-dependent creep and stress relaxation rates. This is most likely caused by the interactions between water and the components of the ECM [14]. Below 4% strain, tendons exhibit elastic behavior, meaning that the tissue returns to its original length after strain release. Above 4% strain, loading causes microscopic and macroscopic failure [47]. The stress–strain curve depicts the viscoelastic behavior of a fibrous tissue (Fig. 15.2). The toe region (1.5–3.0% strain) results from gradual straightening of the crimped areas of the collagen fiber [10, 21]. The crimp pattern allows the tissue to respond rapidly to sudden strain loads and acts as a shock absorber to prevent damage from excessive loading [9, 48]. As strain increases, the tendon or ligament exhibits a linear elastic response to stress. In this region, fibers have become parallel and lose all crimp appearance. The slope created due to the linear stress–strain response is referred to as the Young's modulus and ranges from 1 to 2 GPa [8, 21]. At the end of this region, microfractures of collagen fibers occur. This yield point ranges from 5–7% strain [10, 21]. Beyond the elastic yield point, macroscopic failures of collagen fibers occur in an unpredictable manner in the failure region. Tearing of the fibers is observed around $12-15\%$ strain and results in rupture of the tissue. Failure strength of fibrous tissues ranges from 50–150 MPa [21]. Through animal experimentation, it has been shown that tensile strength, elastic stiffness (Young's modulus), and weight of the tendon can increase in response to greater physical activity [8].

15.3 Injury and Healing

Understanding the types of fibrous tissue injuries and general stages of the healing process is significant because different injuries may require varied tissue engineering approaches that may be employed at specific times during healing to best restore the tissue. The following sections will provide an overview of the classifications of tendon and ligament injuries, the natural healing process, and the current reconstruction procedures and their limitations.

15.3.1 Injuries

Injuries are classified as acute or chronic and direct or indirect [49]. Direct injuries are caused by non-penetrating injuries from accidents resulting in rupture or tearing. On the other hand, indirect injuries are often the result of acute tensile load and chronic overuse and demonstrate repetitive microtrauma [3, 23]. This class of injury is often referred to as tendinosis or tendinopathy in tendons [50].

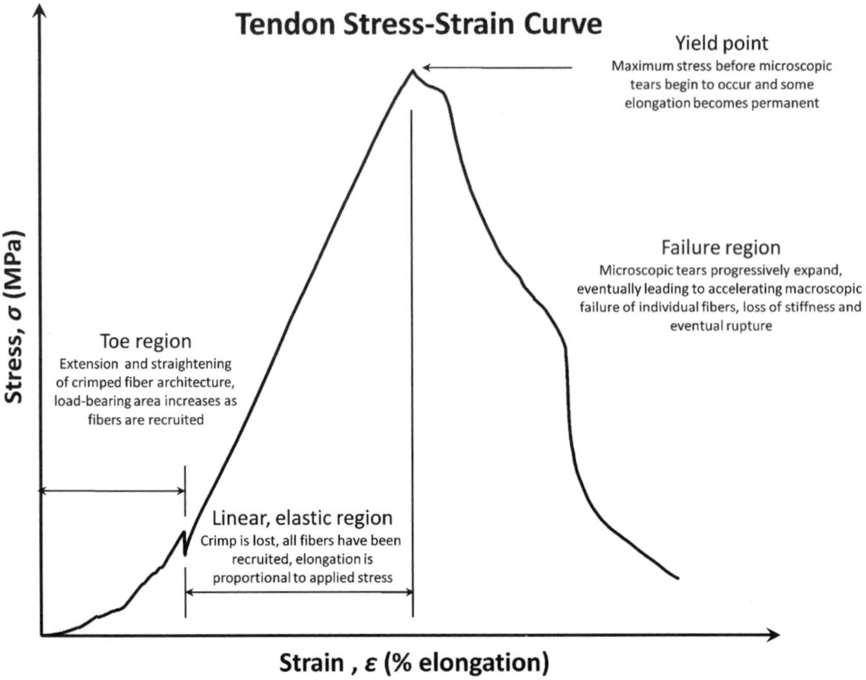

Fig. 15.2 Typical stress–strain curve for bovine patellar tendon. A tendon stress-strain curve exhibits behavior representing the toe region, the linear elastic region, the yield point, and the failure region (plot courtesy of Dr. Yongzhi Qiu)

Acute and chronic injuries are caused by both intrinsic and extrinsic factors. Intrinsic factors include age, gender, biomechanics, systemic diseases, (e.g., rheumatoid arthritis), and genetic factors [51]. Extrinsic factors are external stimuli, such as, physical load, environment, occupation, and training [51].

15.3.2 Healing

Understanding the events of healing in tendons and ligaments is important because tissue engineering techniques attempt to mimic or promote the environment and events of this process. Healing of tendon and ligaments after traumatic injury occurs in three overlapping phases: inflammatory, proliferation, and remodeling [28, 52]. The inflammatory phase occurs immediately after the injury. A hematoma is formed and erythrocytes and leukocytes are recruited. Within the first 24 hours, monocytes and macrophages release pro-inflammatory chemicals to increase vascular permeability, initiate angiogenesis, and attract fibroblasts at the site of injury. An increase in water, collagen type III, glycosaminoglycans, and fibronectin is observed, which stabilizes the formation of new ECM [3].

After a few days, the proliferation phase begins, marked by active fibroblast matrix synthesis [3]. The newly formed ECM exists as a disorganized network; collagen type III formation peaks during this phase and water and glycosaminoglycan concentrations remain high [53]. It is believed that these changes help optimize collagen synthesis and the gradual conversion from collagen type III to collagen type I [42, 54]. The healing tissue can remain in the proliferation stage for up to 6 weeks [52].

The last phase, remodeling, is characterized as having decreased fibroblast size and slowed matrix synthesis. The collagen fibers align themselves along the long axis of the tendon. Collagen type I content and crosslinking increases, and glycosaminoglycan, water, and DNA content have returned to levels of a normal tissue. The healing tissue can take up to a year to develop the functional strength of the uninjured tissue [54, 55].

15.3.3 Current Reconstruction Techniques

The standard treatment for tissue replacement uses autografts [56–58]. This procedure has shown to improve cell proliferation, promote new tissue growth, and initially exhibit sufficient mechanical strength for normal function [4, 23, 59]. However, over time, an anterior cruciate ligament (ACL) autograft is not capable of providing complete stabilization to the knee under torsion loads [28]. This failure may be caused by the lack of revascularization at the injury site, which is necessary for long-term success of the surgical graft. Lastly, there is a scarce availability of tissue because this procedure takes tissue from the injured patient, creating the limitation of donor site morbidity [4, 27, 59–61] Another procedure for tissue replacement uses allografts [27, 60]. Tissues are often taken from cadaver patellar tendon, hamstring tendon, or Achilles tendon [4, 60]. Although this procedure eliminates the limitation of donor site morbidity, it carries the risk for disease transmission and is subject to limited availability [60–62]. Additionally, sterilization of allografts to prevent an immune response alters the mechanical properties of the tissue [4, 60]. Furthermore, graft surgeries do not address replacement of the tendon or ligament to bone interface [63, 64].

15.4 Tissue Engineering of Fibrous Tissues

In response to the aforementioned limitations of tissue grafts, a myriad of means to engineer tendons and ligaments has been developed over the past 15 years. Ideally, tissue engineering methods will regenerate injured tissue to sufficient mechanical strength to restore function and promote cell growth [27]. Approaches examined to date include using varied cell types seeded on both natural and synthetic biomaterials. Additionally, such constructs may be further stimulated with biological and/or mechanical signals. Each of these key aspects in tendon and ligament tissue engineering is discussed in depth in this section.

15.4.1 Cells

A main component of the tissue engineering approach to regeneration of fibrous tissues is the availability of appropriate cells. The presence of cells is imperative to remodeling because they promote proliferation, cell-cell signaling, and ECM formation. Fibroblasts are the main cell type found in tendons and ligaments. Many laboratories have developed fibroblast-seeded scaffolds and have successfully shown that fibroblasts can adhere and proliferate on a variety of materials [65–68]. These cells secrete typical tendon and ligament ECM molecules, such as collagen type I, III, and proteoglycans. One concern with using this cell type is the availability of native tendon and ligament fibroblasts because they are difficult to harvest without using invasive surgery [27].

Another potential cell source for tissue regeneration is dermal fibroblasts. This cell type can be easily obtained from the skin, which eliminates availability issues. It has been shown that these cells can adhere to and proliferate on collagen fiber scaffolds and silk sheets [69–71]. One study has shown that dermal fibroblasts have the ability to proliferate faster than native ligament counterparts when cultured *in vitro* and *in vivo* [68]. Autologous ACL and skin fibroblasts were retrieved from rabbits, labeled, seeded onto a collagen fiber scaffold, and incubated *in vitro*. The results revealed that after 3 days, the number of skin fibroblasts attached to the fiber scaffold was significantly more than the numbers of attached autologous fibroblast, suggesting increased cell proliferation [68]. After incubation, fibroblast-seeded collagen fiber scaffolds were implanted into the knee joints of the rabbits that served as cell donors. Viable dermal fibroblasts remained attached to the scaffold for at least 4 weeks. Dermal fibroblasts have also been shown to upregulate gene expression and secrete tendon and ligament ECM components like collagen type I and III when treated with growth factors [72, 73]. Although experiments involving dermal fibroblasts have shown positive results for cell proliferation and ECM formation [74], concerns remain about whether dermal fibroblasts will behave similarly to native tendon/ligament fibroblasts after transplantation into a new environment.

Stem cells have also been extensively explored for orthopedic tissue engineering applications. For fibrous tissue regeneration, mesenchymal stem cells (MSCs) from bone marrow sources have been widely investigated [9, 75]. MSCs can differentiate into osteoblasts, chondrocytes, myoblasts, and adipocytes, as well as tendon/ligament fibroblasts [76, 77]. One study has shown that a collagen type I construct seeded with bone marrow-derived MSCs had greater structural and material properties than constructs without cell seeding [78]. These constructs were implanted in defect rabbit Achilles tendons and evaluated 4, 8, and 12 weeks later via biochemical analysis and examination of fiber structural organization. Over time, MSC-seeded constructs resulted in better alignment of cells and collagen fibers than the unseeded controls [78]. Another experiment studied the mechanical properties of MSC-seeded collagen type I gels implanted in injured rabbit patellar tendons [75]. Four weeks after implantation, maximum stress, Young's modulus, and strain energy density were significantly increased over the unseeded implant controls. Results also revealed an increased number of tenocytes and the formation of a larger collagen fiber bundle in the MSC-seeded implants [75]. These studies concluded that MSCs delivered to an injury site can improve the biomechanics, structure, and overall function of the tissue [75, 78].

MSCs can also adhere to and proliferate on scaffolds and secrete ECM molecules found in native tendon and ligament tissue [79–82]. Human MSCs seeded on RGD-modified silk scaffold and incubated *in vitro* for 21 days demonstrated upregulation of gene expression for collagen type I, collagen type III, and tenascin-C by day 14 [81]. MSCs have also been shown to improve wound healing, as seen by the increased mechanical properties and increased cell and fiber organization 26 weeks after implantation into a patellar tendon gap defect in a rabbit model [80, 83].

In sum, these findings suggest that MSCs are good candidates for tendon and ligament tissue engineering [84]. However, specific genes and/or surface markers that define a MSC from other stromal-derived cells have not been identified, which may pose problems in confirming purity of cell source [85]. Similarly, before MSCs can be used consistently for tendon/ligament tissue regeneration, specific protocols must be developed to promote MSC differentiation toward a fibroblastic lineage, while suppressing differentiation towards other cell types.

Another cell source for fibrous tissue engineering is MSCs derived from human embryonic stem cells (hESCs) [86]. hESCs are cells from an early embryo that can be expanded nearly indefinitely while in the undifferentiated state and have the ability to develop into any cell type in the body [87]. One study investigated the potential of hESC-derived MSCs (hESC-MSCs) for tendon regeneration [88]. The cells were formed into sheets *in vitro*, creating engineered tendons that were implanted into defect patellar tendons in rats. After 4 weeks, hESC-MSC tendon implants showed more collagen fiber formation than in fibrin-treated controls and the tissue appeared to be dense with higher cell numbers with spindle-like morphologies [88]. Using cell-labeling techniques, hESC-MSCs were seen to be distributed around the injury site 2 weeks after implementation. These cells, under microscopy, were characterized as having spindle-like morphologies and were oriented along the direction of mechanical force. From real time-polymerase chain reaction (RT-PCR) analysis, it was seen that collagen type III, collagen type XIV, and tenascin-C had high gene expression after 2 weeks, indicating that these cells were able to improve tendon repair through upregulation of ECM molecules [88]. Gene expression of two key growth factors for tendon healing, TGF-β3 and basic fibroblast growth factor (bFGF), was also detected 2 weeks after implantation, suggesting that hESC-MSC are able to promote repair in part through expression of soluble factors [88]. One major challenge of using hESCs themselves in fibrous tissue engineering is that their pluripotency and self-renewal causes concern for spontaneous differentiation and the resulting formation of teratomas, a benign tumor composed of various cell types [89]. Therefore, an intermediate step to differentiate hESCs into multipotent cells, such as the MSCs examined in this study, may be required before this cell type can be applied *in vivo*.

15.4.2 *Scaffolds*

Scaffolds may be used to deliver cells and provide a structural support at a site of injury. Scaffolds must allow for cell attachment, contain pores for secretion of appropriate ECM molecules, allow bioactive molecules to access the cells, integrate into the injured tissue area, and have the ability to translate mechanical cues from the environment to the engineered construct [90]. Integration into the tissue is achieved by designing biodegradable materials that degrade at the same rate new tissue is formed [27].

Poly(esters) are a common synthetic scaffold material for tendon and ligament tissue engineering. This class of fibers can be manipulated to form woven matrices that enhance mechanical strength [91]. Polymer degradation is achieved hydrolytically and the byproducts are metabolically removed or remain inert. The most common poly(esters) include poly(lactic acid) (PLA), poly(glycolic acid) (PGA), and poly(lactic-co-glycolic acid) (PLGA) [92]. A study using a twisted PLA scaffold seeded with human MSCs resulted in upregulation of collagen type I, tenascin-C, and decorin gene expression after 15 days in culture [93]. These results suggest that a PLA scaffold allowed for homogenous cell seeding and fibroblastic gene expression, making this material a promising scaffold candidate for ligament tissue engineering. Another study using PGA as a scaffolding material reported the ability to restore mechanical capacity of tendon gap defects in a hen flexor tendon model [94]. After 14 weeks, histology revealed that the engineered PGA scaffold with autologous tenocytes had undistinguishable structure to native tendon tissue and biomechanical analysis demonstrated higher breaking strength of PGA scaffolds comparable to normal tendon strength [94]. Lastly, knitted PLGA seeded with bone marrow stromal cells implanted into an Achilles tendon gap defect in rabbits demonstrated tissue regeneration and improved mechanical properties after 12 weeks [95]. Immunohistochemical assays revealed the formation of collagen type I and collagen type III fibers in regenerated tissue and mechanical testing characterized the scaffold construct as having a tensile modulus similar to that of a normal tendon control [95]. Synthetic polymers are advantageous because the composition of the material can be easily controlled [92]. These biomaterials are easy to tailor for specific applications and are more readily available than natural materials because they can be synthesized in a laboratory setting. However, because synthetic materials are not found in native tissue, they have less ability to direct tissue growth without further biological modification [96].

In contrast, naturally based scaffolds are advantageous over synthetic materials because many are already found in the body, therefore it is believed that these materials may incorporate and be remodeled more like native tissues [92]. In addition, many already possess bioactive molecules that can interact with seeded cells. However, unlike synthetics, one drawback of naturally based materials is that it may be difficult to obtain large enough amounts of pure product for clinical scale-up [96]. Since collagen composes the bulk of fibrous tissues for tendon and ligament applications, natural scaffold materials often utilize collagen fibers in the form of a porous sponge. MSCs seeded on these materials have increased ECM gene expression and protein deposition both *in vitro* and after *in vivo* implantation in rabbit patellar and Achilles tendon [97–99]. However, collagen fibers acquired from animals must be processed to remove foreign pathogens to minimize disease transmission [91]. Collagen can also easily be degraded, which causes the matrix to rapidly lose mechanical strength [91, 100]. Crosslinking can slow down the process of degradation and the rate of mechanical property loss. However, this technique can introduce potential toxic residues in the form of crosslinking agents [91].

Silk, a protein fiber from silkworms, can also be used as a naturally derived scaffold for tendon and ligament tissue engineering. Silk is composed of a fibroin core and a glue-like sericin cover. Silk fibers have high Young's modulus values when compared to PLA and collagen [101] and undergo relatively slow proteolytic degradation *in vivo* [27]. However, over long periods of time, degradation is mediated by a foreign body response. In one study, 12 weeks after silk was implanted in the abdomen wall of a rabbit, tensile strength of the fibers decreased 80% from their original value and histology revealed a decrease in number of fibers over 2 years [102]. While the mechanical properties of silk are promising, there is a concern of the potential negative immune response because it is not a native material found in the body [79, 91].

15.4.3 Exogenous Factors

A number of biochemical and mechanical signals can be used to manipulate cell and scaffold interactions for fibrous tissue engineering. Various exogenous factors have been identified that improve tendon and ligament cell proliferation and matrix formation *in vitro* and *in vivo* [8], which could be harnessed to improve production of engineered tendon/ligaments *in vivo* or *ex vivo*. This section discusses both soluble factors (i.e., growth factors) that improve cellular response and the use of bioreactors to create controlled culture systems for tissue-engineered cell and scaffold constructs.

15.4.3.1 Soluble Factors

TGF-β, platelet-derived growth factor (PDGF), bFGF, and insulin-like growth factor-1(IGF-1) have all shown to upregulate fibroblast proliferation and ECM production [73, 103, 104].

TGF-β: TGF-β increases collagen and proteoglycan gene expression and synthesis in fibroblasts [105–107]. *In vitro* studies have examined the effects of the introduction of TGF-β1 at different concentrations (0.12–25 ng/mL) in culture media [72]. Human dermal fibroblasts showed a significant increase in gene expression of collagen type III after 3 days [72]. In another study, proteoglycan production of canine ligament fibroblast was measured via gel filtration chromatography [107]. After 24 hours, cells cultured with a 1 μg/mL solution of TGF-β1 resulted in significantly higher proteoglycan synthesis than the growth factor-free control [107]. *In vivo* studies have also been performed to evaluate the effects of growth factors on healing of an injured ACL [108]. TGF-β1 was administered to rabbits at the site of an overstretched injury in the right ACL. After 12 weeks, results revealed that the application of 4 ng of TGF-β1 significantly enhanced the healing in the injured site, as seen through increased stiffness of the tissue and increased maximum load values [108]. It is suggested that this is the result of increased collagen type I production in the matrix network.

PDGF: An *in vitro* study with a canine model was performed to examine the effects of single and combined growth factors on cell proliferation and collagen production. Fibroblasts isolated from the intrasynovial flexor tendon were cultured in media containing 10 ng/mL of PDGF and/or 10 ng/mL bFGF. After cell culture for 24 houes, cell proliferation, determined via thymidine incorporation, in the presence of PDGF increased 13-fold when compared to the no-growth factor control [73]. When PDGF and bFGF were combined, both cell proliferation and collagen synthesis, measured by 3H-proline incorporation, increased in a dose-dependent manner from 5 to 40 ng/mL [73].

It has been shown that PDGF increases mechanical properties of ligament tissue *in vivo* [109]. This study used a rabbit model to introduce PDGF at concentrations of 400 ng and 20 μg into the ruptured right medial collateral ligament. After 6 weeks, results demonstrated that both doses of PDGF caused a significant increase in cross sectional area when compared to the negative-growth factor control [109]. Stiffness and ultimate elongation values were significantly higher than the control values for 20 μg dose of PDGF, suggesting that the growth factor enhanced structural properties during healing [109].

bFGF: As evidenced in the study described above, bFGF can stimulate cell proliferation [73]. In addition, bFGF increases migration of rat tendon fibroblasts in an *in vitro* wound model at dosages ranging from 0–50 μg/L. At 10 μg/L, bFGF "wound" closure was most accelerated. Through measurement of 5-bromo-2-deoxyuridine incorporation, the mechanism for this process was identified as cell proliferation [110].

IGF-1: IGF-1 acts to promote matrix synthesis and cell proliferation [111–113]. IGF-1 mRNA and protein levels have been shown to increase at injury sites in soft tissues. This upregulation can help the healing process because IGF-1 increases proliferation activity that is associated with the inflammatory and proliferation stages of healing [104].

Growth factors also play a role in MSC maintenance and differentiation. The previously mentioned growth factors have all shown to increase MSC growth and tendon/ligament ECM production [114–116]. In addition, growth and differentiation factors (GDF) 5, 6 and 7, classified in the bone morphogenetic protein (BMP) family, play a major role in tendon and ligament differentiation.

GDF 5, 6, 7: *In vivo* studies have shown that injection of GDF 5, 6, and 7 improve healing capacity of injured tendons in rats and rabbits [117–120]. In a rat model, GDF 5 and GDF 6 at concentrations of 0, 1, and 10 μg were soaked on a collagen sponge. After 14 days, it was seen that failure loads increased for rat Achilles tendons implanted with the treated sponge when compared to untreated collagen sponge controls. Histology revealed that the application of GDF 5 and GDF 6 resulted in cell-abundant regions distributed around the collagen sponge [117].

The introduction of these factors can also promote new tendon and ligament tissue formation [121]. Another study used GDF 5, 6, and 7 implanted subcutaneously and in the quadriceps muscle of rat models. In the subcutaneous implant, after 21 days, light microscopy and electron microscopy were utilized to observe collagen type I with structure resembling newly formed tendon tissue. Northern blot analysis and PCR revealed mRNA expression of elastin, decorin, and collagen type I [121]. When implanted into the quadriceps muscle, light microscopy images confirmed crimped neotendon-/neoligament-like tissue formation in GDF implants after 10 days [121]. Overall, the results of this study support that GDF 5, 6, and 7 can influence differentiation of connective tissue precursor cells to tendon and ligament cells.

Growth factor experiments have shown success in promoting cell proliferation, differentiation, and matrix production in a variety of both *in vitro* and *in vivo* models of tendon/ligament healing. However, further studies must be undertaken to better understand the specific intracellular pathways involved and the effects of combining different growth factors simultaneously or in a temporally controlled manner before optimal growth factor regimens for improving fibrous tissue production from cell-scaffold constructs can be identified.

15.4.3.2 Bioreactors

To improve tissue formation within cell-scaffold constructs, bioreactor culture systems have been explored for a variety of tissue engineering applications. Bioreactors can be divided into two classes: constructs that can be directly implanted into the body and the *in vivo* environment acts as the bioreactor, or constructs that can be placed in an *ex vivo* cell culture system to control and maintain the biochemical and physical environment [8]. An *in vivo* bioreactor system provides a native environment for cell culture, but fine control of signals is lost and understanding of regulatory pathways is not clear. An *ex vivo* bioreactor allows for the control and introduction of biochemical and physical signals, which can help promote cell proliferation, differentiation, and tissue development. In particular, *ex vivo* tensile stimulation has been reported to induce cellular proliferation, fibroblastic differentiation, cellular alignment, and ECM synthesis and remodeling [122–125]. In addition, this type of bioreactor may, in turn, provide better understanding of tissue development associated mechanosensitive signaling pathways. However, concern remains over scalability of *ex vivo* bioreactors for clinical scale production of engineered constructs.

Cells can respond differently when cultured in a two-dimensional (2D) or a three-dimensional (3D) system [126]. 2D culture allows for confluent and uniform cell seeding, but does not create an environment similar to the native tissue environment, while 3D cultures can more closely mimic natural tissue architecture. In a bioreactor, a 3D environment allows mechanical stimulation to be uniform across and through the scaffold. Mechanical stimulation in the form of cyclic tensile stress has been recently identified as a critical component in the tissue engineering approach for tendon and ligament regeneration [127]. The widely used Tissue Train® culture system is a method for culture that provides tensile loading of cells in a 3D matrix or hydrogel [128]. The system consists of a loading well plate to first seed the matrix or gel and cells on a flexible membrane. The loading well plate is removed and a loading post is attached. When a vacuum is applied to the loading post, the membrane deforms the sides of the flexible membrane and, thus, the construct undergoes uniaxial strain [129]. In one study using this system for tendon/ligament applications, avian tendon fibroblasts were suspended in a collagen type I gel in each well of the culture plates. The loading regimen consisted of uniaxial cyclic strain of 1% at 1 Hz for 1 hour/day up to 11 days. Histological staining revealed cells aligned in the direction of the axial load, similar to what is found in native tendon tissue. Mechanical testing also revealed that the elastic modulus increased over time with strain and the ultimate tensile strength was significantly higher than that of the non-loaded controls [129].

In other experiments using bioreactors for tensile stimulation, human patellar tendon fibroblasts were cultured and seeded on micro-grooved silicone surfaces and subject to uniaxial stretch at 0, 4, and 8% at 0.5 Hz for 4 h. After stretching, cells were incubated statically for 4 hours and then analysis was performed. RT-PCR results revealed that stretching induced increased gene expression of collagen type I and collagen type III. Enzyme-linked immunosorbent assays (ELISA) of proteins released into the media also indicated increases in collagen type I in the media for stretched cells [122]. The results of this study confirm that strain is necessary for fibroblast ECM protein expression. The stimulation of cyclic loading is also necessary for fibroblasts to adopt an elongated spindle shape that is seen in native fibroblasts [123, 130].

MSCs under mechanical strain have also been shown to increase fibrous tissue ECM gene expression and protein production [27, 115, 127, 131, 132]. In one study that applied a 10% translational followed by a 25% rotational strain on collagen gels seeded with bone marrow-derived cells for 14 days, real time RT-PCR results indicated collagen type I, collagen type III, and tenascin-C were upregulated in strained samples when compared to the baseline measurements of the control group and immunostaining images detected the presence of collagen type I and III. In addition, mechanically stimulated constructs did not show an upregulation of typical markers for bone and cartilage (i.e., bone sialoprotein and collagen type II) [132].

15.5 Tissue Engineering of Fibrous Tissue Interfaces with Bone

The enthesis, or site of attachment of the tendon or ligament to the bone, is a common focus of tissue overuse injuries that can lead to rupture [133]. Engineering fibrous tissue-bone interfaces is challenging as constructs must address the required mechanical properties and physiology of two very disparate tissues. The native interfacial tissue's fibrocartilaginous composition also differs significantly from the tissues on either side (tendon/ligament and bone). However, enthesis tissue engineering is similar to regenerating the midsubstance of the tendon or ligament in that cells, scaffolds, and exogenous factors have been explored to recreate the insertion site, although more complex combinations of these basic elements may be required than for regular fibrous tissue engineering. This section will discuss concepts of co-culture of different cell types, phasic and gradient scaffolds, and delivery of soluble factors to regenerate the transition from fibrous tissue to bone.

15.5.1 Cells

Co-culture methods enable the interaction between two different cell populations in a controlled system. Such systems have been proposed to aid interface tissue engineering, as well as understanding the developmental processes resulting in the formation of the fibrous tissue-bone insertion [46]. At the tendon-/ligament-bone insertion site, fibroblasts, chondrocytes, hypertrophic chondrocytes, and osteoblasts have been identified [12, 13, 18, 134]. A study performed using a co-culture of monolayer bovine osteoblasts with a condensed micromass of bovine chondrocytes found that, over 21 days *in vitro*, cell number remained constant over time for both cell types. In addition, there was little glycosaminoglycan deposition present in co-culture experiments when compared to the chondrocyte culture control, and alkaline phosphatase activity remained constant over time, as opposed to increasing over time in the osteoblast-only control. It was shown that co-culture had no effect on osteoblast collagen type I gene expression, but mineralization was delayed [135]. These results suggest that the interactions between the two cell types affect the phenotype of both cells; however, further studies need to be performed to understand the type of specific interactions that are responsible for the alterations observed.

Co-culture experiments have also been performed utilizing bovine ACL fibroblasts and osteoblasts from trabecular bone fragments of neonatal calves [136]. This co-culture model was created in a tissue culture well with a permeable hydrogel divider in the middle. By day 7, fibroblasts and osteoblasts had migrated to the interface region of the hydrogel. Alkaline phosphatase activity in the co-culture peaked at day 14 and decreased through day 28, whereas the osteoblast control culture demonstrated increasing intensity of alkaline phosphatase staining over 28 days. Glycosaminoglycan deposition (measured by Alcian Blue staining) did not change over time in the co-culture and collagen type II and aggrecan expression (measured by RT-PCR) were elevated after 28 days [136]. Mineralization was also observed to remain relatively low levels in the co-culture samples. The results of the study indicate that co-culture may be an important aspect to include for creation of the fibrocartilaginous tissue that is found at the insertion point. However, further experiments examining additional cell types and/or soluble factors to improve the amount and integration of this fibrocartilaginous tissue with juxtaposing bone and fibrous tissues are needed before engineering of a more complete fibrous tissue-bone interface can be achieved.

15.5.2 *Scaffolds*

The scaffold design for an interface region needs to recapitulate the complex structure of the native tendon/ligament to bone insertion site. The scaffold should exhibit a gradient of structural and mechanical properties that mimics the native tissue [137]. A stratified or multi-phased scaffold is able to achieve this characteristic. Scaffold phases must also have the ability to integrate into the native tissue after implantation. This can be achieved by using gradually degradable biomaterials. A study has been performed to develop a triphasic scaffold with co-culture for the ligament-bone interface [138]. This scaffold is modeled after the native structure, in which “Phase A” was designed with a PLGA mesh for fibrous tissue formation and seeded with human fibroblasts, “Phase B” contained PLGA microspheres for fibrocartilage culture, and “Phase C” utilized sintered PLGA and bioactive glass with human osteoblasts for bone formation. After 42 days, fibroblast and osteoblast cells migrated to “Phase B” and increased matrix production similar to the interface region, while cell specific matrices were secreted for “Phase A” and “Phase C” [138]. When a triphasic system with tri-culture of bovine fibroblasts in “Phase A,” chondrocytes in “Phase B,” and osteoblasts in “Phase C” was implanted *in vivo* in a subcutaneous rat model, matrix production compensated for the decrease in mechanical properties of a degrading scaffold and phase specific controlled matrix heterogeneity was maintained 2 months after implantation [139]. These results show that stratified scaffolds have the potential to promote multiple zones of tissue regeneration in a single scaffold system [137].

As an alternative to a construct containing discrete phases, a graded scaffold has also been examined for fibrous tissue-bone interface regeneration [140]. This gradient was achieved by controlling the location of a retrovirus for osteogenic transcription factor Runx2/Cbfa1 on a collagen I scaffold. Dermal rat fibroblasts were seeded on these scaffolds and osteogenic and fibroblastic cell activity was studied. After 42 days of *in vitro* culture, microCT imaging revealed zonal organization of mineral deposition and fibroblastic ECM on the graded scaffold. Quantitative RT-PCR confirmed upregulated expression of osteogenic specific markers in fibroblasts at regions of dense retroviral coating. These constructs were then implanted into ectopic subcutaneous sites of syngeneic rats. After 14 days *in vivo*, microCT imaging revealed mineral deposition was present in areas of high retroviral coating only. This experiment demonstrates proof-of-concept evidence for a means to create a single scaffold that can exhibit properties of a native interface region containing graded mineralization.

Phasic and gradient scaffolds both aim to recreate the tendon/ligament to bone interface. Phasic scaffolds are limited by the lack of continuous transitions between different zones. However, the gradient scaffolds developed to date pose the problem of requiring gene transfection agents to achieve the desired biological outcome. While promising early results have been obtained, for both techniques, reestablishment and regeneration of the interface region has not been successfully shown *in vivo*, therefore additional experiments are required. Effects of biological, physical, and chemical stimulation on these constructs also have not been explored [137]. Therefore, significant further work in this area is required before these approaches could be implemented clinically for interface regeneration.

15.5.3 Soluble Factors

The growth factor BMP-2 has been shown to stimulate tendon-/ligament-bone interface healing [141–143]. BMP-2 was incorporated into a poly(ethylene glycol) (PEG)/hyaluronic acid hydrogel with periosteal progenitor cells to direct fibrocartilaginous attachment and new bone formation in a healing tendon model [141]. This construct was implanted in the knee joints of white rabbits for up to 6 weeks. After this time, RT-PCR revealed that osteogenic markers of collagen type I and osteopontin were present, and the cartilage specific markers of collagen type II and aggrecan were expressed. Histological findings demonstrated that in hydrogels with BMP-2, the graft interface contained organized collagen fibers and Sharpy-like fibers after 3 weeks [141]. This study suggests improved graft fixation may be achieved clinically with a BMP delivered from a PEG-based hydrogel.

Another study aimed to develop a method for improving the integration of grafts for the replacement of ACL. Semitendinosus tendon grafts were infected with a retroviral adenovirus-BMP-2. These tendon grafts were implanted and replaced the native ACLs of rabbits [142]. Over the course of 8 weeks after surgery, a four-zone interface was histologically visible and higher failure loads and stiffness levels when compared to grafts without BMP-2 were observed [142]. Overall, this study demonstrates the potential of BMP-2 gene transfer to improve the integration of tendon grafts to bone after reconstruction surgery.

Delivery of soluble factors has been a recent advance in engineering fibrous tissue interfaces and, as the above studies indicate, holds promise in enhancing current graft fixation and providing possible means to create fully integrated tissue-engineered bone-ligament-bone grafts. However, further experiments are required to better understand the signaling pathways involved and the effects of temporal combinations of growth factors on tissue formation, bone tunnel healing, and graft fixation in order to further optimize these approaches.

15.6 Conclusions

When rupture of tendon or ligaments occurs, graft surgeries can be performed to restore function. However, these grafts are often not able to recreate original mechanical properties, such as ultimate strength and elongation [4]. For this reason, tissue engineering approaches have been investigated that possess the potential to overcome the shortcomings of surgical procedures by fully restoring the native tissue architecture and composition, including the fibrous tissue to bone interface.

Fibrous tissue engineering utilizes cells, scaffolds, and/or exogenous factors in various combinations. Cell types most commonly investigated include autologous fibroblasts, dermal fibroblasts, and MSCs because they have demonstrated secretion of tendon-/ligament-specific matrix molecules under the proper culture conditions [74]. Both natural and synthetic scaffolds can act as cell carriers at a site of injury, but must be optimized to facilitate cell attachment, differentiation, and upregulation and secretion of ECM components while providing sufficient mechanical stability at the defect site. Lastly, exogenous factors, such as growth factors and bioreactor systems, have been explored to enhance cell culture environments and promote tissue regeneration both *in vivo* and *ex vivo*.

While the means to regenerate fibrous tissues has been extensively studied, engineering of the fibrous tissue interface to bone has not been explored in the same depth. Interface tissue engineering has significant implications because current graft surgeries do not restore interface structure or function [63, 64]. Similar to engineering fibrous tissues, interface engineering combines cells, scaffolds, and exogenous factors, although more complex construct designs may be required than for regular fibrous tissue engineering.

Many challenges remain before the ultimate goal of recreating tendon/ligaments and their interfaces can be achieved. In addition to identifying a cell source with appropriate expansion capabilities and a scaffold with proper degradation and biological activity, it is difficult to fully implement a protocol for introducing exogenous factors such as growth factors or mechanical stimulation when understanding of the signaling pathways by which these stimuli act has not been fully elucidated. While results of proof-of-concept experiments are promising, tendon-/ligament-bone interface tissue engineering provides an additional set of design constraints in order to create regions that vary in mechanical properties and composition. Therefore, the current combination of cells and scaffolds must be optimized *in vitro* and further *in vivo* studies must be performed to confirm the efficacy of these methods in restoring the transitional region.

While these challenges may appear daunting, recent advances in scaffold synthesis and fabrication, basic biological understanding of both tendon and ligament development as well as signaling pathways underlying mechanotransduction, and identification of new potential cell sources hold promise to address the limitations of current tissue-engineered constructs. Therefore, continued interdisciplinary research to create the next generation of approaches that harness new findings from such disparate fields as materials science, chemical and mechanical engineering, and cell biology will undoubtedly lead to greatly improved tissue engineering-based therapies for tendon and ligament injuries as well as promote quick and efficient translation for future clinical use.

Acknowledgments The authors would like to thank Dr. Yongzhi Qiu and Dr. Peter J. Yang for their contributions to the figures depicted in this chapter.

References

1. Praemer A, Furner S, Rice D (1999) Musculoskeletal condition in the United States. American academy of orthopaedic surgeons. American Academy of Orthopaedic Surgeons, Parke Ridge, IL
2. Bray RC, Rangayyan RM, Frank CB (1996) Normal and healing ligament vascularity: a quantitative histological assessment in the adult rabbit medial collateral ligament. J Anat 188:87–95
3. Lin T, Cardenas L, Soslowsky LJ (2004) Biomechanics of tendon injury and repair. J Biomech 37(6):865–877
4. Laurencin CT, Freeman JW (2005) Ligament tissue engineering: an evolutionary materials science approach. Biomaterials 26(36):7530–7536
5. Tadokoro K, Matsui N, Yagi M, Kuroda R, Kurosaka M, Yoshiya S (2004) Evaluation of hamstring strength and tendon regrowth after harvesting for anterior cruciate ligament reconstruction. Am J Sports Med 32(7):1644–1650
6. Chiou HM, Chang MC, Lo WH (1997) One-stage reconstruction of skin defect and patellar tendon rupture after total knee arthroplasty—a new technique. J Arthroplasty 12(5):575–579
7. Yang PJ, Temenoff JS (2009) Engineering orthopedic tissue interfaces. Tissue Eng Part B Rev 15(2):127–141
8. Goh JCH, Ouyang H-W, Teoh SH, Chan CKC, Lee EH (2003) Tissue-engineering approach to the repair and regeneration of tendons and ligaments. Tissue Eng 9(Suppl 1):31–44
9. Khatod M, Amiel D (2003) Ligament biochemistry and physiology. In: Pedowitz R, O'Connor JJ, Akeson WH (eds) Daniel's knee injuries, 2nd edn. Lippincott Williams & Wilkins, Philadelphia, PA, pp 31–42
10. Wang JH (2006) Mechanobiology of tendon. J Biomech 39(9):1563–1582
11. Hoffman A, Gross G (2007) Tendon and ligament engineering in the adult organism: mesenchymal stem cells and gene-therapeutic approaches. Int Orthop 31(6):791–797
12. Lim J, Temenoff JS (2009) Tendon and ligament tissue engineering: restoring tendon/ ligament and its interface. In: Meyer U, Handschel J, Meyer T, Wiesmann HP (eds) Fundamentals of tissue engineering and regenerative medicine. Springer, Berlin, pp 254–269
13. Doroski DM, Brink KS, Temenoff JS (2007) Techniques for biological characterization of tissue-engineered tendon and ligament. Biomaterials 28(2):187–202
14. Hammoudi TM, Temenoff JS (2011) Biomaterials for regeneration of tendons and ligaments. In: Burdick JA, Mauck RL (eds) Biomaterials for tissue engineering applications. Springer, Berlin, pp 307–341
15. Birk DE, Mayne R (1997) Localization of collagen types I, III and V during tendon development. changes in collagen types I and III are correlated with changes in fibril diameter. Eur J Cell Biol 72(4):352–361
16. Benjamin M, Ralphs JR (2000) The cell and developmental biology of tendons and ligaments. Int Rev Cytol 196:85–130

17. Riley G (2003) The pathogenesis of tendinopathy: a molecular perspective. Rheumatology 43 (2):131–142
18. Laurencin CT, Ambrosio AMA, Borden MD, Cooper JA (1999) Tissue engineering: orthopedic applications. Annu Rev Biomed Eng 1:19–46
19. McNeilly CM (1997) Tendon cells *in vivo* form a three dimensional network of cell processes linked by gap junctions. J Anat 190:477–478
20. Liu SH, Yang RS, Alshaikh R, Lane JM (1995) Collagen in tendon, ligament, and bone healing—a current review. Clin Orthop Relat Res 318:265–278
21. Martin RB, Burr DB, Sharkey NA (1998) Mechanical properties of ligament and tendon. In: Martin RB, Burr DB, Sharkey NA (eds) Skeletal tissue mechanics. Springer, New York, NY, pp 309–346
22. Wang JHC, Losifidis MI, Fu FH (2006) Biomechanical basis for tendinopathy. Clin Orthop Relat Res 443:320–332
23. Woo SLY, Debski RE, Zeminski J, Abramowitch SD, Saw SSC, Fenwick JA (2000) Injury and repair of ligaments and tendons. Annu Rev Biomed Eng 2:83–118
24. James R, Kesturu G, Balian G, Chhabra A (2008) Tendon: biology, biomechanics, repair, growth factors, and evolving treatment options. J Hand Surg Am 33(1):102–112
25. Yoon JH, Halper J (2005) Tendon proteoglycans: biochemistry and function. J Musculoskelet Neuronal Interact 5(1):22–34
26. Birk DE, Fitch JM, Babiarz JP, Doane KJ, Linsenmayer TF (1990) Collagen fibrillogenesis *in vitro*: interaction of types I and V collagen regulates fibril diameter. J Cell Sci 95 (4):649–657
27. Vunjak-Novakovic G, Altman G, Horan R, Kaplan DL (2004) Tissue engineering of ligaments. Annu Rev Biomed Eng 6(1):131–156
28. Woo SLY, Abramowitch SD, Kilger R, Liang R (2006) Biomechanics of knee ligaments: injury, healing, and repair. J Biomech 39(1):1–20
29. Danielson KG, Baribault H, Holmes DF, Graham H, Kadler KE, Iozzo RV (1997) Targeted disruption of decorin leads to abnormal collagen fibril morphology and skin fragility. J Cell Biol 136(3):729–743
30. McCormick RJ (1999) Extracellular modifications to muscle collagen: implications for meat quality. Poult Sci 78(5):785–791
31. Ezura Y, Chakravarti S, Oldberg A, Chervoneva I, Birk DE (2000) Differential expression of lumican and fibromodulin regulate collagen fibrillogenesis in developing mouse tendons. J Cell Biol 151(4):779–787
32. Border WA, Noble NA, Yamamoto T, Harper JR, Yamaguchi Y, Pierschbacher MD, Ruoslahti E (1992) Natural inhibitor of transforming growth factor-beta protects against scarring in experimental kidney disease. Nature 360(6402):361–364
33. Ruoslahti E, Yamaguchi Y (1991) Proteoglycans as modulators of growth factor activities. Cell 64(5):867–869
34. Elefteriou F, Exposito JY, Garrone R, Lethias C (2001) Binding of tenascin-X to decorin. FEBS Lett 495(1–2):44–47
35. Probstmeier R, Pesheva P (1999) Tenascin-C inhibits beta(1) integrin-dependent cell adhesion and neurite outgrowth on fibronectin by a disialoganglioside-mediated signaling mechanism. Glycobiology 9(2):101–114
36. Chiquet M, Reneda AS, Huber F, Fluck M (2003) How do fibroblasts translate mechanical signals into changes in extracellular matrix production? Matrix Biol 22(1):73–80
37. Chiquet-Ehrismann R, Tucker RP (2004) Connective tissues: signalling by tenascins. Int J Biochem Cell Biol 36(6):1085–1089
38. Grinnell F (1984) Fibronectin and wound healing. J Cell Biochem 26(2):107–116
39. Jozsa L, Lehto M, Kannus P, Kvist M, Reffy A, Vieno T, Jarvinen M, Demel S, Elek E (1989) Fibronectin and laminin in Achilles tendon. Acta Orthop Scand 60(4):469–471
40. Williams IF, McCullagh KG, Silver IA (1984) The distribution of types I and III collagen and fibronectin in the healing equine tendon. Connect Tissue Res 12(3–4):211–227

41. O'Brien M (1997) Structure and metabolism of tendons. Scand J Med Sci Sports 7(2):55–61
42. Woo SLY, Buckwalter JA (1988) AAOS/NIH/ORS workshop—injury and repair of the musculoskeletal soft tissues. Savannah, Georgia, June 18–20, 1987. J Orthop Res 6 (6):907–931
43. Benjamin M, Ralphs JR (1998) Fibrocartilage in tendons and ligaments–an adaptation to compressive load. J Anat 193:481–494
44. Woo SLY, Smith DW, Hildebrand KA, Zeminski JA, Johnson LA (1998) Engineering the healing of the rabbit medial collateral ligament. Med Biol Eng Comput 36(3):359–364
45. Moffat KL, Sun WHS, Pena PE, Chahine NO, Doty SB, Ateshian GA, Hung CT, Lu HH (2008) Characterization of the structure-function relationship at the ligament-to-bone interface. Proc Natl Acad Sci U S A 105(23):7947–7952
46. Lu H, Jiang J (2006) Interface tissue engineering and the formulation of multiple-tissue systems. Adv Biochem Eng Biotechnol 102:91–111
47. Jozsa LG, Kannus P (1997) Human tendons: anatomy, physiology, and pathology. Human Kinetics, Champaign, IL
48. Shrive NG, Thornton GM, Hart DA, Frank CB (2003) Ligament mechanics. In: Pedowitz R, O'Connor JJ, Akeson WH (eds) Daniel's knee injuries, 2nd edn. Lippincott Williams & Wilkins, Philadelphia, PA, pp 97–112
49. Hyman J, Rodeo SA (2000) Injury and repair of tendons and ligaments. Phys Med Rehabil Clin N Am 11(2):267–288
50. Benazzo F, Maffulli N (2000) An operative approach to Achilles tendinopathy. Sports Med Arthrosc 8:96–101
51. Rees JD, Wilson AM, Wolman RL (2006) Current concepts in the management of tendon disorders. Rheumatology 45:508–521
52. Sharma P (2005) Tendon injury and tendinopathy: healing and repair. J Bone Joint Surg Am 87(1):187–202
53. Oakes BW (2003) Tissue healing and repair: tendons and ligaments. In: Frontera WR (ed) Rehabilitation of sports injuries: scientific basis. Blackwell Science, Boston, MA, pp 8–21
54. Gomez MA (1995) The physiology and biochemistry of soft tissue healing. In: Griffin L (ed) Rehabilitation of the injured knee, 2nd edn. Mosby, St. Louis, MO, pp 34–44
55. Buckwalter JA, Hunziker EB (1996) Orthopaedics healing of bones, cartilage, tendons, and ligaments: a new era. Lancet 348(Suppl 2):18
56. Baer GS, Harner CD (2007) Clinical outcomes of allograft versus autograft in anterior cruciate ligament reconstruction. Clin Sports Med 26(4):661–681
57. Carey JL, Dunn WR, Dahm DL, Zeger SL, Spindler KP (2009) A systematic review of anterior cruciate ligament reconstruction with autograft compared with allograft. J Bone Joint Surg Am 91A(9):2242–2250
58. Krych AJ, Jackson JD, Hoskin TL, Dahm DL (2008) A meta-analysis of patellar tendon autograft versus patellar tendon allograft in anterior cruciate ligament reconstruction. Arthroscopy 24(3):292–298
59. Miller R, Azar F (2008) Knee injuries. In: Canale S, Beaty J (eds) Campbell's operative orthopaedics. Mosby Elsevier, Philadelphia, PA, pp 2346–2575
60. Spindler KP, Kuhn J, Freedman K, Matthews C, Dittus R, Harrell FJ (2004) Anterior cruciate ligament reconstruction autograft choice: bone-tendon-bone versus hamstring: does it really matter? A systemic review. Am J Sports Med 32(8):1986–1995
61. Petrigliano FA, McAllister DR, Wu BM (2006) Tissue engineering for anterior cruciate ligament reconstruction: a review of current strategies. Arthroscopy 22(4):441–451
62. Barber F (2003) Should allografts be used for routine anterior cruciate ligament reconstructions. Arthroscopy 19:421
63. Kruegerfranke M, Siebert CH, Scherzer S (1995) Surgical treatment of ruptures of the Achilles tendon: a review of long-term results. Br J Sports Med 29(2):121–125
64. Uhthoff HK, Trudel G, Himori K (2003) Relevance of pathology and basic research to the surgeon treating rotator cuff disease. J Orthop Sci 8(3):449–456

65. Huang D, Chang TF, Aggrawal A, Lee RC, Ehrlich HP (1993) Mechanism and dynamics of mechanical strengthening in ligament-equivalent fibroblast-populated collagen matrices. Annu Rev Biomed Eng 21:289
66. Dunn MG, Liesch JB, Tiku ML, Zawadsky JP (1995) Development of fibroblast-seeded ligament analogs for ACL reconstruction. J Biomed Mater Res 29(11):1363–1371
67. Goulet F, Germain L, Rancourt D, Caron C, Normand A, Auger FA (1975) Tendons and ligaments. In: Lanza RP, Langer R, Chick WL (eds) Principles of tissue engineering. R.G. Landes Academic, Austin, TX, pp 639–664
68. Bellincampi LD, Closkey RF, Prasad R, Zawadsky JP, Dunn MG (1998) Viability of fibroblast-seeded ligament analogs after autogenous implantation. J Orthop Res 16:414–420
69. Gentleman E, Lay AN, Dickerson DA, Nauman EA, Livesay GA, Dee KC (2003) Mechanical characterization of collagen fibers and scaffolds for tissue engineering. Biomaterials 24 (21):3805–3813
70. Gentleman E, Livesay GA, Dee KC, Nauman EA (2006) Development of ligament-like structural organization and properties in cell-seeded collagen scaffolds *in vitro*. Ann Biomed Eng 34(5):726–736
71. Takezawa T, Ozaki K, Takabayashi C (2007) Reconstruction of a hard connective tissue utilizing a pressed silk sheet and type-1 collagen as the scaffold for fibroblasts. Tissue Eng 13(6):1357–1366
72. Fawzi-Grancher S, DeIsla N, Faure F (2006) Optimization of biochemical condition and substrates *in vitro* for tissue engineering of ligament. Ann Rev Biomed Eng 34 (11):1767–1777
73. Thomopoulos S, Harwood FL, Silva MJ (2005) Effects of several growth factors on canine flexor tendon fibroblast proliferation and collagen synthesis *in vitro*. J Hand Surg Am 30 (3):441–447
74. Eijk FV, Saris DBF, Riesle J, Willems WJ, Van Blitterswijk CA, Verbout AJ, Dhert WJA (2004) Tissue engineering of ligaments: a comparison of bone marrow stromal cells, anterior cruciate ligament, and skin fibroblasts as cell source. Tissue Eng 10(5/6):893–903
75. Awad HA, Butler DL, Boivin GP, Smith FNL, Malaviya P, Huibregtse B, Caplan AI (1999) Autologous mesenchymal stem cell-mediated repair of tendon. Tissue Eng 5(3):267–277
76. Caplan AI (1991) Mesenchymal stem-cells. J Orthop Res 9(5):641–650
77. Caplan AI (1994) The mesengenic process. Clin Plast Surg 21(3):429–435
78. Young RG, Butler DL, Weber W, Caplan AI, Gordon SL, Fink DJ (1998) Use of mesenchymal stem cells in a collagen matrix for Achilles tendon repair. J Orthop Res 16(4):406–413
79. Altman GH, Horan RL, Lu HH, Moreau J, Martin I, Richmond JC, Kaplan DL (2002) Silk matrix for tissue engineered anterior cruciate ligaments. Biomaterials 23(20):4131–4141
80. Butler DL, Awad HA (1999) Perspective on cell and collagen composites for tendon repair. Clin Orthop Relat Res 367(Suppl 3):324–332
81. Chen J, Altman GH, Karageorgiou V (2003) Human bone marrow stromal cell and ligament fibroblast responses on RGD-modified silk fibers. J Biomed Mater Res 67(2):559–570
82. Cristino S, Grassi F, Toneguzzi S (2005) Analysis of mesenchymal stem cells grown on a three-dimensional HYAFF 11-based prototype ligament scaffold. J Biomed Mater Res 73 (3):275–283
83. Awad HA, Boivin GP, Dressler MR, Smith FNL, Young RG, Butler DL (2003) Repair of patellar tendon injuries using a cell-collagen composite. J Orthop Res 21(3):420–431
84. Ge ZG, Goh JCH, Lee EH (2005) Selection of cell source for ligament tissue engineering. Cell Transplant 14(8):573–583
85. Steinert AF, Kunz M, Prager P, Barthel T, Jakob FJ, Noeth U, Murray MM, Evans C, Porter RM (2011) Mesenchymal stem cell characteristics of human anterior cruciate ligament outgrowth cells. Tissue Eng Part A 17(9–10):1375–88
86. Chen JL, Yin Z, Shen WL, Chen X, Heng BC, Zou XH, Ouyang HW (2010) Efficacy of hESC-MSCs in knitted silk-collagen scaffold for tendon tissue engineering and their roles. Biomaterials 31(36):9438–9451

87. Pera MF, Reubinoff B, Trounson A (2000) Human embryonic stem cells. J Cell Sci 113:5–10
88. Chen X, Song XH, Yin Z, Zou XH, Wang L-L, Hu H, Cao T, Zheng M, Ouyang HW (2009) Stepwise differentiation of human embryonic stem cells promotes tendon regeneration by secreting fetal tendon matrix and differentiation factors. Stem Cells 27:1276–1287
89. Amit M, Gerecht-Nir S, Itskovitz-Eldor J (2005) Culture, subcloning, spontaneous and controlled differentiation of human embryonic stem cells. In: Bongso A, Lee EH (eds) Stem cells: from bench to bedside. World Scientific, Singapore
90. Caplan AI (2005) Mesenchymal stem cells: cell-based reconstructive therapy in orthopedics. Tissue Eng 11(7–8):1198–1211
91. Vieira AC, Guedes RM, Marques AT (2009) Development of ligament tissue biodegradable devices: a review. J Biomech 42(15):2421–2430
92. Liu Y, Ramanath HS, Wang D (2008) Tendon tissue engineering using scaffold enhancing strategies. Trends Biotechnol 26(4):201–209
93. Heckmann L, Schlenker HJ, Fiedler J, Brenner R, Dauner M, Bergenthal G, Mattes T, Claes L, Ignatius A (2006) Human mesenchymal progenitor cell responses to a novel textured poly (L-lactide) scaffold for ligament tissue engineering. J Biomed Mater Res B Appl Biomater 81(1):82–90
94. Cao Y, Liu Y, Liu W, Shan Q, Buonocore SD, Cui L (2002) Bridging tendon defects using autologous tenocyte engineered tendon in a hen model. Plast Reconstr Surg 110 (5):1280–1289
95. Ouyang HW, Goh JCH, Thambyah A, Teoh SH, Lee EH (2003) Knitted poly-lactide-co-glycolide scaffold loaded with bone marrow stromal cells in repair and regeneration of rabbit Achilles tendon. Tissue Eng 9(3):431–439
96. Temenoff JS, Mikos A (2009) Biomaterials: the intersection of biology and materials science. Pearson Prentice-Hall, Upper Saddle River, NJ
97. Juncosa-Melvin N, Boivin GP, Galloway MT, Gooch C, West JR, Butler DL (2006) Effects of cell-to-collagen ratio in stem cell-seeded constructs for Achilles tendon repair. Tissue Eng 12(4):681–689
98. Juncosa-Melvin N, Shearn JT, Boivin GP, Gooch C, Galloway MT, West JR, Nirmalanandhan VS, Bradica G, Butler DL (2006) Effects of mechanical stimulation on the biomechanics and histology of stem cell-collagen sponge constructs for rabbit patellar tendon repair. Tissue Eng 12(8):2291–2300
99. Juncosa-Melvin N, Matlin KS, Holdcraft RW, Nirmalanandhan VS, Butler DL (2007) Mechanical stimulation increases collagen type I and collagen type III gene expression of stem cell-collagen sponge constructs for patellar tendon repair. Tissue Eng 13(6):1219–1226
100. Shearn JT, Juncosa-Melvin N, Boivin GP, Galloway MT, Goodwin W, Gooch C, Dunn MG, Butler DL (2007) Mechanical stimulation of tendon tissue engineered constructs: effects on construct stiffness, repair biomechanics, and their correlation. J Biomech Eng 129 (6):848–854
101. Altman GH, Diaz F, Jakuba TC, Horan RL, Chen J, Lu H, Richmond JC, Kaplan DL (2003) Silk-based biomaterials. Biomaterials 24(3):401–416
102. Postlethwait RW (1969) Tissue reaction to surgical sutures. In: Dumphy JE, Van Winkle W (eds) Repair and regeneration. McGraw-Hill, New York
103. Fu SC, Wong YP, Cheuk YC (2005) TGF-beta1 reverses the effects of matrix anchorage on the gene expression of decorin and procollagen type I in tendon fibroblasts. Clin Orthop Relat Res 431:226–232
104. Molloy T, Wang Y, Murrell GA (2003) The roles of growth factors in tendon and ligament healing. Sports Med 33(5):381–394
105. Murphy PG, Loitz BJ, Frank C, Hart DA (1994) Influence of exogenous growth factors on the synthesis and secretion of collagen types I and III by explants of normal and healing rabbit ligaments. Biochem Cell Biol 72(9–10):403–9
106. Marui T, Niyibizi C, Georgescu HI, Cao M, Kavalkovich KW, Levine RE, Woo SLY (1997) Effect of growth factors on matrix synthesis by ligament fibroblasts. J Orthop Res 15(1):18–23

107. DesRosiers EA, Yahia L, Rivard CH (1996) Proliferation and matrix synthesis response of canine anterior cruciate ligament fibroblasts submitted to combined growth factors. J Orthop Res 14:200–208
108. Kondo E (2005) Effects of administration of exogenous growth factors on biomechanical properties of the elongation-type anterior cruciate ligament injury with partial laceration. Am J Sports Med 33(2):188–196
109. Hildebrand KA, Woo SLY, Smith DW, Allen CR, Deie M, Taylor BJ, Schmidt CC (1998) The effects of platelet-derived growth factor-BB on healing of the rabbit medial collateral ligament - an *in vivo* study. Am J Sports Med 26(4):549–554
110. Chan B, Chan K, Maffulli N, Lee K (1997) Effect of basic fibroblast growth factor. an *in vitro* study of tendon healing. Clin Orthop Relat Res 342:239–247
111. Banes AJ, Tsuzaki M, Hu PQ, Brigman B, Brown T, Almekinders L, Lawrence WT, Fischer T (1995) PDGF-BB, IGF-I and mechanical load stimulate DNA synthesis in avian tendon fibroblasts *in vitro*. J Biomech 28(12):1505–1513
112. Kang HJ, Kang ES (1999) Ideal concentration of growth factors in rabbit's flexor tendon culture. Yonsei Med J 40(1):26–29
113. Abrahamsson SO, Lohmander S (1996) Differential effects of insulin-like growth factor-I on matrix and DNA synthesis in various regions and types of rabbit tendons. J Orthop Res 14:370
114. Hankemeier S, Keus M, Zeichen J, Jagodzinski M, Barkhausen T, Bosch U, Krettek C, Van Griensven M (2005) Modulation of proliferation and differentiation of human bone marrow stromal cells by fibroblast growth factor 2: potential implications for tissue engineering of tendons and ligaments. Tissue Eng 11(1–2):41–49
115. Moreau JE, Bramono DS, Horan RL, Kaplan DL, Altman GH (2008) Sequential biochemical and mechanical stimulation in the development of tissue-engineered ligaments. Tissue Eng Part A 14(7):1161–1172
116. Moreau J, Chen J, Bramono DS (2005) Growth factor induced fibroblast differentiation from human bone marrow stromal cells *in vitro*. J Orthop Res 23(1):164–174
117. Aspenberg P, Forslund C (1999) Enhanced tendon healing with GDF 5 and 6. Acta Orthop Scand 70(1):51–54
118. Forslund C, Aspenberg P (2001) Tendon healing stimulated by injected CDMP-2. Med Sci Sports Exerc 33(5):685–687
119. Forslund C, Aspenberg P (2003) Improved healing of transected rabbit Achilles tendon after a single injection of cartilage-derived morphogenetic protein-2. Am J Sports Med 31 (4):555–559
120. Forslund C, Rueger D, Aspenberg P (2003) A comparative dose–response study of cartilage-derived morphogenetic protein (CDMP)-1,-2 and-3 for tendon healing in rats. J Orthop Res 21(4):617–621
121. Wolfman NM, Hattersley G, Cox K, Celeste AJ, Nelson R, Yamaji N, Dube JL, DiBlasioSmith E, Nove J, Song JJ, Wozney JM, Rosen V (1997) Ectopic induction of tendon and ligament in rats by growth and differentiation factors 5, 6, and 7, members of the TGF-beta gene family. J Clin Invest 100(2):321–330
122. Yang GG, Crawford RC, Wang JHC (2004) Proliferation and collagen production of human patellar tendon fibroblasts in response to cyclic uniaxial stretching in serum-free conditions. J Biomech 37(10):1543–1550
123. Miyaki S, Ushida T, Nemoto K, Shimojo H, Itabashi A, Ochiai N, Miyanaga Y, Tateishi T (2001) Mechanical stretch in anterior cruciate ligament derived cells regulates type I collagen and decorin expression through extracellular signal-regulated kinase 1/2 pathway. Mater Sci Eng C Biomim Supramol Syst 17(1–2):91–94
124. Henshaw DR, Attia E, Bhargava M, Hannafin LA (2006) Canine ACL fibroblast integrin expression and cell alignment in response to cyclic tensile strain in three-dimensional collagen gels. J Orthop Res 24(3):481–490

125. Hannafin JA, Attia EA, Henshaw R, Warren RF, Bhargava MA (2006) Effect of cyclic strain and plating matrix on cell proliferation and integrin expression by ligament fibroblasts. J Orthop Res 24:149–158
126. Cukierman E (2001) Taking cell-matrix adhesions to the third dimension. Science 294 (5547):1708–1712
127. Brenhardt HA, Cosgriff-Hernandez EM (2009) The role of mechanical loading in ligament tissue engineering. Tissue Eng Part B Rev 15(4):467–475
128. Banes AJ, Qi J, Anderson DS, Maloney M, Sumanasinghe R (2009) Tissue train culture system. Culturing cells in a mechanically active environment. Hillsborough Business Center, Hillsborough, NC
129. Garvin J, Qi J, Maloney M, Banes AJ (2003) Novel system for engineering bioartificial tendons and application of mechanical load. Tissue Eng 9:967–979
130. Park SA, Kim IA, Lee YJ, Shin JW, Kim CR, Kim JK, Yang YI (2006) Biological responses of ligament fibroblasts and gene expression profiling on micropatterned silicone substrates subjected to mechanical stimuli. J Biosci Bioeng 102(5):402–412
131. Doroski DM, Levenston ME, Temenoff JS (2010) Cyclic tensile culture promotes fibroblastic differentiation of marrow stromal cells encapsulated in poly(ethylene glycol)-based hydrogels. Tissue Eng Part A 16(11):3457–3466
132. Altman GH, Horan RL, Martin I, Farhadi J, Stark PRH, Volloch V, Richmond JC, Vunjak-Novakovic G, Kaplan DL (2001) Cell differentiation by mechanical stress. FASEB J 15 (14):270–272
133. Benjamin M, McGonagle D (2009) Entheses: tendon and ligament attachment sites. Scand J Med Sci Sports 19(4):520–527
134. Sharma P, Maffulli N (2005) Basic biology of tendon injury and healing. Surgeon 3(5):309–316
135. Jiang J, Nicoll SB, Lu H (2003) Effects of osteoblast and chondrocyte co-culture on chondrogenic and osteoblastic phenotype *in vitro*. In: Transactions of the 49th annual meeting of the Orthopaedic Research Society New Orleans, LA
136. Wang INE, Shan J, Choi R, Oh S, Kepler CK, Chen FH, Lu HH (2007) Role of osteoblast-fibroblast interactions in the formation of the ligament-to-bone interface. J Orthop Res 25 (12):1609–1620
137. Moffat K, Wang I, Rodeo S, Lu H (2009) Orthopedic interface tissue engineering for the biological fixation of soft tissue grafts. Clin Sports Med 28(1):157–176
138. Spalazzi JP, Doty SB, Moffat KL, Levine WN, Lu H (2006) Development of controlled matrix heterogeneity on a triphasic scaffold for orthopedic interface tissue engineering. Tissue Eng 12(12):3497–3508
139. Spalazzi JP, Dagher E, Doty SB, Guo XE, Rodeo SA, Lu HH (2008) *In vivo* evaluation of a multiphased scaffold designed for orthopaedic interface tissue engineering and soft tissue-to-bone integration. J Biomed Mater Res A 86A(1):1–12
140. Phillips JE, Burns KL, Le Doux JM, Guldberg RE, Garcia AJ (2008) Engineering graded tissue interfaces. Proc Natl Acad Sci 105(34):12170–12175
141. Chen CH, Liu HW, Tsai CL, Yu CM, Lin IH, Hsiue GH (2008) Photoencapsulation of bone morphogenetic protein-2 and periosteal progenitor cells improve tendon graft healing in a bone tunnel. Am J Sports Med 36(3):461–473
142. Martinek V, Latterman C, Usas A, Abramowitch S, Woo SLY, Fu FH, Huard J (2002) Enhancement of tendon-bone integration of anterior cruciate ligament grafts with bone morphogenetic protein-2 gene transfer–a histological and biomechanical study. J Bone Joint Surg Am 84A(7):1123–1131
143. Rodeo SA, Suzuki K, Deng XH, Wozney J, Warren RF (1999) Use of recombinant human bone morphogenetic protein-2 to enhance tendon healing in a bone tunnel. Am J Sports Med 27(4):476–488

Chapter 16
Synthesis of Layered, Graded Bioscaffolds

Daniel W. Weisgerber, Steven R. Caliari, and Brendan A.C. Harley

16.1 Introduction

The extracellular matrix (ECM) is a complex 3D structure of matrix proteins and proteoglycans that defines the extrinsic environment surrounding cells. Biomaterials are often designed to explicitly mimic distinct features of this microenvironment. Approaches to design "monolithic" biomaterials—uniform 3D structures that present a defined combination of structural, compositional and biomolecular cues—have improved markedly, and are responsible for many fundamental advances in our understanding of how cells interrogate and respond to their microenvironment. For example, previous canonical works have established the significance of biomaterial composition [2, 3] and soluble factor supplementation [4–6] as critical regulators of cell behavior, stem cell fate, and biomaterial regenerative potential. However, with these advances has also come an increasing understanding that in many cases monolithic structures are insufficient. Notably, many tissues in the body contain a degree of heterogeneity or patterning. A critical class of such is found in tissues containing interfaces. In this chapter we concentrate on the design and development of two distinct biomaterial composites for orthopedic tissue engineering. First, the

D.W. Weisgerber
Department of Materials Science and Engineering, University of Illinois at Urbana-Champaign, Urbana, IL, USA
e-mail: weisger3@illinois.edu

S.R. Caliari
Department of Chemical and Biomolecular Engineering, University of Illinois at Urbana-Champaign, Urbana, IL, USA
e-mail: caliari1@illinois.edu

B.A.C. Harley (✉)
Department of Chemical and Biomolecular Engineering, Institute for Genomic Biology, University of Illinois at Urbana-Champaign, Urbana, IL, USA
e-mail: bharley@illinois.edu

S. Thomopoulos et al. (eds.), *Structural Interfaces and Attachments in Biology*,
DOI 10.1007/978-1-4614-3317-0_16,

native osteochondral (cartilage-bone) interface provided the motivation for creating techniques to fabricate multi-compartment collagen-glycosaminoglycan (GAG) scaffolds (CG scaffolds); this structure contains region-specific compartments as well as gradients of ECM proteins and soluble biomolecules (growth factors, proteins, cytokines) across the interface. Second, the development of a tendon regeneration strategy has required implementation of bioinspired composite structures to generate bioactive, porous scaffolds that maintain sufficient mechanical integrity. Although focused on orthopedic tissue engineering, the methods discussed here have broader applicability to many other tissue systems. Critically, both case studies provide valuable information regarding the integration of defined layers, compartments, and gradations into a single biomaterial structure.

16.2 Collagen-GAG Scaffolds: History of Applications

The ECM is a fibrillar network of structural proteins (collagens, proteoglycans, etc.), specialized proteins for cell adhesion (fibronectin, laminin, etc.), and other tissue-specific materials such as hydroxyapatite in bone [7]. The ECM defines the physical morphology of tissues and the local environment in which cells reside. Tissue engineering scaffolds are used as 3D analogs of the native ECM to heal or modify tissues in a controlled manner. In order to be successful, these scaffolds must be able to recapitulate integral aspects of the ECM microenvironment while supporting a range of physiological cell processes.

As analogs of the native ECM, collagen-GAG materials possess several vital characteristics for successful tissue engineering scaffolds, including a 3D microstructure with a high degree of pore interconnectivity, tunable degradation and resorption rates, surface ligands for cell adhesion, and mechanical integrity [7, 8]. CG biomaterials were first developed in the 1970's through a collaborative effort between Dr. Ioannis Yannas, a professor at Massachusetts Institute of Technology, and John F. Burke, a surgeon at Massachusetts General Hospital. Originally developed for regenerative repair of full-thickness skin wounds, CG biomaterials have been utilized in a plethora of tissue engineering studies, both *in vivo* as regenerative templates for skin, peripheral nerves, conjunctiva, and a range of orthopedic tissues (bone, cartilage, tendon, intervertebral disk) [9–12] as well as *in vitro* as 3D microenvironments to probe more fundamental questions about cell behaviors and cell–matrix interactions [13–15]. Scaffold microstructure (porosity, mean pore size, pore shape, interconnectivity, specific surface area) [9, 12, 15–23] and mechanical properties (Young's modulus, yield stress) [24–33] have been shown to be key factors that can influence cell behaviors such as adhesion, motility, contraction, stem cell differentiation, gene expression, and overall bioactivity [9].

CG scaffolds are traditionally created from a suspension consisting of co-precipitated collagen (typically type I) and glycosaminoglycan content in a weak acetic acid solution [9]. The collagen backbone of this scaffold provides

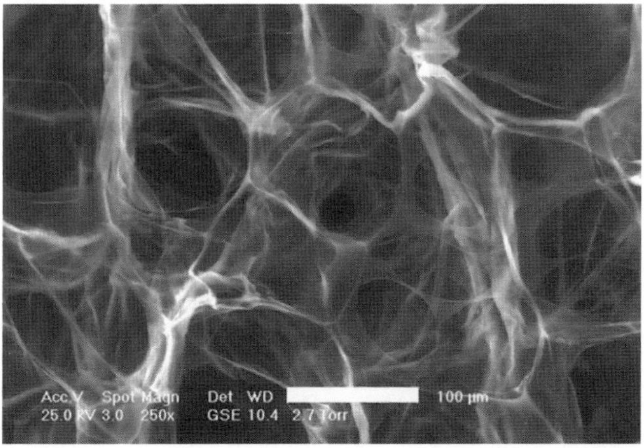

Fig. 16.1 ESEM image of the pore structure of the CG scaffold ($T_f = -40°C$). Scale bar: 100 μm. (Reproduced, with permission, from Pek et al. [38])

controllable biodegradation rates and products, native ligands to aid cell attachment, and relatively weak antigenicity/immunogenicity [34, 35]. GAGs were added to the collagen material for several reasons beyond that of ECM biomimicry. First, the co-precipitation of collagen with GAG increased the open-cell nature of the scaffold, facilitating cell penetration and subsequent metabolic support; the CG composite was also more resistant to degradation, thereby reducing the need for heavy crosslinking that would otherwise leave the material brittle [35]. Not surprisingly, the addition of GAG was also shown to significantly improve material mechanical integrity [35]. While chondroitin sulfate remains the primary GAG constituent, additional GAGs can be added for tissue-specific reasons, such as the generation of a collagen-hyaluronic acid (HA) scaffold for cartilage tissue engineering [36]. Homogenization and acidic co-precipitation (pH <3.2) of the collagen with GAG content also destroys collagen's quaternary structure (without denaturing the collagen). This resulted in unique hemostatic properties for CG materials through the limitation of platelet aggregation *in vivo* normally associated with collagen materials [35]. CG scaffolds are typically fabricated from a suspension containing between 0.5 and 1% w/v collagen and 0.05–0.1% w/v GAG [7]. These values were selected so that the resultant scaffolds have high porosities to enable rapid cellular infiltration and diffusive transport processes, but also because of the inherent difficulty in processing collagen-GAG suspensions with higher solids content without denaturing the collagen due to the increased temperature and shear stresses required for complete mixing.

The scaffold structure is created via lyophilization [7]. Briefly, the CG suspension is frozen at a specified temperature and rate [19, 37], resulting in a continuous, interpenetrating network of ice crystals surrounded by fibers of CG co-precipitate termed struts. Sublimation of the ice crystals at a low vacuum

(<200 mTorr) produces a highly porous scaffold where the scaffold pore size and shape is defined by the size and shape of the ice crystals formed during solidification (Fig. 16.1) [38]. Modifying suspension freezing rate, final freezing temperature, and inclusion of annealing steps have all been shown to significantly alter final scaffold pore structure [19, 37, 39]. These scaffolds resemble low-density, open-cell foams, with an interconnected network of struts and are typically fabricated with relative densities (ρ^*/ρ_s) significantly less than 5% (porosities greater than 95%).

Recently, CG fabrication schemes have been modified to enable integration of calcium phosphate (CaP) mineral content into the prototypical CG scaffold [40–42], including control over the mineral to organic ratio (CaP mass fraction) of the collagen-GAG-CaP (CGCaP) triple co-precipitates (0–80 wt%) in order to cover a range that includes the mineral content of developing osteoid and natural (cortical) bone (75 wt% CaP) [40, 43]. CGCaP scaffolds are of particular interest for orthopedic applications due to their potential to mimic the native biochemistry of bone, notably the creation of an interpenetrating collagenous matrix (organic) and CaP (mineral) network, as well as the significant improvement in overall mechanical properties of the CGCaP scaffolds relative to non-mineralized CG scaffolds [44–46]. The addition of a mineral phase to the classic CG scaffold archetype enabled the development of composite materials with the requisite biochemical and biomechanical properties for bone and interfacial tissue engineering. CGCaP scaffold technology has been used as the basis for creating multiphase collagen scaffolds for the repair of interfacial tissues, notably osteochondral defects [40, 41, 47].

16.3 Multi-compartment Scaffolds for Interfacial Tissue Engineering

Tissue interfaces are found throughout the body; they link distinct tissue compartments with a stable interface most often containing gradients in ECM content (i.e., collagens, GAGs, CaP) and soluble biomolecules (i.e., growth factors, proteins, cytokines) across the interface. Notably, articular joint surfaces contain two distinct tissue types, bone and articular cartilage, meeting at a smooth, stable interface (the "tidemark"). A major contributing factor to the stability of the osteochondral interface is the smooth compositional transition between mineralized bone and unmineralized cartilage [48] that occurs as CaP content gradually decreases from the levels found in the subchondral bone plate (~75 wt%) across a zone of calcified cartilage to zero in articular cartilage. Over this same transition, type II collagen content dramatically increases from zero in the subchondral bone to the levels found in native cartilage. Most significantly, collagen fibrils extend across this tidemark from each side, ensuring a continuous organic phase [49–51]. Here we describe integration of CG and CGCaP scaffold technologies to develop a multi-compartment collagen scaffold for the repair of orthopedic interfaces.

16.3.1 Fabrication of Osteochondral CG-CGCaP Multi-compartment Scaffolds

In designing a multi-compartment scaffold, important factors to control include the chemical and microstructural composition of each compartment and the interfacial region. A *liquid phase co-synthesis* method was developed to enable fabrication of multi-compartment CG scaffolds for osteochondral tissue engineering. This multi-compartment scaffold was designed to be a single biomaterial construct containing distinct osseous (bone) and cartilagenous (cartilage) regions (compartments), each with distinct microstructural, chemical, and mechanical properties that are connected via a continuous interface [47]. The osseous compartment for subchondral bone regeneration was made from type I collagen, chondroitin sulfate, and CaP while the cartilagenous compartment for cartilage regeneration was composed of type II collagen and chondroitin sulfate. Using this new fabrication scheme, distinct CG and CGCaP suspensions are created containing ECM components representative of each tissue compartment.

The continuous interface is created by layering the cartilagenous compartment and the osseous compartment suspensions in a conventional freeze-drying mold, but then incorporating a processing step to enable partial diffusive mixing between the two suspensions near their interface. Once the region of interdiffusion was created between the suspension layers, freeze-drying was used to form the final multi-compartment scaffold microstructure (Fig. 16.2) [47]. This fabrication method prevents complications often observed in layered scaffolds containing abrupt interfaces such as those created when suturing or gluing distinct phases together post-fabrication. In these cases delamination due to stress concentrations, foreign body contamination (from glue or other adhesive), and inefficient cellular transport between scaffold phases can be a significant problem [47]. The differential chemistry, microstructure, and mechanics of the osseous and cartilagenous compartments enable these layered scaffolds to exhibit compressive deformation behavior that mimics behavior observed in natural articular joints [47, 52]. The continuous interface between scaffold regions may also be critical for the recapitulation of native interfacial physiology for tissues such as ligament and tendon [47].

16.3.2 Methods of Characterizing Multi-compartment CG-CGCaP Scaffolds

It is imperative to develop quantitative analysis techniques to consider the biophysical, compositional, and biomechanical properties of multi-compartment scaffolds. Experimental characterization of multi-compartment CG scaffold properties such as chemical composition, pore morphology (size/shape), relative density, permeability, and mechanics have been used to describe distinct scaffold features. Experimental characterization has also been supplemented by modeling approaches that enable a more complete understanding of the microenvironment presented by the

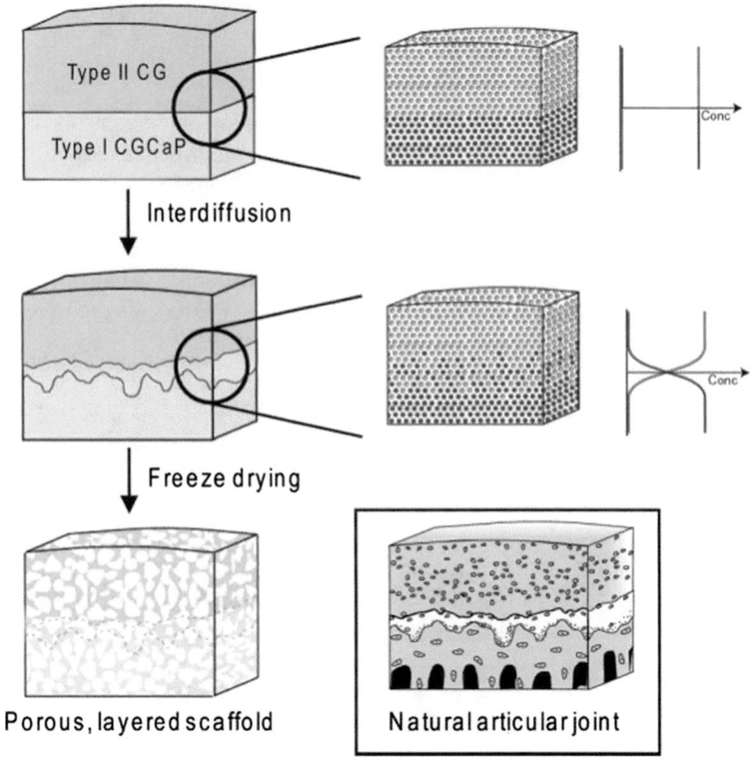

Fig. 16.2 Schematic of liquid phase co-synthesis scheme. Type II collagen-GAG (CG) suspension (*blue*) is carefully layered on top of collagen-GAG-CaP (CGCaP) suspension (*tan*) and allowed to interdiffuse. Interdiffusion followed by freeze-drying creates a gradient interface between the two compartments that mimics the physiology of natural articular joints. (Reproduced, with permission, from Harley et al. [47])

CG structure to distinct cells or populations of cells. While it is possible to mechanically separate the multi-compartment scaffold and perform analysis on individual compartments, methods that enable simultaneous analysis of discrete regions from within a single gradient or multi-compartment scaffold are especially useful.

Scaffold composition can be assessed by a number of analytical tools, notably dimethylmethylene blue (DMMB) assay to determine GAG content, hydroxyproline assay to determine collagen content, and mass subtraction to determine CaP content [40]. Further, CaP phase can be determined via subsequent X-ray diffraction (XRD) analysis of the scaffold regions [40, 41]. In order to qualitatively describe the distribution of CaP mineral content within the multi-compartment scaffold, combined SEM imaging and energy dispersive X-ray spectroscopy (EDX) can be used to show both the local pore microstructure at the interface and to determine the mineral content and spatial distribution of mineral within the scaffold (Fig. 16.3) [47].

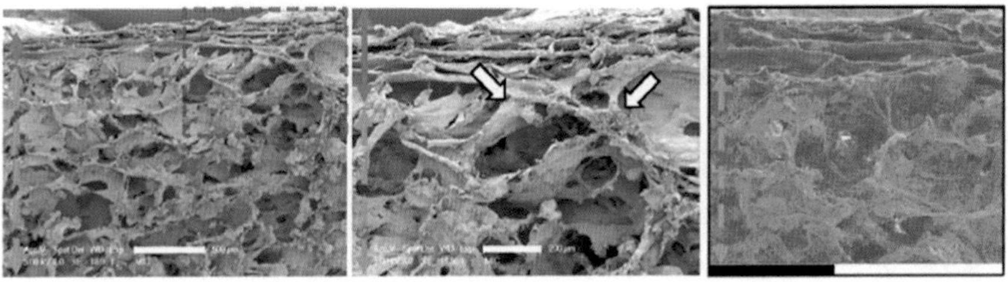

Fig. 16.3 *Left, middle*: SEM shows the continuity of collagen fibers at the interface between the CG (*blue line*) and CGCaP (*tan dashed line*) compartments. Scale bars: 500 μm (*left*), 200 μm (*middle*). *Right*: energy dispersive X-ray spectroscopy (EDX) superimposed on SEM image of the multi-compartment CG-CGCaP scaffold demonstrates the localization of Ca and P mineral content in the CGCaP (bone) compartment. (Reproduced, with permission, from Harley et al. [47])

CG microstructure (pore size and morphology) is best quantified via a stereological approach. Longitudinally and transversely oriented scaffold samples are embedded in glycolmethacrylate, sectioned, stained, and observed using optical microscopy. A linear intercept approach can resolve a best-fit ellipse representation of the pore morphology. Dimensions of the ellipse (major and minor axes) allow calculation of both an equivalent mean diameter and a mean pore aspect ratio [14, 19, 37, 53]. Micro-computed tomography (microCT) has also been used to analyze pore microstructure [14, 19, 37, 54], though it often requires significant use of contrast agents to enable accurate visualization of the non-mineralized CG content. For subsequent discussion of mechanics and permeability in this chapter, a model multi-compartment scaffold variant (CG compartment mean pore size: 219 ± 27 μm; CGCaP compartment: 200 ± 42 μm; Interface region: 208 ± 20 μm) will be described.

Cellular solids modeling approaches have proven to be useful tools in the description and characterization of CG scaffold pore geometry and microstructural properties (e.g., pore shape, specific surface area) [55, 56]. CG scaffolds have been primarily modeled as low density, open-cell foams using a tetrakaidecahedral (14-sided polyhedron) unit cell. Application of modeling approaches using the tetrakaidecahedral unit cell with CG scaffolds has led to estimations of a number of key microstructural features of the CG scaffolds, notably scaffold-specific surface area (surface area divided by the volume of the scaffold) [19, 21], mechanical behavior [57], strut geometry and deformation [14, 15], and permeability (SA/V) [58]. A key parameter used in these analyses is the relative density (ρ^*/ρ_s) of the scaffold, which is also equivalent to (1−% porosity). Relative density (ρ^*/ρ_s) is defined as the ratio of the density of the scaffold (ρ^*) divided by the density of the solid material the scaffold was fabricated from (ρ_s).

Mechanical testing has been performed to determine both the standalone moduli of individual scaffold compartments and the behavior of the multi-compartment scaffolds. Results have demonstrated that these scaffolds possess nonlinear stress–strain behavior with three distinct regions (linear, collapse plateau, and densification) as is characteristic of low density open-cell foams (Fig. 16.4) [47].

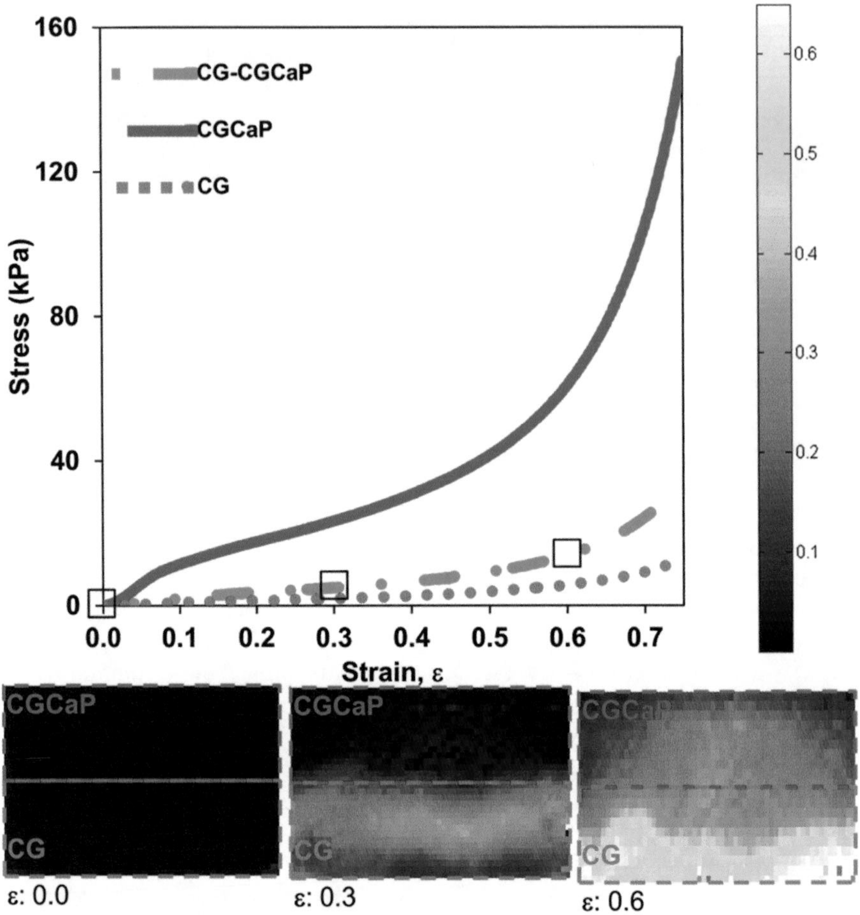

Fig. 16.4 *Top*: Stress–strain curves of CG, CGCaP, and CG-CGCaP ($T_f = -10°C$) scaffolds, each demonstrating the distinct linear, collapse plateau, and densification regimes characteristic of low density open-cell foams. *Bottom*: Ultrasound elastography images, corresponding to applied strains of 0.0, 0.3, and 0.6, illustrate the local strain experienced in the CG-CGCaP scaffold

Further, the elastic modulus of the individual struts that define the scaffold network has also been characterized [57]; scaffold modulus has also been shown to remain consistent in orthogonal planes of isotropic scaffolds [57], but vary significantly between orthogonal planes of anisotropic scaffold variants [53]. The mechanical behavior of CGCaP scaffolds under compression as well as the modulus of the individual mineralized struts have also been evaluated [41, 46]. These results offer insight to the mechanical properties of a standardized set of CG materials. For the model multi-compartment scaffold, the CG compartment exhibited a modulus of 9 ± 1 kPa, while the CGCaP compartment possessed a modulus of 155 ± 17 kPa.

Analysis of the multi-compartment scaffold showed a modulus of 23 $\pm$ 2 kPa, with the low modulus suggestive of compartmentalization of all scaffold deformation in the softer CG region. Serial microCT analysis has been used to depict the behavior of individual compartments within the multi-compartment osteochondral scaffold; the softer cartilagenous compartment experienced more deformation compared to the osseous compartment (negligible strain) [47]. Recently, ultrasound elastography approaches have been used to depict local strain in the discrete scaffold compartments of a multi-compartment scaffold, confirming localized scaffold deformation in the non-mineralized region under compressive loads (Fig. 16.4).

Scaffold permeability varies significantly across the multi-compartment CG scaffold. Permeability of tissue engineering scaffolds is a critical design parameter to be controlled as it influences the diffusion of cytokines, nutrients, and waste throughout the scaffold prior to material vascularization; further, biomaterial permeability has also been shown to significantly impact cell migration processes and scaffold biodegradation rates, amongst others [59]. Material permeability also affects fluid pressure fields and shear stresses within the construct, additional potential stimuli for functional adaptation [60]. Permeability of tissue engineering scaffolds is dictated by a variety of microstructural characteristics including porosity, pore size and orientation, pore interconnectivity, fenestration size and shape, specific surface area, and applied strain. Cellular solids approaches have been utilized to build descriptive models of scaffold permeability that accurately capture the effect of scaffold pore size, relative density, and applied strain on overall scaffold permeability [58]. When examining the model multi-compartment scaffold, the permeability of each compartment was found to behave as predicted by the previously described cellular solids model; however, the permeability of the entire multi-compartment scaffold was found to match that of the mineralized layer. Here, the mineralized compartment provided the limiting resistance due to its smaller pore size and higher relative density. The findings that multi-compartment scaffold mechanical properties match the CG compartment while the bulk permeability matches the CGCaP compartment, while not surprising, underscore the importance of continuing to develop methods to quantitatively analyze region-specific properties within heterogeneous biomaterials.

16.3.3 Clinical Application of Multi-compartment CG-CGCaP Scaffolds

The weak antigenicity/immunogenicity of the collagen/GAG content within the CG scaffold as well as its controllable biodegradability, previous FDA-approval, and overall history in clinical applications [34, 35] make CG scaffolds an attractive target for clinical translation. Multi-compartment CG-CGCaP scaffolds are currently being developed and tested for orthopedic interface regeneration applications. The first generation multi-compartment CG-CGCaP scaffold is currently undergoing clinical trials as an osteochondral regeneration template after successful *in vitro* and preclinical trials demonstrated that these scaffolds can successfully integrate into bone defects and show preliminary bony substitution and mineralization as well as improved chondrogenesis in the CG compartment [61, 62]. Additionally, the *liquid-phase co-synthesis* technique holds promise for the regeneration of not only osteochondral defects, but also other physiological interfaces such as the tendon-bone junction.

16.4 Core-Shell Composites for Orthopedic Tissue Engineering

Connective tissues such as tendon and ligaments transmit mechanical loads and enable normal locomotion. These tissues are also commonly injured with over 17 million injuries occurring each year with annual costs in the tens of billions of dollars in the United States alone [63]. The most serious injuries require surgical intervention; such tendon and ligament injuries are responsible for hundreds of thousands of surgical procedures each year in the United States [8, 63].

One of the key challenges of orthopedic tissue engineering is to create scaffolds that are bioactive and can support tissue regeneration while remaining mechanically competent. The most common biomaterial designs for tendon and ligament tissue engineering are electrospun or woven polymer mats [64–66]. While these constructs can be designed with tensile moduli approaching the level of tendon, electrospun mats are dense and essentially 2D materials with inadequate permeability, porosity, and biodegradability. Highly porous scaffolds are alternative biomaterials that could potentially supersede many of these drawbacks. Porous scaffolds have excellent permeability and can be fabricated from natural, biodegradable materials. However, these types of materials are typically orders of magnitude too weak for tendon applications. To attempt to overcome this limitation, there are several common methods of scaffold mechanical enhancement that do not have adverse effects on construct bioactivity. For tendon and ligament scaffolds these include the creation of aligned microstructure to mimic the native tissue architecture [65, 67] and mechanical stimulation of cell-seeded scaffold constructs [68–71]. While these methods can marginally improve construct mechanical properties, they have not been successful in reaching levels of native tendon.

While the multi-scale properties of tendon cannot be replicated by current biomaterials technologies, composite materials have shown promise for complex tissue engineering applications. Nature provides an alternative design scheme for tendon tissue engineering applications: core-shell composites. Plant stems combine a porous core with a dense shell to aid osmotic transport (core) while maintaining sufficient tensile/bending stiffness (shell); many bird beaks also combine a dense shell and porous core to enhance compressive strength and mechanical efficiency [72]. This type of material has also been utilized to engineer high strength metal tubing [73]. Mauck et al. have recently fabricated composites for intervertebral disk tissue engineering consisting of an agarose gel mimicking the central nucleus

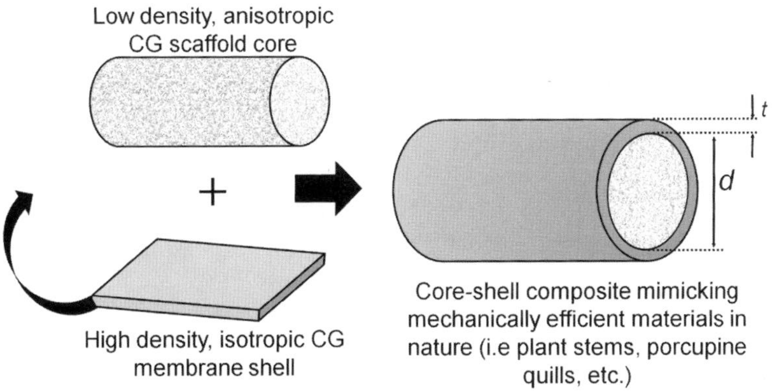

Fig. 16.5 Schematic of CG core-shell composite design

pulposus integrated with layered, aligned nanofiber mats mimicking the annulus fibrosus region [74, 75].

The CG scaffold-membrane composite paradigm was developed to avoid the typical tradeoff for porous tissue engineering scaffolds between mechanical properties (Young's modulus: E^*) and bioactivity (permeability: k and porosity: ε). Briefly, previous experimental and cellular solids modeling studies have shown that scaffold modulus increases with $(\rho^*/\rho_s)^2$ (and is not affected by pore size) but that scaffold permeability increases as $(1-(\rho^*/\rho_s))^{3/2}$ [57, 58]. Hence, to increase CG scaffold elastic modulus by the two or three orders of magnitude necessary for tendon applications (minimum 100 MPa hydrated modulus), the corresponding increase in relative density would have adverse effects on overall scaffold bioactivity (permeability and porosity). Taking inspiration from core-shell structures in nature [56], the scaffold-membrane composite design can help overcome these limitations.

16.4.1 Fabrication of Aligned CG Scaffold-Membrane Composites via Liquid–Solid Phase Co-synthesis

The core-shell CG composite paradigm was implemented using the same technologies developed to create multi-compartment CG scaffolds for osteochondral tissue engineering. Here a high density (high tensile strength) CG membrane was combined with a low density (porous) aligned CG scaffolds into a single biomaterial via a liquid–solid phase co-synthesis method [1, 47] (Fig. 16.5). As a precursor for using these composites for tendon repair, the scaffold core contained a longitudinally aligned, anisotropic pore microstructure fabricated using a recently developed directional freeze-drying approach [53]. The aligned microstructure was hypothesized to improve construct regenerative capacity by increasing the modulus in the direction of alignment and by providing contact guidance cues to cells. Scaffold cores were fabricated from a suspension of type I microfibrillar collagen and chondroitin sulfate [53].

The composite shell was created from a novel CG membrane fabricated via an evaporative process from the same precursor suspension as the CG scaffold. Briefly, degassed CG suspension was pipetted into Petri dishes and allowed to air dry in a fume hood, resulting in a dense CG sheet with thickness on the order of tens to hundreds of microns [1]. The amount of CG content within the suspension, mediated by either total suspension volume or suspension density, correlated to the thickness of the resultant membrane [1]. CG membranes displayed a consistent relative density (75%) significantly larger than that of the scaffold core (0.6%); membrane stiffness could be further modulated via post-fabrication crosslinking procedures.

Scaffold-membrane constructs were created via liquid–solid phase co-synthesis [1, 47] while degree of scaffold core anisotropy was separately modulated via a directional solidification approach. Membrane pieces were cut to size, rolled, and placed directly into a PTFE mold containing a copper bottom used to induce directional solidification [53]. The CG suspension was then pipetted inside the rolled membrane and allowed to hydrate the membrane [1]. The degree of membrane incorporation can be tuned by adjusting the hydration time of the membrane in the scaffold suspension prior to freeze-drying. The mold was then placed on a precooled freeze-dryer shelf where the significant disparity in thermal conductivities ($k_{Cu}/k_{PTFE} \sim 1{,}600$) promoted unidirectional heat transfer through the copper bottom during lyophilization. Conventional sublimation was then used to remove the ice content from the frozen CG suspension, resulting in core-shell CG composites containing an aligned pore microstructure [53]. The porous CG core and dense CG shell are integrated into a single continuous biomaterial that combines excellent porosity, permeability, and bioactivity with increased mechanical competence necessary for tendon applications. SEM analysis of the scaffold core shows elongated, aligned pores in the scaffold longitudinal plane as a result of unidirectional heat transfer; in contrast, pores in the scaffold transverse plane are circular and more isotropic (Fig. 16.6). The CG membrane displays a dense network of fibrillar collagen content and shows excellent integration with the CG scaffold in scaffold-membrane composites. Additionally, the membrane does not delaminate from the scaffold core during the freeze-drying process or after hydration [1].

16.4.2 Characterization of CG Membrane Physical and Mechanical Properties

CG membranes were fabricated via an evaporative process with thicknesses varying over an order of magnitude (23–240 μm) (Fig. 16.7) [1]. The thickness could be adjusted by changing the amount of solid collagen-GAG material used during fabrication. Despite differences in thickness, the relative density was consistently in the 0.75–0.80 range (CG scaffold relative density: 0.006). Swelling ratio tests revealed that all membrane variants were at least 90% hydrated after 30 min in PBS

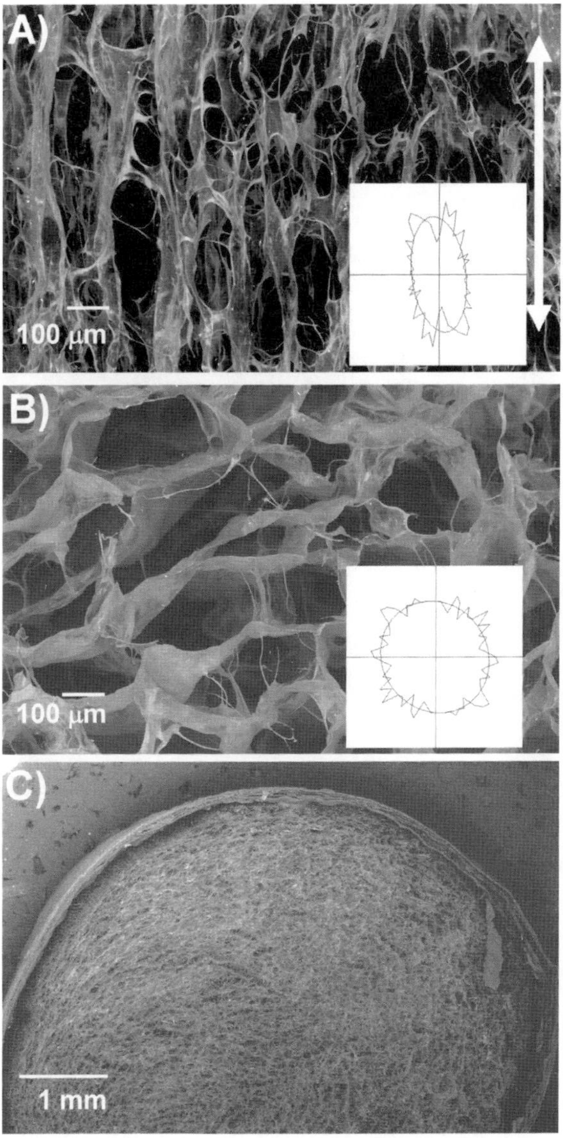

Fig. 16.6 (**a**) SEM of longitudinal CG scaffold section displaying aligned, elongated pore structure. Scale bar: 100 µm. (**b**) SEM of transverse CG scaffold section displaying round, isotropic pore structure. Scale bar: 100 µm. (**c**) SEM of scaffold-membrane interface showing integration of two materials. Scale bar: 1 mm. (Reproduced, with permission, from Caliari et al. [1])

(data not shown). Mechanically, membranes are isotropic in plane and both physical (dehydrothermal: DHT) and chemical (1-ethyl-3-[3-dimethylaminopropyl] carbodiimide hydrochloride: EDAC) crosslinking methods can be used to further crosslink the membranes [1]. As expected, significantly crosslinking was introduced via EDAC treatment. Notably, the highest crosslinked CG membrane displayed ~7–10-fold increases in modulus over non-crosslinked controls [1], comparable to increases seen for CG scaffolds treated with the same crosslinking strategies [57].

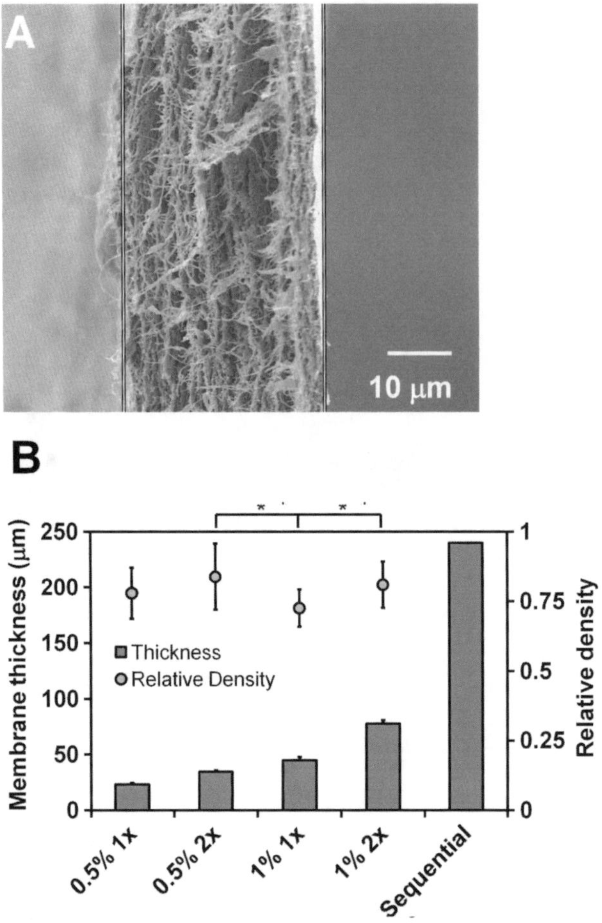

Fig. 16.7 (**a**) SEM of membrane cross-section illustrating dense, layered fibrillar organization. Scale bar: 10 μm. (**b**) Membranes can be produced over a wide range of thicknesses (23–240 μm) with consistent relative density (0.75–0.80) ($n = 17$). Error bars: Mean ± SD. (Reproduced, with permission, from Caliari et al. [1])

16.4.3 CG Scaffold-Membrane Composites: Experimental and Theoretical Results

Following successful fabrication of aligned CG scaffold-membrane composites, the mechanical properties of these materials were described using experimental and theoretical techniques. The aligned CG scaffold core demonstrated superior mechanical properties in the direction of alignment compared to isotropic controls [1], a result consistent in the literature and that correlated with modeling analyses of anisotropic cellular solids [56, 65, 67].

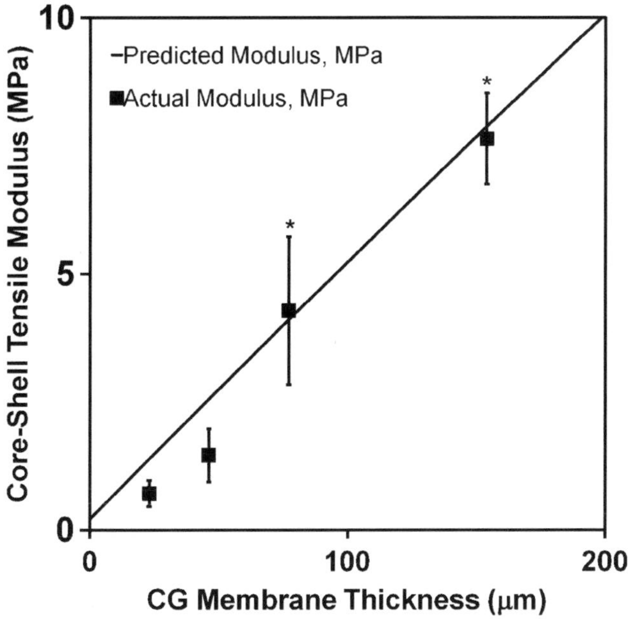

Fig. 16.8 Core-shell composite Young's modulus ($n = 6$) compares favorably to layered composites theoretical prediction. The close agreement is indicative of integration of the membrane shell with scaffold core. Shell thicknesses: 23, 45, 78, and 155 μm. Error bars: Mean ± SD. (Reproduced, with permission, from Caliari et al. [1])

After separate mechanical characterization of aligned CG scaffolds and CG membranes, CG scaffold-membrane composites were fabricated and characterized using membranes ranging in thicknesses from 23 μm (0.5% 1×) to 155 μm (1% 2× wrapped twice around scaffold). These scaffolds demonstrated dramatically increased tensile moduli over CG scaffold controls (no membrane shell) with a 36-fold increase observed for the 155 μm membrane thickness. Experimental results were compared to predictions from layered composites theory. Layered composites theory has previously been used to accurately predict the tensile properties of multicomponent materials based on the relative size of the individual components and their separate moduli [1]. CG core-shell composite Young's modulus ($E^*_{\text{composite}}$) can be predicted by the rule of mixtures as a function of scaffold core Young's modulus (E^*_{scaffold}), membrane shell Young's modulus E^*_{membrane}, composite radius (r), and membrane thickness (t) [1]:

$$E^*_{\text{composite}} = E^*_{\text{scaffold}}\left(\frac{(r-t)^2}{r^2}\right) + E^*_{\text{membrane}}\left(1 - \frac{(r-t)^2}{r^2}\right) \tag{16.1}$$

Experimental results correlate well with theoretical predictions, especially for composites with the two thicker membranes (78, 155 μm) (Fig. 16.8). The close

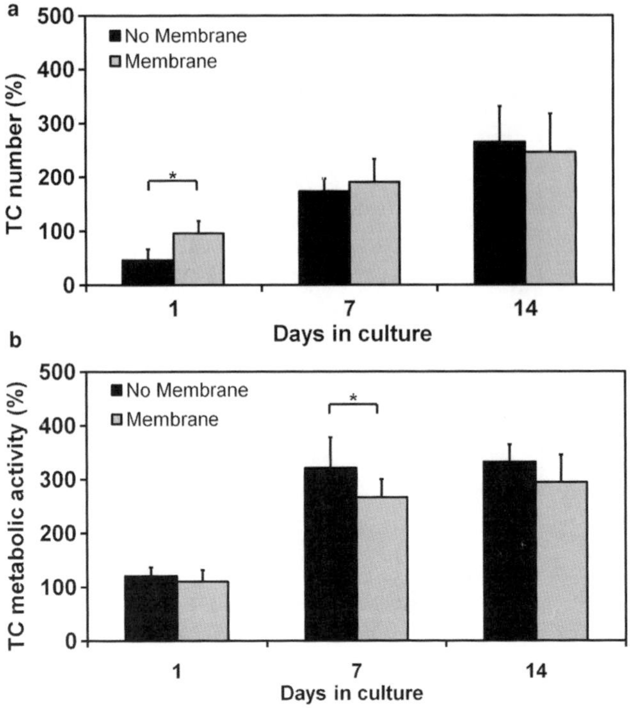

Fig. 16.9 (**a**) CG-membrane scaffolds support significantly higher TC number at day 1 ($n = 6$) and similar cell number at days 7 and 14 ($n = 6$) compared to CG scaffolds. Both groups show large increases in TC number from day 1 to day 7 and from day 7 to day 14. (**b**) CG scaffolds display higher TC metabolic activity at day 1 ($n = 18$), significantly higher bioactivity at day 7 ($n = 12$), and higher TC metabolic activity at day 14 ($n = 6$). Both groups show large increases in TC metabolic activity from day 1 to day 7. Error bars: Mean ± SD. (Reproduced, with permission, from Caliari et al. [1])

agreement of the experimental results with the theoretical predictions indicates that the core-shell scaffolds behave like layered composites, implying adequate integration of the membrane with the scaffold (Fig. 16.6c) [1].

Finally, the capability of CG scaffold-membrane composites to support tendon cell (TC) attachment, proliferation, and long-term viability was assessed. TC metabolic activity and number were measured over a 14-day *in vitro* culture period in aligned CG scaffolds with (CG-membrane) and without (CG) membrane shells (Fig. 16.9) [1]. Early (1 day) results demonstrated that addition of the membrane shell did not significantly affect metabolic activity ($p = 0.10$) (Fig. 16.9b). Interestingly, cell number was significantly increased in CG-membrane scaffolds (Fig. 16.9a). This is likely due to the effect of the dense membrane shell in preventing the cell solution from leaking out of the porous scaffold after seeding. This hypothesis is corroborated by previous work demonstrating that collagen membrane wraps can effectively keep nutrients and soluble factors localized to the wound site *in vivo* [76, 77]. Both groups showed dramatic increases in cell number and metabolic activity at day 7. After 14 days of culture there were no significant differences between the groups in tendon cell proliferation or metabolic activity (Fig. 16.9a–b), indicating that the core-shell constructs have adequate permeability to support the nutrient and metabolite transport necessary for sustained cell viability and proliferation.

16.5 Conclusions

Porous, 3D biomaterials have been used extensively for a variety of tissue engineering applications, primarily as analogs of the ECM capable of inducing regeneration of damaged tissues and organs. CG scaffolds are an important class of these materials that have been applied as regeneration templates for a wide variety of wounds. Here, two new classes of CG scaffolds were described. First we described multi-compartment CG scaffolds, where distinct regions of the scaffold can contain distinct compositional, mechanical, and microstructural properties. Notably, a liquid phase co-synthesis method has been created to allow these distinct scaffold compartments to be linked via a continuous interface. The second class of materials are scaffold-membrane CG composites; here CG membrane structures were integrated into the scaffold structure in order to significantly improve the mechanical competence of a CG scaffold without sacrificing scaffold porosity. In both cases, modeling frameworks were introduced in order to better understand the observed changes in microstructural and mechanical parameters. Additionally, in the case of the first class of composites it was important to explore methodologies that allow regional characterization of the scaffold due to the heterogeneous nature of the material. Both classes of materials should also be amenable to integration with photolithographic techniques recently developed in our laboratory to immobilize distinct groups of biomolecules within CG scaffolds in a spatially defined manner [78]; this approach is expected to facilitate creation of gradient and compartment-specific biomolecular (i.e., growth factors, ligands) patterns within these and other CG scaffold variants. Overall, the materials described here provide an exciting basis for future experiments targeted at developing regeneration templates for orthopedic interfaces as well as other classes of gradient and interfacial tissues.

Acknowledgments This work was supported in part by the NSF IGERT 0965918 (DWW), the Chemistry-Biology Interface Training Program NIH NIGMS T32GM070421 (SRC), the Chemical and Biomolecular Engineering Dept. (DWW, SRC, BAH), and the Institute for Genomic Biology (DWW, SRC, BAH) at the University of Illinois at Urbana-Champaign. We wish to acknowledge the assistance of Rebecca Yapp, Yue Wang, and Dr. Michael Insana (UIUC) for assistance with ultrasound elastography-based analyses as well as Manuel Ramirez for assistance in CG membrane fabrication and characterization. Research described in this manuscript was carried out in part at the Frederick Seitz Materials Research Laboratory Central Facilities, University of Illinois, which are partially supported by the US Department of Energy under grants DE-FG02-07ER46453 and DE-FG02-07ER46471.

References

1. Caliari SR, Ramirez MA, Harley BAC (2011) The development of collagen-GAG scaffold-membrane composites for tendon tissue engineering. Biomaterials 32(34):8990–8998
2. Yannas IV, Burke JF, Huang C, Gordon PL (1975) Suppression of *in vivo* degradability and of immunogenicity of collagen by reaction with glycosaminoglycans. Polymer Prepr 16 (2):209–214
3. Yannas IV, Burke JF, Gordon PL, Huang C, Rubenstein RH (1980) Design of an artificial skin II: control of chemical-composition. J Biomed Mater Res 14(2):107–132
4. Ker EDF, Chu B, Phillippi JA, Gharaibeh B, Huard J, Weiss LE, Campbell PG (2011) Engineering spatial control of multiple differentiation fates within a stem cell population. Biomaterials 32(13):3413–3422
5. Sahoo S, Toh SL, Goh JC (2010) A bFGF-releasing silk/PLGA-based biohybrid scaffold for ligament/tendon tissue engineering using mesenchymal progenitor cells. Biomaterials 31 (11):2990–2998
6. Park A, Hogan MV, Kesturu GS, James R, Balian G, Chhabra AB (2010) Adipose-derived mesenchymal stem cells treated with growth differentiation factor-5 express tendon-specific markers. Tissue Eng Part A 16(9):2941–2951
7. Harley BAC, Gibson LJ (2008) *In vivo* and *in vitro* applications of collagen-GAG scaffolds. Chem Eng J 137(1):102–121
8. Liu Y, Ramanath HS, Wang DA (2008) Tendon tissue engineering using scaffold enhancing strategies. Trends Biotechnol 26(4):201–209
9. Yannas IV (2001) Tissue and organ regeneration in adults. Springer, New York
10. Yannas IV (1990) Biologically-active analogs of the extracellular-matrix—artificial skin and nerves. Angew Chem Int Ed Engl 29(1):20–35
11. Harley BA, Spilker MH, Wu JW, Asano K, Hsu HP, Spector M, Yannas IV (2004) Optimal degradation rate for collagen chambers used for regeneration of peripheral nerves over long gaps. Cells Tissues Organs 176(1–3):153–165
12. Yannas IV, Lee E, Orgill DP, Skrabut EM, Murphy GF (1989) Synthesis and characterization of a model extracellular matrix that induces partial regeneration of adult mammalian skin. Proc Natl Acad Sci U S A 86(3):933–937
13. Farrell E, O'Brien FJ, Doyle P, Fischer J, Yannas I, Harley BA, O'Connell B, Prendergast PJ, Campbell VA (2006) A collagen-glycosaminoglycan scaffold supports adult rat mesenchymal stem cell differentiation along osteogenic and chondrogenic routes. Tissue Eng 12(3):459–468
14. Harley BA, Freyman TM, Wong MQ, Gibson LJ (2007) A new technique for calculating individual dermal fibroblast contractile forces generated within collagen-GAG scaffolds. Biophys J 93(8):2911–2922
15. Harley BAC, Kim HD, Zaman MH, Yannas IV, Lauffenburger DA, Gibson LJ (2008) Microarchitecture of three-dimensional scaffolds influences cell migration behavior via junction interactions. Biophys J 95(8):4013–4024
16. Wake MC, Patrick CW Jr, Mikos AG (1994) Pore morphology effects on the fibrovascular tissue growth in porous polymer substrates. Cell Transplant 3(4):339–343
17. Nehrer S, Breinan HA, Ramappa A, Young G, Shortkroff S, Louie LK, Sledge CB, Yannas IV, Spector M (1997) Matrix collagen type and pore size influence behaviour of seeded canine chondrocytes. Biomaterials 18(11):769–776
18. Zeltinger J, Sherwood JK, Graham DA, Mueller R, Griffith LG (2001) Effect of pore size and void fraction on cellular adhesion, proliferation, and matrix deposition. Tissue Eng 7 (5):557–572
19. O'Brien FJ, Harley BA, Yannas IV, Gibson LJ (2005) The effect of pore size on cell adhesion in collagen-GAG scaffolds. Biomaterials 26(4):433–441
20. Jaworski J, Klapperich CM (2006) Fibroblast remodeling activity at two- and three-dimensional collagen-glycosaminoglycan interfaces. Biomaterials 27(23):4212–4220

21. Murphy CM, Haugh MG, O'Brien FJ (2010) The effect of mean pore size on cell attachment, proliferation and migration in collagen-glycosaminoglycan scaffolds for bone tissue engineering. Biomaterials 31(3):461–466
22. Tierney CM, Jaasma MJ, O'Brien FJ (2009) Osteoblast activity on collagen-GAG scaffolds is affected by collagen and GAG concentrations. J Biomed Mater Res A 91(1):92–101
23. Tierney CM, Haugh MG, Liedl J, Mulcahy F, Hayes B, O'Brien FJ (2009) The effects of collagen concentration and crosslink density on the biological, structural and mechanical properties of collagen-GAG scaffolds for bone tissue engineering. J Mech Behav Biomed Mater 2(2):202–209
24. Pelham RJ Jr, Wang Y (1997) Cell locomotion and focal adhesions are regulated by substrate flexibility. Proc Natl Acad Sci U S A 94(25):13661–13665
25. Grinnell F, Ho CH, Tamariz E, Lee DJ, Skuta G (2003) Dendritic fibroblasts in three-dimensional collagen matrices. Mol Biol Cell 14(2):384–395
26. Grinnell F, Ho CH, Lin YC, Skuta G (1999) Differences in the regulation of fibroblast contraction of floating versus stressed collagen matrices. J Biol Chem 274(2):918–923
27. Freyman TM, Yannas IV, Gibson LJ (2001) Cellular materials as porous scaffolds for tissue engineering. Prog Mater Sci 46(3–4):273–282
28. Torres DS, Freyman TM, Yannas IV, Spector M (2000) Tendon cell contraction of collagen-GAG matrices *in vitro*: effect of cross-linking. Biomaterials 21(15):1607–1619
29. Engler A, Bacakova L, Newman C, Hategan A, Griffin M, Discher D (2004) Substrate compliance versus ligand density in cell on gel responses. Biophys J 86(1 Pt 1):617–628
30. Jiang H, Grinnell F (2005) Cell-matrix entanglement and mechanical anchorage of fibroblasts in three-dimensional collagen matrices. Mol Biol Cell 16(11):5070–5076
31. Peyton SR, Putnam AJ (2005) Extracellular matrix rigidity governs smooth muscle cell motility in a biphasic fashion. J Cell Physiol 204(1):198–209
32. Yeung T, Georges PC, Flanagan LA, Marg B, Ortiz M, Funaki M, Zahir N, Ming W, Weaver V, Janmey PA (2005) Effects of substrate stiffness on cell morphology, cytoskeletal structure, and adhesion. Cell Motil Cytoskeleton 60(1):24–34
33. Zaman MH, Trapani LM, Sieminski AL, Mackellar D, Gong H, Kamm RD, Wells A, Lauffenburger DA, Matsudaira P (2006) Migration of tumor cells in 3D matrices is governed by matrix stiffness along with cell-matrix adhesion and proteolysis. Proc Natl Acad Sci U S A 103(29):10889–10894
34. Lynn AK, Yannas IV, Bonfield W (2004) Antigenicity and immunogenicity of collagen. J Biomed Mater Res B Appl Biomater 71(2):343–354
35. Yannas IV, Burke JF (1980) Design of an artificial skin. I. Basic design principles. J Biomed Mater Res 14(1):65–81
36. Tang SQ, Vickers SM, Hsu HP, Spector M (2007) Fabrication and characterization of porous hyaluronic acid-collagen composite scaffolds. J Biomed Mater Res A 82A(2):323–335
37. O'Brien FJ, Harley BA, Yannas IV, Gibson L (2004) Influence of freezing rate on pore structure in freeze-dried collagen-GAG scaffolds. Biomaterials 25(6):1077–1086
38. Pek YS, Spector M, Yannas IV, Gibson LJ (2004) Degradation of a collagen-chondroitin-6-sulfate matrix by collagenase and by chondroitinase. Biomaterials 25(3):473–482
39. Haugh MG, Murphy CM, O'Brien FJ (2010) Novel freeze-drying methods to produce a range of collagen-glycosaminoglycan scaffolds with tailored mean pore sizes. Tissue Eng Part C Methods 16(5):887–894
40. Lynn AK, Best SM, Cameron RE, Harley BA, Yannas IV, Gibson LJ, Bonfield W (2010) Design of a multiphase osteochondral scaffold. I. Control of chemical composition. J Biomed Mater Res A 92(3):1057–1065
41. Harley BA, Lynn AK, Wissner-Gross Z, Bonfield W, Yannas IV, Gibson LJ (2010) Design of a multiphase osteochondral scaffold. II. Fabrication of a mineralized collagen-glycosaminoglycan scaffold. J Biomed Mater Res A 92(3):1066–1077

42. Al-Munajjed AA, O'Brien FJ (2009) Influence of a novel calcium-phosphate coating on the mechanical properties of highly porous collagen scaffolds for bone repair. J Mech Behav Biomed Mater 2(2):138–146
43. Lynn AK, Bonfield W (2005) A novel method for the simultaneous, titrant-free control of pH and calcium phosphate mass yield. Acc Chem Res 38(3):202–207
44. Kanungo BP, Gibson LJ (2010) Density-property relationships in collagen-glycosaminoglycan scaffolds. Acta Biomater 6(2):344–353
45. Kanungo BP, Gibson LJ (2009) Density-property relationships in mineralized collagen-glycosaminoglycan scaffolds. Acta Biomater 5(4):1006–1018
46. Kanungo BP, Silva E, Van Vliet K, Gibson LJ (2008) Characterization of mineralized collagen-glycosaminoglycan scaffolds for bone regeneration. Acta Biomater 4(3):490–503
47. Harley BA, Lynn AK, Wissner-Gross Z, Bonfield W, Yannas IV, Gibson LJ (2010) Design of a multiphase osteochondral scaffold III: Fabrication of layered scaffolds with continuous interfaces. J Biomed Mater Res A 92(3):1078–1093
48. Mow VC, Ateshian GA, Spilker RL (1993) Biomechanics of diarthroidal joints—a review of 20 years of progress. J Biomech Eng 115(4):460–467
49. Li BH, Aspden RM (1997) Mechanical and material properties of the subchondral bone plate from the femoral head of patients with osteoarthritis or osteoporosis. Ann Rheum Dis 56 (4):247–254
50. Poole AR, Kojima T, Yasuda T, Mwale F, Kobayashi M, Laverty S (2001) Composition and structure of articular cartilage—a template for tissue repair. Clin Orthop Relat Res 391: S26–S33
51. Cohen NP, Foster RJ, Mow VC (1998) Composition and dynamics of articular cartilage: structure, function, and maintaining healthy state. J Orthop Sports Phys Ther 28(4):203–215
52. Genin GM, Kent A, Birman V, Wopenka B, Pasteris JD, Marquez PJ, Thomopoulos S (2009) Functional grading of mineral and collagen in the attachment of tendon to bone. Biophys J 97 (4):976–985
53. Caliari SR, Harley BAC (2011) The effect of anisotropic collagen-GAG scaffolds and growth factor supplementation on tendon cell recruitment, alignment, and metabolic activity. Biomaterials 32(23):5330–5340
54. Jungreuthmayer C, Jaasma MJ, Al-Munajjed AA, Zanghellini J, Kelly DJ, O'Brien FJ (2009) Deformation simulation of cells seeded on a collagen-GAG scaffold in a flow perfusion bioreactor using a sequential 3D CFD-elastostatics model. Med Eng Phys 31(4):420–427
55. Gibson LJ, Ashby MF (1997) Cellular solids: structure and properties, 2nd edn. Cambridge University Press, Cambridge
56. Gibson LJ, Ashby MF, Harley BA (2010) Cellular materials in nature and medicine. Cambridge University Press, Cambridge
57. Harley BA, Leung JH, Silva EC, Gibson LJ (2007) Mechanical characterization of collagen-glycosaminoglycan scaffolds. Acta Biomater 3(4):463–474
58. O'Brien FJ, Harley BA, Waller MA, Yannas IV, Gibson LJ, Prendergast PJ (2007) The effect of pore size on permeability and cell attachment in collagen scaffolds for tissue engineering. Technol Health Care 15(1):3–17
59. Agrawal CM, McKinney JS, Lanctot D, Athanasiou KA (2000) Effects of fluid flow on the *in vitro* degradation kinetics of biodegradable scaffolds for tissue engineering. Biomaterials 21 (23):2443–2452
60. Prendergast PJ, Huiskes R, Soballe K (1997) ESB Research Award 1996. Biophysical stimuli on cells during tissue differentiation at implant interfaces. J Biomech 30(6):539–548
61. Getgood AMJ, Kew SJ, Brooks R, Aberman H, Simon T, Lynn AK, Rushton N (2012) Evaluation of early-stage osteochondral defect repair using a biphasic scaffold based on a collagen-glycosaminoglycan biopolymer in a caprine model. The Knee 19(4):422–430
62. Vickers SM, Squitieri LS, Spector M (2006) Effects of cross-linking on chondrogenesis by adult canine and caprine chondrocytes in type II collagen-GAG scaffolds. In: International Cartilage Repair Society Symposium, San Diego, CA

63. Butler DL, Juncosa-Melvin N, Boivin GP, Galloway MT, Shearn JT, Gooch C, Awad H (2008) Functional tissue engineering for tendon repair: a multidisciplinary strategy using mesenchymal stem cells, bioscaffolds, and mechanical stimulation. J Orthop Res 26(1):1–9
64. Li X, Xie J, Lipner J, Yuan X, Thomopoulos S, Xia Y (2009) Nanofiber scaffolds with gradations in mineral content for mimicking the tendon-to-bone insertion site. Nano Lett 9 (7):2763–2768
65. Moffat KL, Kwei AS, Spalazzi JP, Doty SB, Levine WN, Lu HH (2009) Novel nanofiber-based scaffold for rotator cuff repair and augmentation. Tissue Eng Part A 15(1):115–126
66. Pham QP, Sharma U, Mikos AG (2006) Electrospinning of polymeric nanofibers for tissue engineering applications: a review. Tissue Eng 12(5):1197–1211
67. Shang S, Yang F, Cheng X, Walboomers XF, Jansen JA (2010) The effect of electrospun fibre alignment on the behaviour of rat periodontal ligament cells. Eur Cell Mater 19:180–192
68. Juncosa-Melvin N, Shearn JT, Boivin GP, Gooch C, Galloway MT, West JR, Nirmalanandhan VS, Bradica G, Butler DL (2006) Effects of mechanical stimulation on the biomechanics and histology of stem cell-collagen sponge constructs for rabbit patellar tendon repair. Tissue Eng 12(8):2291–2300
69. Saber S, Zhang AY, Ki SH, Lindsey DP, Smith RL, Riboh J, Pham H, Chang J (2010) Flexor tendon tissue engineering: bioreactor cyclic strain increases construct strength. Tissue Eng Part A 16(6):2085–2090
70. Chokalingam K, Juncosa-Melvin N, Hunter SA, Gooch C, Frede C, Florert J, Bradica G, Wenstrup R, Butler DL (2009) Tensile stimulation of murine stem cell-collagen sponge constructs increases collagen type I gene expression and linear stiffness. Tissue Eng Part A 15(9):2561–2570
71. Kuo CK, Tuan RS (2008) Mechanoactive tenogenic differentiation of human mesenchymal stem cells. Tissue Eng Part A 14(10):1615–1627
72. Gibson LJ (2005) Biomechanics of cellular solids. J Biomech 38(3):377–399
73. Utsunomiya H, Koh H, Miyamoto J, Sakai T (2008) High-strength porous copper by cold-extrusion. Adv Eng Mater 10(9):826–829
74. Nerurkar NL, Baker BM, Sen S, Wible EE, Elliott DM, Mauck RL (2009) Nanofibrous biologic laminates replicate the form and function of the annulus fibrosus. Nat Mater 8 (12):986–992
75. Nerurkar NL, Sen S, Huang AH, Elliott DM, Mauck RL (2010) Engineered disc-like angle-ply structures for intervertebral disc replacement. Spine (Phila Pa 1976) 35(8):867–873
76. Guda T, Walker JA, Kim S, Oh S, Appleford MR, Ong JL, Wenke JC (2010) Guiding hydroxyapatite scaffold based bone regeneration *in vivo* with collagen membranes. In: Society for Biomaterials Annual Meeting, Seattle, WA
77. Kimura Y, Hokugo A, Takamoto T, Tabata Y, Kurosawa H (2008) Regeneration of anterior cruciate ligament by biodegradable scaffold combined with local controlled release of basic fibroblast growth factor and collagen wrapping. Tissue Eng Part C Methods 14(1):47–57
78. Martin TA, Caliari SR, Williford PD, Harley BA, Bailey RC (2011) The generation of biomolecular patterns in highly porous collagen-GAG scaffolds using direct photolithography. Biomaterials 32(16):3949–3957

Index

S. Thomopoulos et al. (eds.), *Structural Interfaces and Attachments in Biology*,
DOI 10.1007/978-1-4614-3317-0,

B

C

F

R

S

Printed by Printforce, the Netherlands